Pattern Recognition
Neuroradiology

Pattern Recognition Neuroradiology

Neil M. Borden, MD
Associate Professor of Radiology, Department of Radiology,
Medical College of Georgia at the Georgia Health Sciences University,
Augusta, Georgia

Scott E. Forseen, MD
Assistant Professor of Radiology, Department of Radiology,
Medical College of Georgia at the Georgia Health Sciences University,
Augusta, Georgia

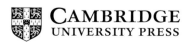
CAMBRIDGE
UNIVERSITY PRESS

CAMBRIDGE UNIVERSITY PRESS
Cambridge, New York, Melbourne, Madrid, Cape Town,
Singapore, São Paulo, Delhi, Tokyo, Mexico City

Cambridge University Press
The Edinburgh Building, Cambridge CB2 8RU, UK

Published in the United States of America by
Cambridge University Press, New York

www.cambridge.org
Information on this title: www.cambridge.org/9780521727037

First published 2011

Printed in the United Kingdom at the University Press, Cambridge

A catalog record for this publication is available from the British Library

Library of Congress Cataloging-in-Publication Data

Borden, Neil M.
    Pattern recognition neuroradiology / Neil M. Borden, Scott E. Forseen.
        p. ; cm.
    Includes bibliographical references and index.
    ISBN 978-0-521-72703-7 (Paperback)
1. Nervous system–Radiography.   2. Diagnosis, Differential.   I. Forseen,
Scott E.   II. Title.
    [DNLM: 1. Brain Diseases–radiography.   2.   Diagnosis, Differential.
3. Neuroradiography–methods.   4. Spinal Cord Diseases–radiography.
WL 141]
RC349.R3B67 2011
616.8′047572–dc23

2011013007

ISBN 978-0-521-72703-7 Paperback

Contents

Abbreviations

ABC   aneurysmal bone cyst

AD   Alzheimer's dementia

ADC map   apparent diffusion coefficient map

ADEM   acute disseminated encephalomyelitis

AIDP   acute inflammatory demyelinating polyradiculoneuropathy

ALL/PLL   Anterior/posterior longitudinal ligament

ALS   amyotrophic lateral sclerosis

AML   acute myeloid leukemia

AT/RT   atypical teratoid/rhaboid tumor

(d)AVF   (dural) arteriovenous fistula

AVM   arteriovenous malformation

BBB   blood brain barrier

C0/1/2/3–7   occiput/atlas/axis/third to seventh cervical vertebra

CADASIL   cerebral autosomal dominant arteriopathy with subcortical infarcts and leukoencephalopathy

CBF   cerebral blood flow

(r)CBV   (relative) cerebral blood volume

CIDP   chronic inflammatory demyelinating polyradiculoneuropathy

CMV   cytomegalovirus

CN   cranial nerve

CNS   central nervous system

CP angle   cerebellopontine angle

CPP   cerebral perfusion pressure

CSF   cerebrospinal fluid

CT   computed tomography

DAI   diffuse axonal injury

DDM   Dyke–Davidoff–Masson (syndrome)

DISH   diffuse idiopathic skeletal hyperostosis

DLB   dementia with Lewy bodies

DNET   dysembryoplastic neuroepithelial tumor

DNL   disseminated necrotizing leukoencephalopathy

DPS   dilated perivascular spaces

DSC   dynamic susceptibility contrast

DVA   developmental venous anomaly

DWI   diffusion weighted imaging/images

EBV   Epstein–Barr virus

EDH   epidural hematoma

FA map   fractional anisotropy map

FLAIR   fluid attenuated inversion recovery pulse sequence

FMD   fibromuscular dysplasia

FSE   fast spin echo (image)

GBM   glioblastoma multiforme

GCT   giant cell tumor

GM   gray matter

GRE   gradient recalled echo (image)

HHT   hereditary hemorrhagic telangiectasia

HIV   human immunodeficiency virus

HTLV-1   human T-cell leukemia virus – type 1

HU   Hounsefield unit

IAC   internal auditory canal

ICP   intracranial pressure

IVH   intraventricular hemorrhage

JNA   juvenile nasopharyngeal angiofibroma

JPA   juvenile pilocytic astrocytoma

L(1–5)   lumbar vertebra (first to fifth)

LCH   Langerhans cell histiocytosis

MELAS   mitochondrial myopathy, encephalopathy, lactic acidosis, and stroke-like syndrome

MERRF   myoclonic epilepsy with ragged red fibers syndrome

MISME   multiple inherited/intracranial schwannomas, meningiomas, and ependymomas

MR(I)(A)(V)   magnetic resonance (imaging) (angiography) (venography)

MS   multiple sclerosis

MSA   multisystem atrophy

MTT   mean transit time

NAA   N-acetyl aspartate

NF-1   neurofibromatosis – type 1

NF-2   neurofibromatosis – type 2

NMO   neuromyelitis optica (Devic's disease)

NPH   normal pressure hydrocephalus

OPCA   olivopontocerebellar atrophy

OPLL   ossification of the posterior longitudinal ligament

PA   primary angiitis

PACS   picture archiving and communications systems

PD   Parkinson's disease

PET   positron emission tomography

PF   posterior fossa

PKAN   pantothenate kinase-associated neurodegeneration

PML   progressive multifocal leukoencephalopathy

PNET   primitive neuroectodermal tumor

PRES   posterior reversible encephalopathy syndrome

PSP   progressive supranuclear palsy

PXA   pleomorphic xanthoastrocytoma

RA   rheumatoid arthritis

rCBF   relative cerebral blood flow

rCBV   relative cerebral blood volume

RCC   renal cell carcinoma

RF   radiofrequency

S(1–4)   sacral vertebrae/sacrum

SAH   subarachnoid hemorrhage

SCIWORA   spinal cord injury without radiographic abnormality

SDH   subdural hematoma

SEGCA   subependymal giant cell astrocytomas

SLE   systemic lupus erythematosus

SPECT   single photon emission computed tomography

SSPE   subacute sclerosing panencephalitis

STIR   short tau inversion recovery pulse sequence

T(1–12)   thoracic vertebra (first to twelfth)

TB   tuberculosis

TIA   transient ischemic attack

TOF time-of-flight

TPN total parenteral nutrition

TR repetition time

V1 first division of the trigeminal nerve

V2 second division of the trigeminal nerve

VA vertebral artery

VHL von Hippel–Lindau syndrome

VR spaces Virchow–Robin spaces

(T1, T2, PD)WI (T1, T2, proton density) weighted image(s)

WM white matter

Foreword

Less than a half a dozen years ago, Dr. Borden requested that I provide him a foreword to his stunning three-dimensional angiographic atlas, which I was happy to do. He has now honored me with the same request for his new and equally impressive text *Pattern Recognition Neuroradiology*, written with his coauthor Scott Forseen, MD. Both authors, I am proud to note, are alumni of Barrow Neurological Institute. That Dr Borden assembled this latest text, with its hundreds of images and unique perspective on interpreting magnetic resonance (MR) images and computed tomographic (CT) scans in such a brief time since his last tome, is evidence enough of his immense commitment to professional education. Nothing else need be said in that respect!

However, much remains to be said about this fine volume and its novel approach to diagnosing neurological disorders. The volume is divided into two major sections, the first devoted to the brain and the second to the spinal cord. Each section begins with a chapter devoted to basic concepts and terminology. The chapter on the brain first summarizes how MR images and CT scans are produced and how the different signals interact with brain tissues. It also defines basic neurological terms needed to interpret neuroradiological images. These chapters will be especially helpful for trainees.

The next chapters in both sections, however, should be read by all because they present Dr. Borden's unique approach to image analysis of the brain and spinal cord.

His structured approach is useful for both novice and seasoned practitioners alike. His emphasis on a repetitive approach to analysis is designed to decrease errors of omission and to increase the efficiency of reading diagnostic studies. He even has thoughtfully provided dictation templates based on his systematic approach in the Appendix. Some might argue that interpretation is as much of an art as a skill, and I would not disagree. But skill can certainly be developed and Dr. Borden's approach should facilitate the acquisition thereof.

The chapters that follow in both sections categorize neurological diseases and their locations and can be referred to as needed. The final chapters before the image gallery in both sections outline differential diagnoses to consider based on lesion location or morphology and again can be referred to as needed.

The brief, conversational text does no more than it should: provide readers a reference for the richness of images that follows and that rightly composes the majority of the volume. The abundance of images offers a comprehensive look at neurological lesions, both common and rare. Readers, whether neuroradiologists, neurosurgeons, or neurologists. regardless of their level of expertise, will not be disappointed, and this volume belongs on the bookshelf of all of these clinicians.

Robert F. Spetzler, MD
Phoenix, Arizona
July 2011

Acknowledgment for Dr. Borden

This book was written from my desire to provide a simplified educational format that includes didactic information in addition to a philosophy and new approach for anyone interested in beginning their mastery of Neuroradiology.

As always this would not be possible without the support and love of my wife Nina and my children Rachel and Jonathan.

This acknowledgement would not be complete without a special thanks to the many talented neuroradiologists at the Barrow Neurological Institute as well as Dr. Cameron McDougall who provided me with an invaluable experience and an unforgettable time in my life while training at the BNI. My awe and tremendous respect for Dr. Spetzler has been an inspiration that has been a shining light and role model to aspire to.

Acknowledgment for Dr. Forseen

None of my endeavors would be possible or worthwhile without my beautiful and understanding wife, Caralee. The terrific training I received at the Barrow Neurological Institute was only possible because of her selflessness. I could not have envisioned the joy and amazement that comes from watching my two sons, Brendan and Mathias, develop and learn to navigate their worlds. I could not be more proud of the two of them. Special thanks go to my mother for setting me on the glide path to success, notwithstanding the occasional gentle and not-so-gentle "repositioning" of the path I had set for myself. Thank you goes to my father for continually demonstrating to me how to achieve excellence through persistence, hard work, and refusal to accept limitations placed on me by other people. I have been very fortunate to have top flight mentors at all levels of my training. I attempt to walk in the footsteps of these individuals and incorporate their skills into my work each day. Finally, I would like to acknowledge the many medical students, residents, and fellows that make the daily practice of medicine interesting, entertaining, and challenging. It is my sincere hope that the contents of this book will be considered useful.

Introduction

To me, the phrase pattern recognition infers not only the ability to match the appearance of a new image to a previously imprinted image pattern in our brains but to use additional cognitive clues that are known to arrive at a differential diagnosis or, in certain instances, an exact diagnosis. Pattern recognition is not solely dependent on the visual appearance of the image, although it is vitally important. Having appropriate clinical information is also vitally important when analyzing images. Unfortunately it is not uncommon to review imaging studies without this information. Pattern recognition includes incorporation of all of the following so that an accurate and plausible differential diagnosis can be provided. This includes: (1) location of the lesion(s) – intra- versus extra-axial and specific anatomic region, (2) patient's age, (3) clinical history, (4) morphology of lesion(s) such as shape, demarcation, signal intensity or density, enhancement pattern, diffusion characteristics, and other less commonly used magnetic resonance (MR) characteristics such as perfusion and spectroscopy.

I also believe that creating a standard sequence of image analysis and having dictation templates permits your brain to incorporate a different type of pattern of thinking that will become innate over time, like a reflex, which will also enhance your interpretive skills.

After having performed thousands of diagnostic cerebral angiograms and performing neuroendovascular procedures, I have been asked by novices how do you know how to arrive at a specific location within the brain with the catheter. The answer is the same as if someone had asked you how you know how to get to your house, your parents' house, and your grandparents' house. The answer is simple. You have traveled those routes before and after having done so for a period of time you simply follow the pattern (route) that has been imprinted in your brain.

I believe the field of radiology is a specialty certain types of individuals excel at and others do not. The cognitive requirements in radiology can be learned by all but to be a good radiologist requires an inherent ability in visual–spatial recognition, which is not present in all. Each of our brains is unique in some way, but I believe that the ability to excel at working with images or the ability to excel at working with written language may not be present in all of us. I speak from experience. I live in a world of pictures/images. My own brain deals with images in a more primary role. I can learn and assimilate new information more quickly and efficiently than written language. I am a true believer in the phrase "a picture is worth a thousand words." This is not to say that written language is not important but in my world it takes a back seat.

Practicing neuroradiology (or other subspecialty in radiology) is a task requiring repetition with incorporation of image patterns with basic cognitive cues/clues. The cues (or clues) helping you arrive at a reasonable differential diagnosis based upon the image pattern include: location of abnormality, patient's age, a knowledge of what normal macro-/microanatomy exists at this location, and a basic knowledge of neuropathologic entities.

Although the number of different pathologies that can involve the body is vast, you must always remember that common pathologies occur commonly. Never forget the phrase "unusual manifestations of a common disorder are more frequent than a common manifestation of an unusual disorder." In addition to this it is very important to realize that sometimes lesions that fit a certain imaging pattern become localized to unusual locations not typical for that lesion. If you begin your career learning the basic pathologies pertinent to each region of the body, with time and looking at more and more cases you will begin to assimilate the less common appearances of these lesions in addition to less frequently encountered lesions.

The goal of this book is to present the basics of neuroradiology in a type of outline format that allows the reader to learn and efficiently incorporate these concepts into their practice of neuroimaging whether the reader is a resident, fellow, or general radiologist. This book is not intended to provide an exhaustive compendium of neuroradiology. The information contained in this book is not new but hopefully the way it is presented will benefit the reader in ways other textbooks have not.

Neil M. Borden, MD

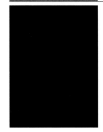

How to use Section 1

The intent of this book is to provide a reference for the interpretation of brain and spine related disorders. I have tried to simplify the presentation of this material into a structured/outline framework. I truly believe that the first step in becoming a good radiologist is to build a routine pattern of image analysis that should closely align with a structured method of dictation/reporting.

Step 1

Learn/know the basic concepts/terminology in chapter 1. This information will provide some basic building blocks that will allow you to optimize the learning experience in this book and are often questions that will be asked of you as a resident.

Step 2

Review Chapter 2, which provides a basic approach toward image analysis.

Step 3

Build/create dictation templates/macros based upon a logical way you find to analyze the image. I have provided sample dictation templates in the appendix, which I have incorporated into my daily work. These templates should include both pertinent positives as well as pertinent negatives. You can use or modify my templates or create a template that works better for you. After a short period of time of using these templates, your mind will have converted this pattern of dictation into a pattern of image analysis. This is why it is important to start with good templates discussing the major anatomic regions and structures. Errors of omission and misdiagnosis will be minimized with this approach.

Step 4

Chapters 3, 4, and 5 provide, in outline form: (1) a generalized categorization of disease processes (chapter 3), (2) a simplified listing of differential diagnosis by location (chapter 4), and (3) an approach to lesion characterization by imaging appearance such as enhancement, density (on computed tomography [CT]), and signal intensity (on MR) (chapter 5). Utilize this outline presentation to help compartmentalize and categorize your understanding of the various pathologies you will encounter. Images in chapter 6 will be cross referenced with the text in chapters 1 and 3.

Step 5

Chapter 6 provides examples of the typical appearances of many of the lesions described in chapters 3, 4, and 5, with brief descriptions. The images should provide you with the basic building blocks for improving your pattern recognition of neurologic lesions.

Chapter 1

Basic concepts: definitions, terminology, and basics of brain imaging

Biologic basis of magnetic resonance image (MRI) production

MR images represent the distribution of mobile hydrogen nuclei (protons) in the body. Mobile hydrogen nuclei are present in the body primarily in the form of water molecules and fat molecules. To produce MR images, the patient is placed in a strong, static magnetic field. Radiofrequency (RF) energy is used to excite protons (hydrogen nuclei). Following excitation, protons return to a relaxed state through two characteristic relaxation processes, T1 relaxation (spin lattice or longitudinal relaxation) and T2 relaxation (spin-spin relaxation). During relaxation, signals from the magnetization of the protons are recorded. Tissues have differing combinations of the T1 and T2 relaxation rates. The contrast in MR images (variation in signal intensities) is often described as T1 weighted, T2 weighted, or proton density weighted. The spatial localization that depicts the signal strength from each picture element of the image (pixel) is accomplished through the application of gradient magnetic fields. Gradient magnetic fields are used to perturb the magnetic fields in the patient's body from left to right, anterior to posterior, and inferior to superior. The purpose of the magnetic gradients is to slightly alter the Larmor frequencies that provide spatial localization information. The gradients produce systematic changes in the frequency of the detected signal according to the position of tissues within the image. A two-dimensional Fourier transformation is used to decompose an interference pattern from many frequencies into their individual component frequencies, which are spatially localized through the application of the gradients. The signal strength of tissues on T1 weighted images (T1WI) depends upon how much longitudinal relaxation occurs between each TR, the repetition time for RF excitations. Tissues with short T1 relaxation times have higher signal strength on T1WI. Fat and subacute blood are typical materials with short T1 relaxation times and therefore appear bright (white) on T1WI. Water has a long T1 relaxation time therefore it appears dark on T1WI. The signal strength of tissues on T2 weighted images (T2WI) depends upon the loss of phase coherence of the spinning protons. Tissues that lose phase coherence slowly have prolonged T2 relaxation times and demonstrate more signal strength (are brighter or whiter) than tissues that lose phase coherence more quickly. Water is typical of a material with a prolonged T2 relaxation time. Most (not all) pathology results in an increase in the water content of the abnormality, which prolongs both T1 and T2 relaxation times of the abnormal tissue and therefore appears dark on T1WI and bright on T2WI, similar to the expected appearance of water (or CSF) on these sequences. The signal strength of tissues on proton density weighted images (PDWI) depends upon the physical density of mobile protons in each pixel. On PDWI, tissues are relatively isointense as soft tissues have similar proton densities. Hard tissues, such as compact or cortical bone, produce very little signal and appear quite dark in MR images.

When you talk about MR images always remember to use the term signal intensity, not density (which is only appropriate for CT).

Biologic basis of MR vascular flow imaging: magnetic resonance angiography and magnetic resonance venography

There are two major concepts in vascular flow imaging:

1. Velocity induced signal loss, which results in the hypointense appearance of flowing blood (black blood).
2. Flow related enhancement on T1 weighted gradient echo imaging secondary to the entrance of fully magnetized blood into the imaging slice, resulting in the bright (white) appearance of flowing blood. Static tissue in the slices of a T1 weighted gradient echo sequence experience many RF pulses, which reduce the detected signal from static tissues. Flowing blood is bright on T1 weighted gradient echo sequences because the

signal from fully magnetized blood is greater than the signal from static tissues. This technique is called time-of-flight (TOF). The technique of TOF intracranial MR angiography (MRA) and MR venography (MRV) is essentially the same. Both the MRA and MRV sequences use gradient echo T1WI. What determines whether you create arterial or venous images is the placement of a saturation band/pulse, which is positioned parallel to the acquired slice to eliminate signal from blood flowing in the opposite direction. In the case of MRA the saturation band is placed above the acquired slice to eliminate venous flow, and for MRV the band is placed inferior to the slice to eliminate inflow of arterial blood.

Different acquisition modes for TOF MRA:

(i) 2D TOF technique: all of the data from individual slices in the volume of interest are acquired before sequential acquisition of data from other slices in the volume to be scanned. One slice is acquired at a time before moving on to the next. This technique is more sensitive to slow flow.
(ii) 3D TOF technique: the entire volume of interest is excited repeatedly and the individual slices are phase encoded. As you move deeper into the 3D volume of tissue, saturation effects occur as the protons flowing further into the volume are exposed to multiple RF pulses. The effect is that the flow related enhancement diminishes the further you go into the 3D slab. This technique is more sensitive to fast flow.

Signal strength in magnetic resonance angiography

The greatest signal strength of flowing blood occurs when the flow is perpendicular to the imaging slice. Therefore, axial image acquisition results in the greatest signal when the direction of blood flow is inferior to superior, such as occurs in neck MRA. The smallest signal strength of flowing blood occurs when the plane of flow is in the same plane as the imaging plane. This occurs for instance when the upper cervical vertebral artery passes over the posterior arch of C1, which is in the same plane as that in which the axial imaging is taking place. This is because protons are exposed to multiple RF pulses while flowing within the imaging plane, which results in saturation of the signal from blood flowing within the imaging plane. Remember that the signal strength on T1WI is related to the amount of longitudinal relaxation that occurs between each TR. If the protons are exposed to repetitive RF pulses then the degree of longitudinal relaxation occurring between each TR is minimized and therefore the signal strength is reduced.

Diffusion weighted (DW) MRI

This set of MR images exploits the ability of water to diffuse within the intercellular and intracellular environment of the brain. Because water diffuses more freely along cerebral white matter (WM) tracts than across WM tracts, water has enhanced diffusion along the direction of these tracts. This is an example of anisotropic diffusion, diffusion preferentially in one direction. Cerebral gray matter (GM) is not organized in tracts, thus diffusion in GM is an example of isotropic diffusion, diffusion showing no preferred direction. Three different contrasts can be produced in diffusion imaging; diffusion trace images, apparent diffusion coefficient (ADC) maps, and fractional anisotropy (FA) maps. Diffusion trace images represent a geometric average of diffusion in all three orthogonal directions. ADC maps are pseudo-quantitative maps indicating the magnitude of diffusion in each image voxel. FA maps are maps that demonstrate the relative amount of anisotropic diffusion in each image voxel. Diffusion imaging uses different diffusion gradient strengths, called the B value. It is typical to acquire diffusion images using B values of 0, 500, and 1000. With greater B values you enhance your ability to identify areas of altered diffusion. While diffusion imaging is used mainly in the evaluation of stroke, to differentiate an acute/subacute infarct (increased signal on diffusion trace images and decreased signal on the ADC map) from an older infarct (greater than 7–10 days), other pathologies will also demonstrate restricted diffusion. In pathology, extracellular water is often incorporated into cells, which increases the proportion of water having restricted diffusion space resulting in increased signal on diffusion trace images and decreased signal on ADC maps. (Refer to Chapter 5 for a listing of the various causes of diffusion restriction.) Restricted diffusion (which looks bright on diffusion trace images and dark on the ADC maps) is typical in areas of cytotoxic edema or when there is tight packing of cellular elements such as in certain hypercellular tumors. Diffusion of water in the intercellular space on the other hand is enhanced (looks bright on diffusion trace images and the ADC map) with vasogenic edema and is an example of T2 shine through. Diffusion weighted images (DWI) have inherent T2 weighting. The ADC map allows you to decide if the brightness seen on the diffusion trace image is a result of restricted diffusion or merely increased T2 signal (called T2 shine through). You should never interpret the diffusion trace images without the ADC map images for comparison.

Magnetic susceptibility

This is a characteristic of all tissues. It is an indication of how magnetized a tissue becomes when placed in a strong magnetic field. There are four descriptions of the magnetic susceptibility:

1. Diamagnetic – the characteristic of tissue to be resistant to being magnetized and to produce a small magnetic field in the opposite direction to the applied field. Most body tissues are diamagnetic. Air and bone have almost zero susceptibility.
2. Paramagnetic – materials and tissues that have a stronger ability to become magnetized and produce a magnetic field in the same direction as the main applied field. Gadolinium (MR contrast agent), deoxyhemoglobin, and methemoglobin are examples.
3. Superparamagnetic – materials with the ability to become magnetized being intermediate between that of paramagnetic and ferromagnetic tissues. Examples are iron oxide particles (MR contrast agent), ferritin, and hemosiderin.
4. Ferromagnetic – materials with the ability to become strongly magnetized and experience a large force when placed in an external magnetic field. These include metals containing nickel, iron, and cobalt.

Magnetic susceptibility signal loss

At the boundaries of various tissues tiny magnetic field gradients exist owing to differences in their magnetic susceptibility. This results in loss of phase coherence of the precessing protons, which will result in the loss of signal at these interfaces. This signal loss is especially prominent in gradient echo sequences and results in a black line around the various tissues.

Helical CT image production

Helical CT uses a thinly collimated x-ray beam rotating around the body in association with an array of x-ray detectors. Multidetector helical CT involves continuous movement of the scanning table/patient through the gantry in association with the rotating detector units. It is the electron density of the various tissues and their ability to attenuate the x-ray beam that is the primary characteristic resulting in the final appearance of the CT image. By convention water has a Hounsefield unit (HU) of zero, bone has an HU of $+1000$, acute blood has an HU of approximately 50–90, air has an HU of -1000, and fat has an HU of -50 to about -100.

When talking about CT images always use the terms density or attenuation rather than signal, which is appropriate only in MRI.

Use of stroke and subdural windows and levels
(see Figure 6.192, page 198)

It has been shown that using variable CT window widths and levels increases the ability to detect subtle, early cerebral infarcts in addition to small hyperdense extracerebral (subdural and epidural) hematomas adjacent to the inner table. With the wide usage of picture archiving and communications systems (PACS), the radiologist can easily alter these viewing parameters. Precise windows and levels should be interactively chosen by the radiologist to optimize/accentuate GM–WM differentiation when assessing for acute strokes (narrowing the window width and level/gray scale) and in the assessment of subdural hematomas (widening the window width and level/gray scale) to provide easier detection of extra-axial (subdural or epidural) hematomas. The standard CT examination should be viewed in four different window widths and levels: (1) standard brain parenchymal windows, (2) bone windows, (3) stroke windows, and (4) subdural windows. This is easily accomplished at the PACS workstation.

Blood brain barrier (BBB)

The blood brain barrier (BBB) is a specialized system of capillary endothelial cells that excludes harmful substances from the central nervous system (CNS) and allows the passage of required nutrients. Areas of the brain that normally lack the BBB will demonstrate contrast enhancement and include: (1) the pineal gland, (2) pituitary gland and stalk (infindibulum), and insertion at the median eminence of the hypothalamus, (3) choroid plexus, (4) dura – you normally see short segments of dural enhancement, and (5) circumventricular organs (named for their close association with the ventricular system) including the area postrema (at the transition of the fourth ventricle into the central canal), organum vasculosum of the lamina terminalis (anterior wall of the third ventricle), and subfornical and subcommissural organ. Pathologic processes such as tumor and infection/inflammation can result in the breakdown of the BBB, which we identify on imaging as areas of contrast enhancement.

Normal cerebral cortex

The cerebral cortex is normally six layered but the hippocampus is three. The hippocampus may appear slightly brighter than other cortical areas on fluid attenuated inversion recovery pulse sequence (FLAIR) images, which may be related to this difference in cortical development.

Cerebrospinal fluid (CSF)

Eighty percent of CSF is produced in the choroid plexus of the lateral and fourth ventricles. The remainder is produced in the interstitial space and ependymal lining. Normal volume is 150 mL in the adult (50% intracranial and 50% intraspinal) and 50 mL in the neonate. CSF is produced at a rate of 3 cc/min. Normal pressure in the adult is 7–15 cm H_2O (abnormal is >18 cm H_2O).

Ependymitis granularis on MRI

Focal areas of increased water content (increased T2 signal) in WM anterior to the frontal horns is secondary to focal breakdown of the frontal horn ependymal lining. This is a normal finding and seen with increased frequency and prominence with advancing age.

Dilated perivascular spaces (Virchow–Robin spaces)

These are pial-lined, interstitial fluid-filled spaces accompanying perforating vessels. They do not have a direct communication with the subarachnoid space.

When small (typical), they are considered normal variants and are found at all ages. Rarely, they can become giant in size. Certain pathologic entities can be associated with unusually large and more numerous Virchow–Robin (VR) spaces such as mucopolysaccharidoses (Hurler and Hunter disease), chronic microvascular ischemic disease with concomitant atrophy (etat crible), and cryptococcal meningitis with gelatinous pseudocysts occupying VR spaces.

Magnetic resonance images

Dilated perivascular spaces (DPSs) are hypointense on T1, isointense on intermediate weighted (you do not see them), and hyperintense on T2WI. They appear as well-circumscribed round, oval, or linear foci of signal intensity similar to CSF. The configuration depends upon the orientation of the DPS relative to the imaging plane. There is an increase in their prominence and number with advancing age, and they are most common in the inferior basal ganglia (at the level of the anterior commisure), high convexity, and deep and subcortical WM. To differentiate DPSs from lacunar infarcts, note that lacunes usually have increased signal intensity on FLAIR images surrounding the lacunes whereas DPSs usually do not but occasionally can have such changes in signal intensity.

Computed tomography images

The spaces appear as well-circumscribed round, oval, or linear foci of decreased density (attenuation) similar to CSF. The configuration depends upon the orientation of the DPS relative to the imaging plane.

Arachnoid granulations (Pacchionian granulations)
(see Figure 6.48, page 95)

These granulations are specialized regions where the arachnoid projects into the dural venous sinus(es) where CSF is reabsorbed into the venous system. They are often round or oval and you may see veins coursing into them. Typically they appear hypodense, like CSF on CT, and follow CSF on T1WI and T2WI. They may appear as filling defects in the venous sinuses but are typically round, not linear or string-like (i.e. if it were an intraluminal clot). Arachnoid granulations can cause an erosive or a scalloped appearance along the inner table and are often seen in the occipital bone to either side of the midline. They may be present in unusual locations, simulating an aggressive, destructive process. They may be present near the sphenoid sinus and occasionally result in CSF leaks/rhinorrhea if they erode into the sphenoid sinus, or CSF otorrhea if they are located along the posterior aspect of the petrous ridge and erode into mastoid air cells.

Concept of brain myelination

The process of myelination begins during fetal development and continues after birth in a predetermined sequence. Immature myelin has a higher water content than mature myelin, therefore unmyelinated WM looks darker on T1WI and brighter on T2WI, just as water behaves. As myelin matures the water content diminishes and there is an increase in brain cholesterol and glycolipids. This increase in lipid content and decrease in water content with maturation of myelin results in the WM looking brighter on T1WI and darker on T2WI. As a rule of thumb, myelination proceeds from inferior to superior, posterior to anterior, and central to peripheral. The adult pattern of myelination occurs earlier on T1WI (at about one year of life) than on T2WI (at about two years of life). Sensory fibers myelinate prior to motor fibers, and projection pathways myelinate before association pathways. The T1 weighted appearance of the brain at birth is similar to the adult brain on T2WI and the appearance of the newborn brain on T2WI is similar to the adult brain on T1WI.

Basic myelination milestones to identify
Myelination, as shown by increased signal
on T1 weighted images

Medulla, dorsal midbrain, and cerebellar peduncles at birth;

Cerebellar WM – progresses from birth to three months of age (looks like the adult);

Pons progressively myelinates from three to six months of age;

Decussation of the superior cerebellar peduncles, ventrolateral thalamus, and posterior limb of the internal capsule at birth;

Pre- and postcentral gyri by one month; motor tracts have matured by three months of age;

Optic nerves, tracts, and radiations before three months; myelination into the occipital WM around the calcarine fissure at three months of age;

Anterior limb of the internal capsule from two to three months of age;

Corpus callosum – splenium at four months, and progresses anteriorly with the genu by six months of age;

Subcortical WM begins at three months progressing from posterior to anterior and continues to increase until about 11 months.

Myelination, as shown by decreased signal intensity on T2WI

Inferior and superior cerebellar peduncles at birth;

Middle cerebellar peduncles by month two or three;

Peripheral extension of myelination of the cerebellum begins at eight months and is complete by about 18 months of age;

Ventrolateral thalamus, decussation of the superior cerebellar peduncles, and patches in the posterior limb of the internal capsule show low signal at birth;

Patches in centrum semiovale by two months of age;

Optic tracts begin at one month and extend along the optic radiations to the calcarine cortex by four months of age;

Internal capsule – the more anterior portion of the posterior limb by seven months and the anterior limb by 11 months of age;

Corpus callosum – splenium at six months and progressing anteriorly to the genu at eight months of age;

Subcortical WM is the last part of the brain to myelinate from occipital (nine months) to frontal (14 months) regions. Remember terminal zones of myelination are in the subcortical frontotemporoparietal regions with frontal and temporal areas complete by about 40 months of age.

Terminal zones of myelination

Terminal myelination zones were believed to be in the peritrigonal regions but there is evidence that the true terminal zones are in the subcortical WM – in the frontotemporoparietal WM. Frontal and temporal subcortical WM progressively myelinates and this is complete by about 40 months. The parietal subcortical WM completes myelination earlier, at about 23 months.

The persistence of high T2 signal in the peritrigonal regions may be related to perivascular spaces imaged on high resolution T2 sequences.

The muddy waters of white matter disease on MRI

A large number of pathologic processes, which can have a similar appearance, manifest as lesions in the WM. Clinical information, age of the patient, and morphologic pattern are all necessary to help distinguish many of these pathologies, which can look alike and still be indistinguishable despite all of this information.

You will often find a few small foci of increased T2/FLAIR signal in the WM (subcortical or deep) in otherwise healthy individuals and find yourself scratching your head about their significance/etiology. These are the so-called UBOs (unidentified bright objects). In the absence of known systemic disease, risk factors for vascular disease such as hypertension, hyperlipidemia, or diabetes, and no significant prior history for trauma or clinical neurologic dysfunction, these are considered entirely nonspecific but may represent gliosis related to a prior subclinical infection or a prior indeterminate event. The vast majority of these UBOs are of no clinical significance and do not evolve into clinically significant pathology.

White matter

WM makes up 60% of the volume of the brain.

Main components

Axons with their envelope of myelin;

Neuroglial cells in WM are oligodendrocytes and astrocytes;

Myelin is formed and maintained by oligodendrocytes;

Myelin – short T1 and T2 signals owing to high lipid content.

Diseases that diminish myelin result in increased water content, leading to decreased T1 and increased T2 signals.

Microvascular ischemic changes (see Figure 6.224, page 218)

WM supplied by long arteries and arterioles that become narrowed by arteriosclerosis and lipohyaline deposits over time results in chronic ischemia with impaired maintenance and formation of myelin,

myelin pallor, associated gliosis, and increased interstitial fluid. You will see faint decreased T1 and increased T2 signal without diffusion restriction, enhancement, or mass effect. Frank necrosis/cavitation of this type of WM injury does not occur unless there is a specific event leading to acute profound reduction in blood flow, as in abrupt vascular occlusion or hypotensive episodes. Risk factors include hyperlipidemia, hypertension, and diabetes. These changes are seen with increased frequency with advancing age. Areas susceptible to microvascular ischemic changes are: (1) the basal ganglia, (2) thalamus, (3) periventricular and subcortical WM, (4) centrum semiovale, and (5) central mid- and upper pons. Areas protected by this process are supplied by short, less than 8 mm arterioles, or have a collateral supply, and include: (1) cortical GM, (2) central corpus callosum, (3) medulla, (4) midbrain, and (5) subcortical U-fibers. You may consider a region of signal abnormality in the WM as an area of old, frank infarction if there is a cystic/necrotic focus. If however there are only areas of decreased T1 and increased T2 signal without frank cavitation then it is more likely chronic WM ischemia. If there is diffusion restriction then consider acute/subacute infarct.

Multiple sclerosis (see Figure 6.176, page 188)

The etiology of multiple sclerosis (MS) is not certain; possibly viral or autoimmune. MS results in perivenular inflammation leading to destruction of myelin. The perivenular location gives rise to linear zones of signal abnormality referred to as Dawson's fingers – perpendicular to the long axis of the lateral ventricles. Deep and subependymal veins are oriented perpendicular to the long axis of the lateral ventricles, giving this appearance. Areas of active inflammation/demyelination may show contrast enhancement indicative of BBB breakdown. Enhancement (nodular or ring) can last 8–12 weeks. In the chronic phase, this leads to atrophy of WM with ex vacuo enlargement of ventricles. Some acute MS lesions show diffusion restriction. Common locations are the periventricular regions with a predilection in periatrial regions, the corpus callosum, along the pial surface of the brainstem, in the pons near the root entry zone of the trigeminal nerves, the cerebellar peduncles, and WM. In the corpus callosum, look for a linear, striated pattern of abnormal signal with involvement of the under-surface near the callosal septal interface. Visual pathways are commonly involved. Posterior fossa lesions are often better seen on fast spin echo (FSE) T2 sequences than on FLAIR, and supratentorial lesions are usually best seen on FLAIR images.

Acute disseminated encephalomyelitis (see Figure 6.166, pages 178–179)

This is thought to be immune mediated, occurring several weeks after a childhood viral illness or vaccination. It appears as a monophasic course in contrast to MS. Lesions are found in WM with a greater tendency for involvement of the basal ganglia and thalami (which may be symmetric). It is less commonly periventricular than MS, and there are bilateral, asymmetric, poorly margined, WM lesions. Contrast enhancement of lesions can occur.

Progressive multifocal leukoencephalopathy (see Figure 6.163, page 176)

Progressive multifocal leukoencephalopathy (PML) is caused by reactivation of a commonly carried virus, the JC virus, and is usually of no harm unless immunosuppressed. It is often found in subcortical WM, more in the parieto-occipital lobes. As the disease progresses, the WM involvement extends deeper. The corpus callosum is less commonly affected than in MS. Cerebellar and brainstem involvement occurs in about 30% of cases and may initially present as solitary lesions in these sites, which are patchy, round, or oval at first and progress to larger, confluent regions; the pattern is often asymmetric with involvement of peripheral WM extending to the GM–WM junction, giving a scalloped appearance. There is generally no contrast enhancement or mass effect.

Human immunodeficiency viral encephalitis (see Figure 6.165, page 177)

The human immunodeficiency virus (HIV) is a neurotrophic retrovirus and causes subacute encephalitis of WM in 30% of patients with AIDS. The images show bilateral, diffuse, patchy and/or confluent, increased T2 signal with poor delineation of lesions. The disease may affect the brainstem, cerebellum, and cerebral hemispheres with subtle, hazy, dirty looking WM and no enhancement. It can remain stable or even improve with drug therapy.

Post-radiation

The extent of involvement depends on the amount of brain in port. Pathologic changes result in obliterative endarteritis over time. There is a latent period with imaging studies first showing changes about 6–8 months after therapy and progressing over several years. When the whole brain is involved you will see diffuse, symmetric, high T2 signal changes in periventricular WM. The corpus callosum and subcortical regions are not involved at first. With time, peripheral extension to the subcortical regions occurs along with atrophy. There is relative sparing of the posterior fossa and internal capsules. High-dose localized radiation can result in radiation necrosis with severe, focal edema with mass effect and enhancement. Differentiation from treated but active tumor may be difficult and may be differentiated by MR spectroscopy and MR perfusion imaging. MR spectroscopy in active tumor shows elevated choline peak and there is increased MR perfusion relative to radiation necrosis.

Post-chemotherapy

Acute effects can produce transient, diffuse, bilateral increase T2 in the WM. More chronic/delayed effects (weeks to months) with patchy to confluent high T2 signal may occur in the periventricular WM, becoming more extensive and confluent with time, with eventual atrophy. Usually there is no enhancement or mass effect unless very severe, which may calcify (mineralizing microangiopathy) especially in children receiving both chemotherapy and radiation. WM damage is intensified with combined chemotherapy and radiation especially in patients with leukemia. This has been called disseminated necrotizing leukoencephalopathy (DNL).

Posterior reversible encephalopathy syndrome (see Figure 6.260, page 241)

Numerous etiologies with the common denominator appearing to be hypertension are seen with medications including immunosuppressive drugs such as cyclosporine, hypertension, chronic renal disease, preeclampsia, eclampsia, and systemic lupus erythematosus (SLE). The high T2 signal in the posterior cerebral subcortical WM may extend frontally; there is usually no diffusion restriction and any enhancement is minimally patchy. It is usually reversible. The posterior circulation is most commonly involved, and this is theorized to be because of the diminished capacity of vascular autoregulation. Rarely there may be diffusion restriction, which leads to permanent foci of signal abnormality (still pathologically and clinically posterior reversible encephalopathy syndrome [PRES] but not reversible).

Metabolic disorders involving white matter (leukodystrophies)

This is a diverse group of disorders including metachromatic leukodystrophy, adrenal leukodystrophy, Alexander's disease, Canavan's disease, Pelizaeus–Merzbacher disease, and more. These are characterized by enzymatic defects resulting in faulty production of and/or maintenance of the WM. These occur in children and are often characterized by an extensive, bilateral, symmetric, and confluent pattern of abnormality. Enhancement can be seen in some of these disorders along the advancing edge of demyelination/dysmyelination.

Vasculitis

There are a wide variety of vasculitic processes that can result in multifocal regions of abnormal signal in the WM and may be limited to the CNS such as primary angiitis of the CNS (PACNS), or part of a more systemic process such as collagen vascular disease, granulomatous disease, polyarteritis nodosa, rheumatoid arthritis, or related to certain drugs. You may see deep WM lesions and/or cortical lesions depending upon the size of the vessels involved.

Traumatic white matter lesion

Small focal areas of abnormal increased T2/FLAIR signal may be seen as the sequelae of previous closed head injury. These may represent the evolution of cerebral contusions (small areas of hemorrhagic bruising of the brain), often found near sites of impact with adjacent bone or other barriers including dural reflections, such as the inferior frontal lobes above the orbital roofs, adjacent to the frontal bone, in the anterior temporal lobes just posterior to the sphenoid wings, adjacent to the pterion, in the mid-temporal lobes just above the petrous ridges, or adjacent to the falx cerebri or tentorium cerebelli. Other WM lesions may represent shear type injuries also referred to as diffuse axonal injury (DAI). These small WM lesions occur secondary to rapid deceleration and occur as a result of rotational/torque forces upon portions of the brain where there is a transition between GM and WM, which have slight differences in composition/density, resulting in the tearing/shearing of axons. These are often seen at the GM–WM junction, in the corpus callosum, and dorsal midbrain. In past decades where high field imaging utilized 1.5 T MRI systems, shear injuries were most often felt to be non-hemorrhagic. However, with the advent of 3T or higher MRI, small areas of magnetic susceptibility (look black) are seen in these regions using gradient echo T2/susceptibility weighted imaging, which is essential in the evaluation of post-trauma patients, especially when the neurologic status of the patient does not match the imaging findings on routine brain MRI without the use of gradient echo T2 images.

Chronic migraines

Multifocal periventricular WM hyperintensities, which can resemble deep WM ischemia or vasculitis, may be seen.

Central pontine myelinolysis (osmotic demyelination) (see Figure 6.185, page 195)

This condition is most common in the central pons but may be extrapontine. It is found most often in alcoholics but is seen in patients with electrolyte disturbances, such as rapid correction of hyponatremia, and in liver transplant patients. You see ovoid, triangular/trident configurations of decreased T1 and increased T2 signal, which may show diffusion restriction acutely but which can reverse. These usually do not enhance but severe cases can show peripheral enhancement of lesions.

Diffuse periventricular high T2 signal (smooth, continuous rind)

This may be seen in association with deep WM ischemic changes of aging, transependymal resorption of CSF in hydrocephalus (see Figure 6.275, page 250), and ventriculitis.

Miscellaneous conditions resulting in white matter lesions

Lyme disease (caused by the gram-negative spirochete *Borrelia burgdorferi*), sarcoidosis (the parenchymal form via extension through DPSs), and collagen vascular diseases (i.e. SLE).

Metabolic disorders of the brain

The metabolic disorders of the brain are a diverse group of disorders characterized by enzymatic defects and associated abnormalities of cellular organelles that can be grouped into lysosomal, peroxisomal, and mitochondrial disorders. For a simpler categorization, they can be divided into the following groups:

1. Disorders primarily involving WM – leukodystrophies
2. Disorders primarily involving GM – many involve lysosomal enzyme defects with failure to degrade certain materials, resulting in storage diseases such as Tay–Sachs Disease and other lipid storage disorders, mucopolysaccharidoses, and glycogen storage disorders
3. Disorders that affect both WM and GM – typical of this group are the mitochondrial and peroxisomal disorders such as Leigh's disease; mitochondrial myopathy, encephalopathy, lactic acidosis, and stroke syndrome (MELAS); myoclonic epilepsy with ragged red fibers syndrome (MERRF), and Kearns–Sayre syndrome
4. Basal ganglia disorders – Huntington disease, Wilson disease, Fahr's disease, and Hallervorden–Spatz disease.

Cerebral perfusion pressure (CPP)

Cerebral perfusion pressure is mean arterial pressure minus intracranial pressure (CPP = MAP – ICP). Normal CPP in adults is >50 mm Hg.

Brain perfusion

Cerebral blood flow:

Normal CBF: 50–60 mL/100 g/min of brain tissue to maintain normal metabolic rate
Ischemic penumbra: ~15–30 mL/100 g/min
Irreversible ischemia: below ~15 mL/100 g/min

Ischemic penumbra

This represents the ischemic tissue at risk for infarction lying outside of the core of infarction. It correlates with diffusion/perfusion mismatch on MRI. This is present when the perfusion deficit (CBF, mean transit time [MTT]) is larger than the diffusion deficit. On CT the mismatch is indicated by the discrepant size in the cerebral blood volume (CBV), which is the CT correlate for the diffusion deficit (infarcted tissue) because you cannot measure diffusion on CT and the CBF. This at risk tissue is the target for stroke therapy.

Watershed zones of ischemia
(see Figures 6.226b, 227c, 230, pages 219, 220, 222)

These areas are the junctional zones between the distal branches of different vascular territories. As such they are prone to ischemic injury, particularly in the setting of hypotension or low states of oxygenation; for instance, near drowning.

CT signs in acute ischemic infarction (stroke)
(see Figures 6.226a, 227a, 232a, pages 219, 220, 223)

> Dense middle cerebral artery sign – intraluminal thrombus, which can be seen in the M1 and/or M2 segments
> Insular ribbon sign – loss of normal high density of the insular cortex from cytotoxic edema
> Sulcal effacement
> Loss of normal GM–WM differentiation – look in the basal ganglia/internal capsule region and along the gray–white interface in the cortical/subcortical regions of the cerebral and cerebellar hemispheres; secondary to cytotoxic edema
> Mass effect – peaks from three to five days
> Enhancement of cerebral infarcts: rule of 3's – enhancement generally starts at about 3 days, peaks at 3 weeks, and is gone by 3 months.

MRI in acute ischemic infarction (stroke)
(see Figures 6.225, 227b, 228d, 230, 237b, 238a–c, pages 219–222, 225, 226)

Diffusion restriction in the setting of cerebral ischemia is considered an indication of irreversible ischemic injury/infarction. Restricted diffusion persists for approximately 7–10 days. While the signal on the ADC map will normalize after this time, increased signal can persist on the diffusion trace image for some time secondary to T2 shine through. Areas of signal abnormality in acute stroke should conform to known vascular territories. You may also see asymmetric vascular enhancement on post-contrast images owing to slow flow. Look for normal flow voids in the major proximal intracranial arterial vascular pedicles. Be aware that diseases other than acute stroke can demonstrate restricted diffusion, such as certain highly cellular tumors and infection. If you are unsure whether you are looking at an acute stroke, obtain a short-term follow-up examination in approximately 2–3 weeks.

Crossed cerebellar diaschesis/atrophy

This is a phenomenon in which there is hypometabolism/reduced blood flow within the cerebellum contralateral to a supratentorial cerebral hemispheric lesion such as infarction, hemorrhage, or tumor. In addition, structural atrophy within the cerebellum contralateral to a cerebral hemispheric insult may also occur (crossed cerebellar atrophy).

Monro–Kellie doctrine

The intracranial contents are enclosed in a rigid shell (the skull). There are three major components of the intracranial structures: (1) brain tissue, (2) arterial and venous blood, and (3) CSF. A state of dynamic equilibrium is maintained in normal situations. If one of these components increases in volume, there must be a decrease in the others to maintain normal equilibrium otherwise the ICP will increase. Normal ICP in adults is less than 10–15 mm Hg. Intracranial hypertension is considered when the ICP is greater than 18–20 mm Hg. Normal ICP is lower in young children and infants. This concept has relevance in the entity of intracranial hypotension when there is a CSF leak resulting in decreased intracranial CSF pressure. With the loss of CSF in the intracranial compartment there is a concomitant increase in the intracranial volume of venous blood resulting in meningeal enhancement, distention of the dural venous sinuses, the appearance of numerous venous collaterals, generalized prominence of intracranial veins, and enlargement of the pituitary gland because of venous engorgement. Intracranial hypotension is also associated with the development of subdural hematomas and hygromas.

Differential diagnosis of white matter hypodensity on CT and decreased T1/increased T2 MRI signal

> Edema – increased water content of tissue; includes cytotoxic and vasogenic types (see below). It is

associated with a positive mass effect, and there are many potential causes.

- Encephalomalacia/gliosis – associated with tissue loss/negative mass effect. This is the end result of many types of insults/injuries.
  - Macrocystic encephalomalacia – cavitary, cystic/necrotic regions of the brain behaving like bulk water (similar to CSF). The clue is isointensity to CSF on FLAIR images, unless it contains high protein in which case it will be hyperintense to CSF on FLAIR.
  - Microcystic encephalomalacia – damaged, gliotic brain with increased water content but without overt cavitary necrosis. The clue is increased signal intensity on FLAIR images.
- Tumor infiltration – usually associated with positive mass effect. Not all tumors enhance; tumor cells often extend beyond the margins of visual enhancement. Enhancement only occurs if the BBB is disrupted. Be careful not to attribute non-enhancing CT hypodense or T2 MRI hyperintense areas near the site of the tumor/tumor resection to encephalomalacia, gliosis, or edema as active tumor may be present. This concept is more applicable to primary cerebral tumors. Metastatic tumors are usually encapsulated and do not infiltrate into the surrounding brain beyond the capsule.
- Demyelination – acutely can produce positive mass effect; chronically there is tissue loss/negative mass effect.

Edema

Cytotoxic (intracellular swelling) results from increased intracellular water owing to toxic or anoxic injury with disruption of the normal sodium ATPase pump. It is usually more prominent in GM. On CT this is seen as loss of GM–WM differentiation and sulcal effacement. On MR you may see sulcal effacement and subtle signal changes (decreased T1, increased T2). Etiologies include ischemic infarction and traumatic injury. Early ischemic edema is cytotoxic but as the infarction evolves, vasogenic edema also becomes evident.

Vasogenic edema results from increased water in the extracellular space of the brain owing to disruption of the blood brain barrier. This edema tends to spread and track through the WM where there is more space for this water to accumulate (as opposed to the tighter packing of cells in GM). It appears as hypodensity within the WM on CT imaging and T1 hypointensity and T2 hyperintensity on MRI. Etiologies include primary or metastatic tumors, and infection/inflammation. This type of edema responds to steroids.

Intracranial hemorrhage
Computed tomography
Acute (approximately 1 hour to 3 days)
The hemorrhage is hyperdense with HU varying from approximately 50 to 90. You may or may not see surrounding edema early on, but this will develop over time. Look for positive mass effect.

Subacute (4 days to 3 weeks)
The hyperdensity of blood gradually decreases and becomes less discrete. It will pass through a stage where blood is isodense with the brain. Surrounding edema becomes more prominent. Subacute hematomas will often show peripheral rim enhancement (2–6 weeks).

Chronic (more than 3 weeks)
The lesion will continue to become more hypodense to the brain and will demonstrate negative mass effect.

Magnetic resonance imaging
Hyperacute (minutes to 6 hours)
Oxyhemoglobin is present in intact red blood cells and plasma. You see hypointense T1 and hyperintense T2 signal; a nonspecific appearance. Look for developing edema.

Acute (12 hours to 4 days)
There is intracellular deoxyhemoglobin. The appearance is isointense to slightly hypointense on T1 and hypointense on T2 images. Look for increasing surrounding edema and mass effect.

Subacute (approximately 4 days to 1 month)
The early subacute (4–7 days) is hyperintense on T1 and hypointense on T2 owing to intracellular methemoglobin. The late subacute (~1–4 weeks) stage is hyperintense on both T1WI and T2WI because of extracellular methemoglobin. Changes occur from peripheral to central regions. Edema and mass effect diminish after the first week and are usually absent at one month.

Chronic (more than 1 month)

The deposition of hemosiderin begins in the periphery of the clot and progresses centrally. Hemosiderin is hypointense on both T1 and T2 images. There is no edema at this stage. Clot retraction occurs with focal atrophic changes. Central T1 and T2 hyperintensity may last for some time.

Intracranial mass effects

Numerous pathologic processes can result in similar mass effect on intracranial structures. The different types of mass effect include: (1) subfalcine herniation – midline herniation/shift of a cerebral hemisphere underneath the falx cerebri; the posterior falx extends deeper (more inferiorly) into the interhemispheric fissure making it easier for the brain to herniate beneath the falx more anteriorly; (2) uncal herniation – medial displacement of the anteromedial point (uncus) of the temporal lobe into the suprasellar cistern; (3) downward transtentorial herniation – inferior displacement of the hippocampus/parahippocampal gyrus into the tentorial incisura from supratentorial mass effect; (4) upward transtentorial herniation – posterior fossa mass effect displaces the superior vermis/cerebellum upward into the tentorial incisura obliterating the supracerebellar/quadrigeminal plate cisterns. You may see mass effect on the tectal plate; (5) transalar/transphenoidal herniation – inferior herniation of the inferior frontal lobe or superior herniation of the anterior temporal lobe over the sphenoid wing; (6) tonsillar herniation – inferior displacement of the cerebellar tonsil into or below the foramen magnum.

Hydrocephalus – two major types; most are type 1
(see Figures 6.273–278, pages 249–252)
Obstructive hydrocephalus

This type of hydrocephalus can be intraventricular (sometimes called non-communicating) or extraventricular (sometimes called communicating and includes normal pressure hydrocephalus [NPH]).

Intraventricular or non-communicating obstructive hydrocephalus

The pattern of ventricular enlargement depends upon the level of obstruction. If there is obstruction at the foramen of Monroe on one side, you will see unilateral lateral ventricular dilatation. If the foramen of Monroe is obstructed on both sides, you get dilatation of both lateral ventricles with normal sized third and fourth ventricles. If the aqueduct is obstructed, there is dilatation of the third and lateral ventricles and of the aqueduct above the obstruction. With obstruction of the outlet foramina of the fourth ventricle (foramina of Luschka and Magendie) you will see dilatation of the fourth, third, and lateral ventricles. This may be indistinguishable from communicating hydrocephalus.

Extraventricular obstructive hydrocephalus (communicating hydrocephalus)

The most common etiologies are hemorrhage, infection, or tumor with the common denominator that they obstruct the passage of CSF over the convexities, and damage the arachnoid granulations impairing resorption of CSF. The fourth ventricle is normal in size in about 25%–30% of cases.

Normal pressure hydrocephalus

This is a form of communicating hydrocephalus seen in the elderly. It is associated with Hakim–Adams triad of: (1) gait apraxia, (2) incontinence, and (3) dementia. Patients may present with one or all of the symptoms. Patients who do best with shunting are those with little or mild dementia. NPH is often underdiagnosed. Diagnostic clues include disproportionate enlargement of the ventricles relative to the sulci, compression of high convexity sulci against the inner table at the vertex, upward bowing of the corpus callosum, decreased height of the interpeduncular cistern, and confluent periventricular increased T2 signal (transependymal CSF resorption). Sometimes you will see gaping Sylvian fissures with otherwise normal sized sulci. Do not be fooled and write off the disproportionate ventricular enlargement to deep WM atrophy. The Sylvian fissures can act as reservoirs and become quite large in NPH (communicating hydrocephalus) while the remaining sulci are not particularly enlarged.

Non-obstructive hydrocephalus

This is a result of increased production of CSF such as in choroid plexus tumor (papilloma or carcinoma).

Atrophy

The presence of cerebral atrophy on imaging studies can reflect predominant cortical atrophy (neuronal loss), preferential WM atrophy, or a combination of both.

Labeling atrophy as mild, moderate, or severe depends upon the age of the patient. What would be considered normal involutional changes in an 80-year-old would be considered unexpected, significant atrophy were the patient 25 years old.

Normal aging

With the expected volume loss that occurs with aging there is a more selective loss of WM than GM in addition to associated cerebellar volume loss. You should expect a proportionate degree of sulcal widening and enlargement of the ventricular system. Dilated perivascular spaces become more prominent and can be extensive (etat cible). These are the normal, expected, involutional changes of aging and usually begin at around the age of 50 years.

Preferential white matter atrophy (central atrophy)

In patients with underlying diabetes, hypertension, hypercholesterolemia, and atherosclerosis there is often accentuated WM volume loss owing to microvascular ischemic changes (small vessel disease). MS is another entity which, by virtue of its predominant WM involvement, will result in preferential WM atrophy with ventricular enlargement that is disproportionate to the widening of the sulci (from cortical volume loss). This type of atrophy is called central atrophy.

Cortical atrophy

This refers to the predominant involvement of the cortical GM mantle resulting in widening of the sulci out of proportion to ventricular enlargement.

Patterns of atrophy can be used to suggest certain neurodegenerative disorders.

Alzheimer's disease (see Figure 6.261, page 242): peak incidence increases with age; it often results in diffuse atrophy with accentuated volume loss in the hippocampus and parietal lobes. You can see hypoperfusion/hypometabolism in these regions on single photon emission computed tomography (SPECT) or positron emission tomography (PET) scans.

Frontal-temporal dementia (see Figure 6.264, page 243): peak incidence is 55–65 years of age (younger than in Alzheimer's disease); it is a result of deposition of abnormal protein (Tau protein). Dementia is secondary to focal cortical atrophy involving the anterior frontal and temporal lobes. Pick's disease is a pathologic variant. The cortical atrophy is usually asymmetric and may be striking with a knife-blade appearance of the gyri. Increased T2 signal in underlying WM is seen. Three clinical variants are: (1) frontal variant – frontal lobe is most severely involved, (2) semantic dementia (progressive fluent aphasia), and (3) progressive nonfluent aphasia (primary progressive aphasia). These latter two entities are associated with more severe temporal lobe involvement.

Severe alcohol abuse: you often see accentuated cerebellar vermian atrophy, which most severely affects the superior vermis.

Huntington disease: marked atrophy of the caudate nucleus with ballooning of the frontal horns.

Basics of brain tumors

World Health Organization classification of brain tumors

This provides a malignancy scale based on histologic features of the tumor and correlates with biologic behavior/prognosis. The classification provides a parallel grading system for each type of brain tumor. The World Health Organization (WHO) classification divides intracranial tumors into four grades depending upon their biologic behavior and prognosis with grades I and II being considered low-grade and grades III and IV being considered high grade. Grade I tumors are localized, non-aggressive lesions. Grades II, III, and IV are infiltrative tumors. Grade II lesions are low-grade but infiltrative lesions, which are difficult to cure because of infiltrative growth and the tendency toward dedifferentiation over time. Grade III tumors are more aggressive, such as anaplastic astrocytoma or oligoastrocytoma. Grade IV is the most aggressive neoplasm, such as glioblastoma multiforme (GBM), associated with short-term survival.

Advanced brain tumor imaging

Advanced MRI techniques such as dynamic susceptibility contrast (DSC) perfusion imaging and spectroscopy have begun to provide additional tools to add to the predictive value of tumor grading and in differentiating tumors from non-neoplastic lesions. Measurements of relative CBV (rCBV) can often differentiate high-grade from low-grade tumors, using values above 1.75 to be more predictive of high-grade gliomas and maximum rCBV values of 1.5 for low-grade gliomas. An exception to this appears to be oligodendrogliomas, which often demonstrate high rCBV measurements. MR spectroscopy provides additional information to aid in differentiating tumors from non-neoplastic lesions and to grade neoplasms. A typical spectrum obtained from a neoplasm shows elevated levels of choline (owing to rapid turnover of cell membranes), reduced N-acetyl aspartate (NAA, a marker of neuronal health), and possible elevation of lactate and lipid (in tumoral necrosis). Higher choline to NAA ratios are often seen with higher grade tumors. Sampling the peritumoral non-enhancing increased T2 signal can help differentiate a primary infiltrating glioma from a metastasis. A tumor spectrum with elevated choline is found in the peritumoral high T2 signal in gliomas owing to their infiltrative nature, whereas choline levels will be low in these regions surrounding metastatic lesions, which are usually encapsulated and non-infiltrative. In addition diffusion imaging of tumors may provide some predictive value with highly cellular, often more malignant tumors showing diffusion restriction.

Pediatric brain tumors

Birth to three years of age – more supratentorial than infratentorial tumors:

Teratoma – most common
PNET – primitive neuroectodermal tumor
Choroid plexus papilloma/carcinoma
Congenital GBM or anaplastic astrocytoma

Three to 11 years old – greater occurrence of infratentorial than supratentorial tumors.
After 11 years old – equal incidence.

Four tumors account for 95% of posterior fossa tumors in the pediatric population – medulloblastoma, cerebellar astrocytoma, ependymoma, and brainstem glioma.

Adult intra-axial brain tumors
Supratentorial (more common than infratentorial)

The most common intra-axial tumors are GBMs (most common glioma) and metastases (20%–30%).

Gliomas (30%–40% of supratentorial tumors) – most common primary intra-axial tumors.

Low grade – more often in young adults
High grade – more often in older adults

Infratentorial

Metastases are the most common and hemangioblastomas are the second most common intra-axial tumors (although much rarer than metastatic tumors).

Hunt–Hess grading scale for clinical grading of non-traumatic subarachnoid hemorrhage

Grade 1: asymptomatic, mild headache and slight nuchal rigidity
Grade 2: moderate to severe headache, nuchal rigidity, cranial nerve palsy, i.e. CN III
Grade 3: mild focal deficit, lethargy, confusion
Grade 4: stupor, moderate to severe hemiparesis, early decerebrate posturing
Grade 5: coma, decerebrate rigidity, moribund

Spetzler–Martin grading scale for intracranial arterial–venous malformations

This is a grading scale for intracranial arterial–venous malformations (AVMs) that correlates with surgical morbidity and mortality and helps direct treatment of AVMs for individual patients. Three characteristics are utilized:

Size of the arterial–venous malformation

<3 cm = 1
3–6 cm = 2
>6 cm = 3

Pattern of venous drainage

Superficial = 0
Deep = 1

Whether the arterial–venous malformation involves or is in close proximity to eloquent cortex

Yes = 1
No = 0

The higher the score, the greater the surgical risk. Potential scores are from grade 1 (AVM <3 cm, has superficial venous drainage, and found in non-eloquent tissue) to grade 5 (>6 cm, has deep venous drainage, and is found in eloquent tissue). Grade 6 is considered a non-operable AVM.

When to use CT and MRI
Computed tomography

Acute trauma or suspected hemorrhage from other etiology

When identification of calcification is important, i.e. craniopharyngioma, retinoblastoma, cysticercosis

Assessment of bone pathology, including temporal bone disease

Acute stroke – to exclude hemorrhage

Interval assessment of ventricular size in patients with hydrocephalus and shunts

CT angiography – higher resolution than MRA

Contraindications for MRI as with certain implantable medical devices such as cardiac pacemakers, cochlear implants, certain aneurysm clips, deep brain stimulation patients (some institutions are allowing MRI)

Magnetic resonance imaging

With a few exceptions MRI is generally a much more sensitive imaging modality compared with CT

Evaluation and extent of tumor infiltration – MRI has greater ability to differentiate different tissue types

Evaluation of skull base tumors – use of fat suppressed sequences is helpful

Evaluation of the pituitary/hypothalamic regions

Staging of metastatic disease – more sensitive than CT

Evaluation of suspected cranial nerve dysfunction

Evaluation for perineural spread of tumor – MRI is very sensitive where CT is very insensitive

Assessment of the posterior fossa – beam hardening artifact in CT creates difficulty in accurate evaluation

Evaluation for sensorineural hearing loss looking for vestibular schwannoma

Evaluation of the acute stroke patient with DWI; when combined with perfusion MRI can also provide information about ischemic penumbra

Traumatic brain injury – use of gradient echo T2/susceptibility weighted imaging significantly increases detection of shear/DAI injuries and is often positive in the face of a normal CT or routine MRI scans

Noninvasive method of vascular evaluation with 2D and 3D TOF MRA – no contrast is necessary, although it can be used

MR spectroscopy may provide important information regarding chemistry/metabolites of various disorders and help differentiate tumor from non-neoplastic processes

In-patients with severe allergy to iodinated CT contrast agents

Lesion localization
Meninges

These are the dura (pachymeninges), arachnoid, and pia (collectively called leptomeninges).

Intra-axial

The lesion arises beneath the pia, within the substance of the brain. If peripherally located near the cortex, the presence of an acute angle between the lesion and surrounding brain suggests this location.

Extra-axial

The lesion arises outside the substance of the brain (external to the pia). Clues: (1) it buckles GM and WM – the GM–WM junction is displaced centrally, (2) an obtuse angle is found between the lesion and brain, (3) the lesion has a dural/meningeal vascular supply, (4) it displaces pial vessels centrally, (5) look for widening of the subarachnoid space at the edge of the lesion, and (6) you may see a rim of CSF between the lesion and brain.

Intraventricular

The lesion primarily arises in the ventricle or secondarily invades the ventricular compartment.

Pineal region

This is the central intracranial region, posterior to the third ventricle containing the pineal gland and surrounded by deep veins.

Sella turcica region

This is the region of the central skull base containing the pituitary gland and surrounded by the cavernous sinus and its contents, and the suprasellar region and its contents including the optic apparatus and arterial vascular structures.

Cerebellar-pontine angle region

This region is defined by the pons and cerebellum medially and the posterior petrous temporal bone laterally. It encompasses cranial nerves, the internal auditory canals, and various vascular structures.

Foramen magnum

This is the largest bony cranial aperture through which the cervical medullary junction passes. The anterior bony lip is called the basion and the posterior bony lip is called the opisthion.

Subfrontal region

This refers to the extra-axial region beneath the frontal lobes and above the bones of the floor of the anterior cranial fossa. These are common sites for meningiomas, an intracranial extension of sinonasal region lesions such as mucoceles, benign and malignant tumors including esthesioneuroblastoma (olfactory neuroblastoma), and encehaloceles.

Posterior fossa

This is the general term for all of the structures (both intra- and extra-axial) located between the dura of the tentorium cerebelli above, the foramen magnum below, and the petrous ridges and clivus laterally and anteriorly.

Petrous portion of the temporal bone region

This is a triangular-shaped bone; the apex is pointed anteromedially toward the foramen lacerum and the base is pointed posterolaterally toward the tympanic portion. Several bony apertures along the posterior surface include the porus acousticus, and the vestibular and cochlear aqueducts. The arcuate eminence (the bony prominence along the superior surface of the superior semicircular canal) is along the anterior–superior surface. This is a bony landmark for middle cranial fossa surgery.

Petrous apex

This is the anterior medial aspect of the triangular petrous temporal bone.

Supratentorial region

This general term refers to all of the contents lying above the tentorium cerebelli. It contains both intra- and extra-axial structures with the largest structures being both cerebral hemispheres.

Calvarial region

This bony vault surrounding the brain is derived from membranous bone. It contains the frontal, parietal, occipital, and portions of the temporal bones.

Skull base region

The bony structures lying beneath the intracranial contents of the anterior, middle, and posterior cranial fossae are derived from endochondral bone.

Craniovertebral junction

This is a crossroads of anatomic regions where tissues of different compartments join. Included are the cervicomedullary junction (upper cervical spinal cord and medulla), the osseous (skull base, C1/2), and ligamentous supporting structures as well as the nasopharynx anteriorly.

Scalp

This refers to the soft tissue contents external/superficial to the outer table of the skull. It contains galea aponeurosis, subcutaneous fat, skin, and dermal appendages.

Cisterns

These are expansions of the subarachnoid spaces.

Basic approach to image interpretation

Before you can embark on the analysis and interpretation of imaging studies, you must learn the basic anatomy of that region. A repetitive approach in the actual process of image analysis is helpful. By incorporating a particular sequence of image analysis each and every time you look at a case, you will eventually create a type of mind/brain reflex or pattern to image analysis. In addition, this will eliminate errors of omission and free your mind to enhance your analytic/interpretive skills. If you approach each case in a different manner, you will find that your ability to characterize, sort, and analyze a case will take more brain energy and this will lead to more interpretive errors and less efficiency in your use of time, which has become increasingly important in this day and age where the pressures of productivity are in the forefront.

In addition to a repetitive approach toward analyzing a case, you should also attempt to create template types of dictations in your brain. This will provide you with a structured order in image analysis each time you review a case. Again, by incorporating a structured report you will reduce errors of omission and increase your efficiency in case review. Radiologic reports created as a narrative (free association, as I say) will not only impair the interpreter's skill but also make the reports more difficult for the referring clinician to understand. I will provide in the appendix basic dictation templates that I use. You can use these or you may modify them to fit your own needs and what works well with your brain.

I will give you my approach in the next few paragraphs, but if you find that a different approach works better for you then I would encourage that. Each of our brains is unique and works a little differently to others. Do not fool with success. If you find a different approach and it works, use it; but use it each and every time.

Looking for image asymmetry seems to be a simple concept but a powerful one in the process of image interpretation. Another important concept is to remember always that one is more likely to identify an unusual manifestation of a common disorder than a common manifestation of an unusual disorder. If you find an abnormality that has typical findings but is not located in the typical location, do not discard the diagnosis based only on location. This is why it is important to learn the typical appearance and locations of lesions so that when presented with an atypical location, your ability to recognize a typical appearance/morphology will not be ignored.

If you identify an abnormality within your first few looks at the images, try to refrain from focusing all of your attention on the obvious abnormality. Put that aside and focus on it at the end of your analytic process. It is often easy to ignore the rest of the examination when a glaring abnormality is seen within seconds of image viewing. When this is done, often important additional/ancillary findings are ignored, which will ultimately detract from your final interpretation.

Magnetic resonance imaging of the brain

When I interpret MRI brain examinations, I first look at the diffusion weighted trace images in conjunction with the ADC map. I then take a brief look at the sagittal T1 sequence for any obvious abnormality. I proceed by looking at the axial FLAIR and FSE T2 images from the bottom to the top of the head (vertex). I look at the different geographical regions in a set sequence: foramen magnum, skull base, cerebellum, brainstem, fourth ventricle, internal auditory canals (IACs), cerebellopontine (CP) angles, signal from the membranous labyrinth, and finally the mastoid bones and petrous apex. I then change my focus of attention on the supratentorial compartment. I begin centrally near the skull base. I look at Meckel's cave, cavernous sinuses, intrasellar, parasellar, and suprasellar regions.

I look at and analyze the morphology, size, and position of the third and lateral ventricles. My attention moves now toward the anterior and medial temporal lobes, inferior frontal lobes, Sylvian fissures, basal ganglia/internal capsule/thalamic regions, the interhemispheric fissure, the pineal gland, the remainder of the temporal and frontal lobes, and then the parietal and occipital lobes. Assessment of GM–WM differentiation should always be in the back of your mind. Lastly, I look at the extra-axial spaces, the cisterns, and subarachnoid spaces, the dura, calvarium (inner table, diploe, and outer table), and then the scalp. When I am finished with the intracranial compartments, I look at the sinonasal region, nasopharynx, orbital regions, and visualized upper neck/cervical spine.

If coronal images are available, I attempt to evaluate the medial temporal lobes, particularly the hippocampal formations.

If post-contrast images are provided, look at these in detail. Identify normally expected areas of enhancement and carefully search for pathologic sites of enhancement. If artifact partially obscures assessment of certain regions, utilize other imaging planes for additional sources of information.

Lastly, I focus my attention on the details of the sagittal T1 images. Identify the corpus callosum, cingulate gyrus, region of the foramen of Monroe, aqueduct of Sylvius, fourth ventricle, vermis of the cerebellum and cerebellar hemispheres, sella turcica (pituitary gland), suprasellar region, optic chiasm, floor of the third ventricle, tuber cinereum (between the mamillary bodies and infindibulum), infindibular and optic recesses of the third ventricle, tectal (quadrigeminal) plate, and pineal gland.

Never forget about the veins. Cortical vein thrombosis, dural venous thrombosis, and venous infarction are entities that are often overlooked. These abnormalities are some of the most missed entities because we just do not think about them. Venous pathology can have devastating results, and often occurs in young individuals. Frequently the signs and symptoms of these entities are nonspecific and therefore overlooked by the clinicians.

Computed tomography of the brain

My approach toward image analysis of CT head examinations is similar but involves fewer steps because the number of sets of images is fewer and is, in most cases, in the axial plane with the exception of multiplanar (coronal, sagittal) reformats, which are easily obtained with the multidetector helical CT technique. I begin my assessment of the axial images from bottom to top, beginning on the lowest, most inferior axial slices. Analyzing the posterior fossa is usually difficult because of the beam hardening artifact that usually streaks across this region. Because of this, it is imperative that you pay close attention to the location of the fourth ventricle, making sure that it is midline in position. Scrutinize the density of the brainstem and cerebellum even though it is easy to discount alterations as merely artifact. If there are subtle changes that might represent true pathology, you may need to recommend MRI for better assessment. Look for any gross asymmetries. Carefully scrutinize the foramen magnum to exclude inferior tonsillar herniation. Slowly move your attention superiorly through the tentorial incisura into the supratentorial compartment. Begin centrally and then peripherally, starting with the basal cisterns. Are they open? Is the ventricular system normal in morphology, size, and position? Assess the various lobes of both cerebral hemispheres. Look for normal GM–WM differentiation. Look for areas of localized mass effect such as sulcal effacement. Look for subtle signs of an extra-axial mass such as buckling of the GM–WM junction. This could be the only indication of a small extra-axial fluid collection (isodense-subacute subdural hematoma) or mass (such as a meningioma). If contrast has been given, assess for areas of pathologic enhancement, always remembering the normally expected regions of enhancement such as segmental areas of dura, vascular structures, choroid plexus, infindibulum, pituitary gland, and pineal gland. View the brain at four windows: (1) normal brain, (2) subdural window, (3) stroke window, and (4) bone window. This process of viewing the images at these different windows is crucial and will minimize potentially significant errors. The subdural window allows visualization of subtle extra-axial abnormalities adjacent to the inner table, which might not be visible on standard brain windows, such as thin acute subdural hematomas. Stroke windows narrow the gray scale and optimize your ability to detect subtle density abnormalities such as early cytotoxic edema with early infarction. On bone windows look for fractures, and solitary or multifocal bone lesions including lytic and blastic changes. If possible look at 3D volume rendered images of the skull. Sometimes linear skull fractures are more apparent on these reconstructions. Look at the anatomy of the sinonasal and orbital regions, and the portions of the upper neck/cervical spine that are included in the images. You may identify significant unexpected abnormalities in these areas. Never forget about the edges of the images.

All of what I have described here may seem like a daunting task at first. With time and repetition, this approach will become imprinted in your brain as a type of pattern for image analysis. Just like working out at the gym can at first be painful and difficult to keep a regimen/routine, with time it becomes less painful and more pleasurable to keep to a specific schedule. This will make your job fun.

Analytic aproach to differential diagnosis
Things to consider
Location, location, location

How many times have you heard this from your realtor?

> While location is an important clue to the diagnosis, it is only a part of the overall picture. Similar lesions will often exhibit the same or similar imaging characteristics regardless of their location. For instance, a meningioma arising from the supratentorial convexity will have similar imaging characteristics to a meningioma arising from the petrous ridge in the posterior fossa. On the other hand, certain lesions will be diagnosed with a greater emphasis placed on their location. For instance,

Lhermitte–Duclos disease is only present in the cerebellum, amyotrophic lateral sclerosis (ALS) is limited to the corticospinal tracts, certain dementias are characterized by certain locations and, by definition, mesial temporal sclerosis is limited to the medial temporal lobe/hippocampal formations.

Patient's age

What are the normal macro- and microanatomic elements in each location?

If the pathology is diffuse or localized, what pathologic processes should be considered?

Always have in the back of your brain the different categories of pathology. This will follow on subsequent pages.

As there are blind spots in analyzing a chest x-ray, there are also blind spots in the analysis of the brain, which you should always look at:

> Foramen magnum
> Mastoid region
> At juncture points between the intracranial and extracranial compartments
> Midline subfrontal/cribriform plate
> Inferior frontal lobes just above the orbital roofs
> Anterior and inferior middle cranial fossa and anterior temporal lobes
> Just above the petrous bones
> Junction of the skull base and upper neck including the nasopharynx and parotid glands

Generalized categorization of disease: disease process/location

Congenital lesions/malformations

A simple rule of thumb: anytime you see one congenital malformation, look for others.

Disorders of organogenesis

Anencephaly
Cephalocele (see Figure 6.1, page 72)
Chiari malformations (types I–III) (see Figures 6.2, 6.3, page 73)
Corpus callosum anomalies (see Figures 6.4, 6.5, pages 74, 75)
Hydranencephaly (see Figure 6.6, page 75)
Porencephaly

Anencephaly

This is the most severe form of neural tube defect with an absence of brain parenchyma and a variable presence of posterior fossa contents (brainstem and cerebellum) and lack of cranial vault. It is incompatible with life. The pre-natal ultrasound scan shows a frog-eye appearance in the coronal plane. There is marked elevation of alpha fetoprotein and polyhydramnios.

Cephalocele

A defect in the calvarium or skull base through which intracranial contents herniate. These are most often midline defects, classified by location and contents. The meningocele includes meninges and CSF; encephalocele includes meninges and neural tissue (usually dysplastic/gliotic). An occipital location is most common in the Western hemisphere and it is associated with a Chiari malformation (Chiari III). A frontoethmoidal location is most common in Southeast Asia, often seen with craniofacial anomalies. Least common are parietal and sphenoid locations: sphenoid location is occult on clinical examination, resulting in delay in diagnosis; others are usually diagnosed at birth. Identify the location and relationship of dural venous sinuses to the cephalocele and other congenital anomalies. Look for a tract of CSF leading from the brain, deformity/stretching of sulci/gyri toward the bony defect, and pointing of the ventricle toward the defect (tethered look). Imaging studies show a midline defect with sclerotic margins.

Chiari malformation (types I–III)

These show variable degrees of hindbrain malformation. Chiari I consists of inferior cerebellar tonsilar ectopia (displacement). This is generally not associated with other brain malformations but you may see anomalies of the skull base/upper cervical spine such as occipitalization of the atlas and Klippel–Feil anomalies. The normal position of the tonsils is 3 mm or less below the foramen magnum (use McCrae's line); 3–5 mm below the foramen magnum is equivocal and greater than 5 mm is abnormal. Abnormal tonsils often have a pointed/peg-like configuration and may be asymptomatic. Sometimes you see inferior tonsilar ectopia on only one side with a normal position on the other. Phase contrast cine CSF flow imaging may reveal abnormal hemodynamics of CSF flow (reduced biphasic, pulsatile flow) through the foramen magnum and in the posterior fossa/upper cervical canal, which may help you decide the significance of tonsilar ectopia and necessity for surgery (occipital craniectomy and resection of the posterior arch of C1). Syringohydromyelia occurs in 20%–40% of Chiari I. Chiari II is the Arnold–Chiari malformation. The etiology is suspected to be failure of complete closure of the caudal end of the neural tube leading to CSF leakage, which decompresses the ventricular system resulting in lack of induction/development of the posterior fossa. Myelomeningocele occurs in 100% of cases; syringohydromyelia in 50%–90%. Hydrocephalus usually develops within 48 hours after closing the myelomeningocele. Imaging shows inferior displacement of the brainstem and cerebellum into the upper cervical canal and an inferiorly displaced medulla with medullary kink and spur.

Numerous associated imaging abnormalities include the cerebellum wrapping around the lateral margins of the brainstem, enlarged foramen magnum, elongated and inferiorly displaced fourth ventricle, scalloping of the clivus and posterior petrous bones, tectal beaking, enlarged mass intermedia (interthalamic adhesion), hypoplastic tentorium cerebelli with upward towering of the vermis/cerebellum, hydrocephalus with colpocephaly (disproportionate enlargement of the atria and occipital horns), and interdigitation of gyri with fenestrated falx. It is also associated with other anomalies including dysgenesis of the corpus callosum, neuronal migration abnormalities, and Luckenschadel (lacunar skull – mesenchymal dysplasia of the calvarium – usually disappears by six months of age). Chiari III is a Chiari II with a low occipital or high cervical encephalocele (very rare).

Corpus callosum anomalies

The corpus callosum develops in a predetermined timing/order between weeks 12 and 20 of gestation. The genu, body, splenium, and the rostrum form in that order. There can be complete or partial absence of the corpus callosum. When partial, the last areas to form are absent. Therefore, if you see an absent anterior corpus callosum and presence of the splenium, consider other abnormalities such as an acquired destructive process or holoprosencephaly as the cause. An isolated anomaly occurs in 20% and is associated with other malformations in 80% of cases. There may be associated lipoma of the corpus callosum. Owing to lack of crossing WM fibers, the longitudinal bundles of Probst develop and indent the medial margins of the lateral ventricles giving a viking-helmet appearance on coronal images. The ventricles are widely separated and parallel in orientation. The third ventricle can extend superiorly and develop an interhemispheric cyst. Disproportionate enlargement of the occipital horns is called colpocephaly. You may see radially oriented sulci directed toward the third ventricle along the mesial hemisphere. The anterior cerebral arteries ascend vertically rather than around the corpus callosum.

Hydranencephaly

This is a severe malformation characterized by an extensive destructive change involving the cerebral hemispheres with variable sparing of the basal ganglia/thalami, brainstem, and cerebellum. You may see a minimal residual cortex along the falx posteriorly or at the base of the anterior cranial fossa. Hydranencephaly is thought to be a result of intrauterine occlusion of the carotid arteries or an infection. It is important to differentiate it from severe hydrocephalus (you may see improvement with shunting); in hydranencephaly there is no hope for a good clinical outcome regardless of treatment. You may see a thin rim of cortical mantle in severe hydrocephalus. The head is large with hydrocephalus and may be small, normal, or large with hydranencephaly.

Porencephaly

This destructive process which, if it occurs during early fetal development (prior to the late second or early third trimester), results in a cystic cavity with smooth walls with fluid that is isointense to CSF on all pulse sequences. No associated glial reaction is seen. It may communicate with the ventricles or subarachnoid space. You must differentiate it from schizencephaly: porencephaly is lined by WM not GM (as in schizencephaly). Destructive cavities developing when the brain is more mature result in a gliotic reaction with septations within the cavity and increased T2/FLAIR signal in the surrounding brain.

Disorders of neuronal migration and sulcation – usually supratentorial

Patients may have seizure disorders, developmental delay, and mental retardation.

Lissencephaly/pachygyria/polymicrogyria (see Figures 6.7, 6.8, page 76)
Cortical dysplasia (see Figures 6.9, 6.10, page 77)
Heterotopia (see Figure 6.11, page 78)
Schizencephaly (see Figure 6.12, page 78)
Unilateral hemimegalencephaly (see Figure 6.13, page 79)

Germinal matrix neurons begin to develop in the subependymal zones in the seventh week of gestation. They begin to migrate peripherally during the eighth week of gestation toward the cerebral cortex. There is a somatotopic relationship between the cells of the germinal matrix and their eventual location along the cortex, meaning that cells in a certain part of the germinal matrix are destined for a particular cortical location. They migrate along radial glial fibers, which maintain this organized fashion of development. Insults during the process of migration will result in a neuronal migration anomaly where the migration of these neurons is halted. These neurons are normal and therefore they demonstrate normal density/signal as cortex on imaging studies.

Lissencephaly/pachygyria/polymicrogyria

There is a spectrum of neuronal migration anomalies with the most severe form being complete lissencephaly or agyria. Less severe forms are incomplete lissencephaly (partial agyria and pachygyria), primarily pachygyria, polymicrogyria, and GM heterotopias. In complete lissencephaly, the brain is smooth with a thick cortex, decreased WM, and shallow vertically oriented Sylvian fissures. A figure-of-eight appearance is seen on axial images. In pachygyria, see areas of cortical thickening, involving small focal areas or larger areas of the brain. Polymicrogyria occurs when the neurons reach the cortex but are abnormally arranged, resulting in multiple small gyri, likened to the dimples on a basketball. These are often located around Sylvian fissures with clefts. Polymicrogyria is difficult to differentiate from pachygyria on imaging studies. Anomalous veins are often seen near the cortical surface of polymicrogyric clefts; you often see gliotic WM underlying the polymicrogyria.

Cortical dysplasia

Focal cortical dysplasia is a focal abnormality in the lamination of cortical neurons, sometimes with involvement of the underlying WM. The form associated with balloon cells and abnormal signal in underlying WM along radial glial lines, often with a comet-like appearance extending from the cortical surface and tapering to the ventricular margin, is called Taylor balloon cell cortical dysplasia. You may only see focal disorganization/thickening of cortical GM.

Heterotopic gray matter

Any insult that occurs during the migration of neurons from the subependymal germinal matrix to their destined cortical regions can result in arrest of the neurons, resulting in heterotopic GM. Heterotopias can occur anywhere along this route from the subependymal and periventricular region to the subcortical region. This can lead to focal nodular or band-like regions of heterotopic neurons. These regions should be isointense to GM on all sequences, show no surrounding edema, and not have enhancement. Patients often have seizure disorders and may have other associated anomalies.

Schizencephaly

This is characterized by full-thickness clefts of the brain, extending from the subarachnoid space to the ventricle, lined by abnormal GM (pachygyria or polymicrogyria). Clefts can be closed (type I) or open (type II), unilateral or bilateral, and often occur near pre- and postcentral gyri. Look for the pial–ependymal seam (the point where the pia lining the cleft joins the ependyma of the ventricle with which it communicates), which can be difficult with the closed-lip form. Look for the dimple in the lateral ventricle where the seam is located. Schizencephaly is associated with seizures, mental retardation, and developmental delay, which are more severe with the open-lip variety and multiple clefts. Differentiate it from destructive process by the presence of GM lining the cleft. If related to a destructive process, the cleft will be lined by WM. Septo-optic dysplasia is seen in up to a third of cases.

Unilateral hemimegalencephaly

This involves hamartomatous overgrowth of part or all of a cerebral hemisphere, and disorganization of the cortex with areas of pachygyria, polymicrogyria, and GM heterotopias. The cortex is thickened and may demonstrate calcification, there is abnormal underlying WM, and it is associated with vascular, venous anomalies. See enlargement of the lateral ventricle with straightening of the frontal horn pointing anterolaterally. Patients have intractable seizures, hemiplegia, and developmental delay. There may be other associated hemihypertrophy syndromes.

Disorders of diverticulation and cleavage – supratentorial

Holoprosencephaly (see Figure 6.14, page 79)
Septo-optic dysplasia (see Figure 6.15, page 80)
Absence of septum pellucidum

Holoprosencephaly

This is a group of disorders characterized by varying degrees of lack of diverticulation of the prosencehalon (forebrain) into the cerebral hemispheres. The least severe form is septo-optic dysplasia with absence of the septum pellucidum associated with hypoplasia of the optic nerves. The most severe form is alobar holoprosencephaly, with the intermediate form being semilobar holoprosencephaly and lobar holoprosencephaly. There are associated craniofacial anomalies such as hypotelorism and cyclopia in the most severe forms.

Septo-optic dysplasia (De Morsier's syndrome)

This may represent the mildest form of lobar holoprosencephaly. There is an absence or hypoplasia of the septum pellucidum, hypoplasia of the optic nerves, and two-thirds of cases have hypothalamic–pituitary dysfunction (usually seen as growth retardation). The absent septum pellucidum results in a box-like configuration to the frontal horns on coronal images. Associated anomalies are absence of the fornix and corpus callosal dysgenesis. Schizencephaly occurs in about 50% of patients.

Isolated absence of the septum pellucidum

This almost never occurs in the absence of other congenital brain malformations.

Posterior fossa cystic malformations

Dandy-Walker complex (see Figures 6.16, 6.17, pages 80, 81)

Mega cisterna magna (see Figure 6.18, page 81)

Arachnoid cyst (see Figure 6.19, page 81)

These are a spectrum of disorders which, at times, can be difficult to differentiate. Sometimes it is difficult to distinguish between a compressed versus a hypoplastic vermis, contributing to some confusion of diagnosis. Identifying the nine normal lobules of the vermis with forward compression as opposed to rotation and anterosuperior compression helps to differentiate these entities. In addition, mass effect may be present in both a mega cisterna magna and arachnoid cyst, making differentiation difficult.

Dandy-Walker complex

Dandy-Walker malformation includes complete or partial (involves the inferior vermis) absence of the cerebellar vermis and a retrocerebellar cyst, which communicates through the dysgenetic vermis with the fourth ventricle, with enlargement of the posterior fossa. In a partial vermian absence, the dysplastic remnant of the superior vermis is rotated anterosuperiorly and compressed. See elevation of the tentorium and the dural venous sinuses with the torcular above the lambdoid sutures (torcular–lambdoid inversion). The cerebellar hemispheres are usually hypoplastic. Other congenital malformations are associated with this condition in approximately 70% of cases. Dandy-Walker variant has a normal (or near normal) size of the posterior fossa and varying degrees of vermian and cerebellar hypoplasia with retrocerebellar fluid collection, which communicates freely through a prominent vallecula with a normal or minimally dilated fourth ventricle. It is also associated commonly with other congenital malformations.

Mega cisterna magna

The mega cisterna magna refers to expansion of the normal cisterna magna, which communicates freely with the subarachnoid spaces and ventricles with normal cerebellar hemispheres and vermis. The falx cerebelli divides the posterior part of the cisterna magna. See enlargement of the posterior fossa with the high position of the tentorium, occuring in 15% of these patients, which may be very large and may even extend supratentorially through a dehiscence of the tentorium cerebelli. May be asymmetric and produce mild mass effect on the cerebellum and falx cerebelli.

Arachnoid cyst

This cyst is secondary to splitting of the arachnoid membrane and does not freely communicate with subarachnoid or ventricular spaces. The posterior fossa is the second most common location after the middle cranial fossa. The cyst can be located in the region of the cisterna magna, cerebellopontine angle, and prepontine, interpeduncular, and quadrigeminal plate cisterns. Ataxia and calvarial asymmetry may be present from mass effect. Arachnoid cysts are usually large when diagnosed (approximately two-thirds are more than 5 cm in size), and are unilocular; contain fluid nearly identical to CSF; have smooth, well-marginated, and often imperceptible walls; but no pathologic enhancement and associated positive mass effect and no diffusion restriction. They can increase in size, differentiated from the Dandy-Walker spectrum by the morphologically normal appearance of the cerebellum, vermis, and brainstem, except for associated mass effect. Differentiating arachnoid cysts from mega cisterna magna may be difficult and may require cisternography. The arachnoid cyst should not fill with contrast but the mega cisterna magna should readily fill.

Disorders of histogenesis – phakomatoses (neurocutaneous syndromes)

Neurofibromatosis type I (NF-1) – supra- and infratentorial abnormalities (see Figures 6.20, 6.21, pages 82, 83)

Neurofibromatosis type II (NF-2 or MISME) – supra- and infratentorial abnormalities (see Figure 6.22, page 84)

Sturge–Weber syndrome – supratentorial abnormalities (see Figure 6.23, page 84)

Von Hippel–Lindau syndrome – infratentorial more than supratentorial abnormalities (see Figure 6.24, page 85)

Tuberous sclerosis (Bourneville's disease) – primarily supratentorial abnormalities (see Figure 6.25, page 86)

Osler–Weber–Rendu syndrome (hereditary hemorrhagic telangiectasia – HHT) – infratentorial, supratentorial, or both (see Figure 6.26, page 87)

NF-1

This is also called peripheral neurofibromatosis or Von Recklinghausen's disease. It is the most common neurocutaneous syndrome with an incidence of about 1 in 3000 to 5000 people, and has an autosomal dominant inheritance with 50% secondary to sporadic genetic mutation. Associated with an abnormal chromosome 17. Accounts for more than 90% of patients with NF. It is also associated with peripheral/skin manifestations with *café au lait* spots, axillary and inguinal freckling, and cutaneous neurofibromas. CNS lesions include optic pathway gliomas (usually low-grade) and other CNS gliomas. Hamartomatous lesions with increased T2 and sometimes increased T1 signal occur in the basal ganglia, pons, and cerebellar WM. They show no mass effect or pathologic enhancement and often disappear with age. You may see exuberant calcifications of the choroid plexus. Plexiform neurofibromas representing infiltrative and locally aggressive lesions occur. They may develop into neurofibrosarcomas. You may see sphenoid wing dysplasia with pulsating exophthalmus and occipital bone/lambdoid suture defect. Associated with vascular dysplasia and with moyamoya disease and aneurysms. Spinal manifestations with sharp angle scoliosis, scalloping of the posterior vertebral bodies, dural ectasia, lateral thoracic meningoceles, and intraspinal and paraspinal neurofibromas may occur. There is NF-1 associated learning disability in 30%–60% of patients.

NF-2

This type is also called central neurofibromatosis or MISME (multiple inherited/intracranial schwannomas, meningiomas, and ependymomas). Bilateral vestibular schwannomas are pathognomonic of NF-2. It is autosomal dominant with 50% of cases related to new mutations, is associated with an abnormality of chromosome 22, and has an incidence of 1 in 50,000 people. Cutaneous lesions are less common than in NF-1. Spinal manifestations include spinal and paraspinal schwannomas, spinal cord ependymomas, and spinal meningiomas. NF-2 is usually diagnosed at a later age (third decade) than NF-1.

Sturge–Weber syndrome

This is also called encephalotrigeminal angiomatosis. It is a sporadic, congenital, but not inherited disorder characterized by failure of development of the normal cerebral venous system. It is associated with a port-wine stain in the V1 or V2 distribution and leptomeningeal angiomatosis. Patients have intractable seizures, hemiparesis, and mental retardation. Imaging findings include pial angiomatosis (unilateral in 80% of cases) more commonly seen in occipital and parietal regions, seen as gyriform leptomeningeal enhancement. Cortical/subcortical gyriform calcifications secondary to chronic venous ischemia that progressively develops over time (tram-track calcifications) may occur. There may be enlargement of the ipsilateral choroid plexus (alternate venous drainage pattern) and other prominent engorged venous structures representing rerouting of venous drainage. The Sturge–Weber syndrome is associated with the Dyke–Davidoff–Masson (DDM) syndrome, which includes hemiatrophy of a cerebral hemisphere, hemihypertrophy of the ipsilateral calvarium (widening of the diploic space), and enlargement of the ipsilateral paranasal sinuses. DDM can be the result of any insult resulting in hemiatrophy of a cerebral hemisphere.

Von Hippel–Lindau syndrome

This is autosomal dominant, associated with a mutation on chromosome 3. It consists of CNS hemangioblastomas (intracranial, and most common in the cerebellum and brainstem, but rarely found supratentorially; spinal hemangioblastomas also occur), endolymphatic sac tumors, retinal angiomas (hemangioblastomas), renal cell carcinoma, pheochromocytoma, and renal and pancreatic cysts. There are no cutaneous manifestations although it is included in the general category of neurocutaneous syndromes (phakomatoses). Hemangioblastomas are highly vascular tumors which can be cystic with a mural nodule, completely solid, or complex. The mural nodule usually abuts the pial surface. The cyst is not a true epithelium lined cyst but consists of fluid surrounded by non-neoplastic, compressed parenchyma. Spinal hemangioblastomas are often associated with prominent, associated fluid/cystic spaces and/or syringohydromyelia. Endolymphatic sac tumors in these patients are often low-grade papillary or cystic adenocarcinomas, and have a unique appearance involving the posterior portion of the petro temporal bone with areas of T1 shortening with destructive/expansile appearance.

Tuberous sclerosis

This is an autosomal dominant congenital disorder with multiorgan hamartomas. Mutations on chromosome 9 and 16 have been identified. Characterized by the clinical triad of seizures, adenoma sebaceum, and mental retardation; only 30% of patients have all three. CNS lesions consist of cortical and subependymal tubers (hamartomas). WM lesions are also seen along the radial glial tracts – lines of migration. Cortical tubers may enlarge the affected gyrus with an associated abnormal central core of WM (increased T2 signal/decreased density), and 20% of cases have a central depression (eye-of-potato). More than 90% have subependymal nodules, most often along the lateral margins of the lateral ventricles (candle guttering), and about 70%–95% have cortical/subcortical tubers. Subependymal nodules calcify progressively with age (in approximately 50% of patients) from 10 years of age. Subcortical tubers may have increased T1 signal early in life. Non-neoplastic nodules often show enhancement (more easily visible on MRI than CT), which does not always indicate neoplastic transformation; 15% have subependymal giant cell astrocytomas (SEGCA) (WHO, grade I) that occur most often in the lateral ventricle near the foramen of Monro, attached to the head of the caudate nucleus, and may cause hydrocephalus. Consider SEGCA if there is an enlarging mass with prominent enhancement. Subependymal nodules have a similar signal to GM, leading to consideration of GM heterotopias. Heterotopias, however, do not calcify.

Osler–Weber–Rendu syndrome (hereditary hemorrhagic telangiectasia)

Hereditary hemorrhagic telangiectasia (HHT) is autosomal dominant with multisystem vascular dysplastic lesions characterized by mucocutaneous and visceral telangiectasias, pulmonary AVMs and AVFs, CNS vascular lesions such as cerebral and spinal AVMs and AVFs, aneurysms, and slow flow lesions such as cavernous malformations, developmental venous anomalies (DVAs), and capillary telangiectasias. The syndrome may present clinically with recurrent epistaxis, gastrointestinal hemorrhage, chronic anemia, or CNS symptoms. CNS symptoms may be related to complications from pulmonary vascular malformations, such as paradoxical emboli with infarcts or abscesses from a pulmonary AVF, or from intracerebral hemorrhage from an intracranial vascular lesion. Classic AVMs are seen in only approximately 16% of patients with HHT.

Craniosynostosis and head shape

This refers to premature closure of cranial sutures and can involve any of the sutures, alone or in combination. This condition can occur as an isolated anomaly or in conjunction with other congenital anomalies/syndromes such as Crouzon's, Apert's, and Pfieffer syndromes. Craniosynostosis results in an abnormal head/skull shape.

Remember that an abnormal head/skull shape at birth may not be abnormal but a result of fetal head position and birth trauma (molding). Postnatally, infant positioning may present with lambdoid flattening. Parents can be instructed to keep the head off the flattened area and to re-check in 6–8 weeks. If the flattening were positional, it should improve. A rare complication of craniosynostosis can be elevated ICP, which is more common with multiple craniosynostosis.

Sagittal suture craniosynostosis (see Figure 6.27, page 87)

This is the most common and 80% occur in males. It leads to a long and narrow shaped head called dolichocephaly or scaphocephaly.

Coronal craniosynostosis

This condition occurs more in females than males, and can be unilateral or bilateral. The unilateral type results in plagiocephaly (unilateral flattening), with the supra-orbital margin higher than on the normal side leading to the harlequin-eye sign. Bilateral coronal suture synostosis leads to brachycephaly (short head in the anterior to posterior dimension).

Metopic craniosynostosis (see Figure 6.28, page 87)

This leads to trigonocephaly with a pointed forehead and a midline ridge, and is associated with hypoplasia of the frontal sinuses. It may have a chromosome 19p abnormality, with mental retardation.

Lambdoid craniosynostosis

This type is found more in males than females. The right side is involved in 70% of cases, and it can be unilateral or bilateral. If unilateral it results in plagiocephaly (flattening on one side), and if bilateral it causes brachycephaly (short anteroposterior dimension of the skull).

Bilateral coronal and lambdoid craniosynostosis

This leads to turricephaly (tower like).

Clover-leaf skull (kleeblattschadel)

Premature closure of all of the sutures, except the squamosal suture, occurs, leading to a trilobular configuration to the head with constrictions in the Sylvian fissures and bulging temporal regions.

Bathrocephaly (see Figure 6.29, page 88)

This condition is a normal variant characterized by bulging of the interparietal part of the occipital bone. No craniosynostosis is present in this variant of skull shape.

Metabolic disorders

This is a diverse group of rare disorders characterized by enzymatic defects and associated abnormalities of cellular organelles. Some of these disorders demonstrate a specific imaging pattern; however, the imaging findings can overlap and be confusing. They can be grouped into lysosomal, peroxisomal, and mitochondrial disorders. For a simpler categorization they can be divided into the following groups:

  White matter disorders
  Gray matter disorders
  Disorders affecting gray and white matter
  Disorders involving the basal ganglia

White matter disorders

Metachromatic leukodystrophy – most common of these conditions and occurs in about 1 in 40,000 births. There is diffuse WM involvement with sparing of subcortical regions and ventricular enlargement but no enhancement typically.

Adrenoleukodystrophy (X-linked) (see Figure 6.30, page 88) – early, you find symmetric WM involvement in periatrial regions, which moves forward and peripherally. There is enhancement along the advancing edge but the subcortical WM is spared.

Alexander's disease (see Figure 6.31, page 88) – macrocephaly is associated with this condition. Frontal lobe WM is found early in its course, with involvement of subcortical regions, and possibly the basal ganglia. Enhancement may be seen in the basal ganglia and periventricular regions.

Canavan's disease – macrocephaly occurs with diffuse involvement of WM and prominent involvement of subcortical U-fibers. There is relative sparing of the internal capsules and the ventricles are usually normal in size. No enhancement is seen but there is a markedly elevated NAA peak at spectroscopy.

Vanishing white matter disease (see Figure 6.32, page 89) – often follows minor head trauma or infection with rapid deterioration. It is autosomal recessive. There are distinct MRI findings of diffuse, symmetric involvement of WM including arcuate fibers, with progressive replacement of the WM with focal regions of CSF signal.

Pelizaeus–Merzbacher disease – shows diffuse WM involvement, including subcortical fibers, on MR. Look for sparing of WM surrounding penetrating vessels, giving a trigroid or leopard-skin pattern. You may see marked cerebellar atrophy.

Phenylketonuria and amino acid disorders – there are often nonspecific findings on imaging studies.

Gray matter disorders

  Tay–Sachs disease
  Neuronal ceroid-lipofuscinosis
  Glycogen storage disease
  Mucopolysaccharidoses

Mucopolysaccharidoses (see Figure 6.33, page 89) – a lysosomal storage disorder characterized by the inability to degrade and the subsequent accumulation of glycosaminoglycans (mucopolysaccharides), and includes Hurler's, Hunter's, and Sanfilippo syndromes. The mucopolysaccharides are deposited in various organs including the CNS. Leptomeningeal and dural deposition of mucopolysaccharides can lead to cord compression. Mucopolysaccharide deposition in neurons leads to cell degeneration and secondary demyelination with cerebral atrophy. Mucopolysaccharide-containing histiocytes (gargoyle cells) accumulate in DPSs surrounding the penetrating blood vessels. The perivascular spaces are more numerous and larger than normally seen and are most prominent in the corpus callosum, periatrial WM, and in the high convexities and centrum semiovale. There may be increased T2 signal in WM surrounding the DPSs. You may also see communicating hydrocephalus.

Disorders affecting gray and white matter

Mitochondrial encephalopathies – include Leigh's disease, MELAS, and MERFF syndromes: a group of disorders characterized by variable mutations resulting in dysfunction of the mitochondria involved in cellular energy production. Structures with the highest ATP demand are most susceptible to injury, such as the deep cerebral GM nuclei and striated muscle.

Leigh's disease (subacute necrotizing encephalomyelopathy) (see Figure 6.34, page 90) – has bilateral, symmetric, increased T2/FLAIR signal in the putamina, and to a lesser degree the caudate heads, thalami, periaqueductal GM, substantia nigra, dentate nuclei, and periventricular WM. It is usually present by the age of two years and is progressive, with death in childhood often secondary to respiratory failure.

Mitochondrial myopathy, encephalopathy, lactic acidosis, and stroke-like episodes (MELAS) (see Figure 6.35, page 90) – acute stroke-like cortical lesions, which often cross typical vascular territories, occur in this syndrome. They appear, disappear, and new lesions appear elsewhere. They are found more in the parieto-occipital than temporal and parietal lobes and in the basal ganglia. Increased signal on DWI with variable appearance on ADC maps (often normal or slightly decreased) are seen. The child usually appears normal at birth, but early on shows delayed growth, seizures, and recurrent cerebral injury, resembling stroke.

Myoclonic epilepsy with ragged-red fibers (MERRF) – the imaging appearance is similar to that in MELAS syndrome, with multiple stroke-like lesions.

Disorders involving the basal ganglia

Huntington disease – an autosomal dominant progressive neurodegenerative disorder usually with the age of onset in the fourth or fifth decades. The clinical triad of early onset dementia, choreoathetosis, and psychosis is seen. The disease duration averages 15–20 years. There is marked basal ganglia involvement most severely involving the caudate nuclei. Imaging shows cortical and subcortical atrophy with the most salient imaging feature being marked caudate nucleus atrophy, causing ballooning of the frontal horns. In addition, the putamen, globus pallidus, thalamus, substantia nigra, and brainstem can be involved. You may see increased T2/FLAIR signal owing to gliosis or decreased T2/FLAIR signal from iron deposition.

Hallervorden–Spatz disease – now called pantothenate kinase-associated neurodegeneration (PKAN) or neurodegeneration with brain iron accumulation (see Figure 6.36, page 91). It is characterized by abnormal iron accumulation in the globus pallidus interna and the parts reticulata of the substantia nigra. There is progressive extrapyramidal motor dysfunction and the condition is usually fatal. On imaging you see the eye-of-the-tiger sign with foci of increased T2 signal surrounded by hypointensity in the globus pallidus. On T1WI there may be hyperintense or normal signal in the globus pallidi. On CT you see hypodense, hyperdense, or normal globus pallidi.

Fahr's disease – also known as familial idiopathic ferrocalcinosis (see Figure 6.37, page 91). There is symmetric calcification involving the globus pallidus, putamen, caudate nuclei, thalami, dentate nuclei, and cerebral WM. It may be caused by defective iron transport leading to free radicals and tissue injury with secondary calcification. It causes neuropsychiatric illness and movement disorder.

Wilson disease – also known as hepatolenticular degeneration, it is an autosomal recessive disorder of copper metabolism secondary to a deficiency of ceruloplasmin, which is the blood transport protein for copper. There is abnormal accumulation of copper in tissues including the liver, brain, cornea (Kayser–Fleischer rings), bones, and kidneys. Liver deposition leads to cirrhosis and degenerative changes in the basal ganglia. Most cases become symptomatic between the ages of 8 and 16 years. The cerebral lesions are usually bilateral and often symmetric. You see symmetric increased or mixed peripheral increased and decreased T2/FLAIR signal in the putamen (most common) and pons. There is also involvement of the caudate nuclei, globus pallidi, and ventrolateral thalami.

Extracranial lesions
Primary scalp

Pilomatrixoma

Sebaceous cyst (epidermal inclusion cyst) (see
Figure 6.38, page 91)

Basal cell carcinoma

Squamous cell carcinoma (see Figure 6.39, page 92)

Melanoma

Lipoma (see Figures 6.40, 6.41, page 92)

Hemangioma (see Figure 6.42, page 93)

Cellulitis and abscess

Cephalohematoma (see Figure 6.43, page 93), caput
succedaneum, subgaleal hemorrhage

Dermoid (see Figure 6.44, page 94)

Plexiform neurofibroma (see Figure 6.45, page 94)

Five layers of the scalp are:

S = skin: epidermis; dermis containing hair
follicles, sweat glands, sebaceous glands, and
arteries and veins

C = connective tissue (subcutaneous): fibrofatty
with dense connective tissue and adipose tissue;
contains arteries, veins, lymphatics, and
cutaneous nerves

A = galea aponeurosis: tendinous structure that
bridges the occipitofrontalis muscle

L = loose connective tissue (subgaleal): "danger
space" that consists of loose fibroareolar tissue;
avascular. This is the layer used as a surgical
plane for neurosurgical scalp flaps. Owing to the
loose areolar make-up of this layer, blood,
edema, or other abnormalities can dissect into
the subcutaneous structures of the face and neck

P = periosteum

Skin lesions
Pilomatrixoma

This is a benign, often calcified lesion of the head and
neck arising from the hair follicle. It occurs more in
females, and in the first two decades of life.

Sebaceous cyst

This is a movable mass under the skin because of
attachment to the skin. It develops when a swollen
hair follicle obstructs the sebaceous gland. It usually
has low density on CT, and on MRI low T1 and high
T2 signal, but this can be variable depending upon

contents. If it ruptures, you can see an inflammatory
reaction surrounding the cyst.

Basal cell carcinoma

This is the most common skin cancer; usually secondary to exposure to sunlight. It has slow growing,
locally invasive tumors, which can destroy adjacent
bone; local spread to lymph nodes or distant sites is
very rare. It may recur after treatment.

Squamous cell carcinoma

This represents about two out of 10 skin cancers.
Tumors often occur on sun-exposed areas of the skin,
are usually more aggressive than basal cell cancers,
and more often invade underlying subcutaneous fat.
There is a greater tendency (yet still uncommon)
toward metastatic spread to lymph nodes and distant
sites, and this can be around nerves (perineurally).

Melanoma

This is a malignant lesion with a high propensity
toward metastatic spread. Metastases are often hemorrhagic. On MRI, the metastatic melanoma may
show a paramagnetic effect owing to melanin, with
increased T1 and decreased T2 signal intensities.

Subcutaneous layer lesions
Lipoma

This is a fatty mass with encapsulation. If you see
areas of soft tissue density or thickened septations,
you want to exclude liposarcoma. CT density and MR
signal parallel normal fat. The lesion will suppress on
fat suppressed (saturated) MR pulse sequences.

Hemangioma

These are the most common tumors of the head and
neck in infancy and childhood. These masses present
in early infancy, undergo rapid enlargement, and
generally involute before adolescence. They have an
intermediate signal on T1WI that increases on T2WI,
which enhances with contrast. You often see vascular
flow voids.

Cellulitis and abscess

These are inflammatory changes involving the skin and
subcutaneous fat. On CT you often see soft tissue swelling, reticulation, and increased density in the subcutaneous layer of the scalp or face. They may progress from
phlegmon (a non-drainable coalescing inflammatory

mass) to frank abscess formation with a peripheral capsule, demonstrating enhancement with central non-enhancing fluid (often high proteinaceous content).

Galea/subgaleal/periosteal lesions

Cephalohematoma

This is a subperiosteal, traumatic accumulation of blood usually at the vertex, and when birth related may increase in size after birth, although limited by the cranial sutures. It is most often over the parietal bones. Resorption is seen in weeks to months; if it does not resolve, it may calcify around the periphery. Other birth related scalp hemorrhages include caput succedaneum, which is a hemorrhagic edema of the skin and subcutaneous tissue, usually from vaginal delivery. These cross suture lines and usually resolve over several days. Subgaleal hemorrhage is a hemorrhage beneath the galea aponeurosis that may dissect into surrounding subcutaneous tissues owing to its loose areolar composition.

Dermoid

These are congenital inclusions containing ectodermal elements at sites of closure during development, which are often midline and associated with suture lines. They contain skin and epidermal appendages (hair, sebum, sebaceous and apocrine glands). On CT you see areas of low attenuation (fat density), and on MRI this is hyperintense on T1WI. They may have a connection with intracranial contents or skin through a sinus tract.

Plexiform neurofibroma

These are infiltrative, locally aggressive nerve sheath tumors usually seen in NF-1. They are cord-like, heterogeneous infiltrative lesions with contrast enhancement. They often infiltrate multiple, contiguous compartments such as the scalp and orbit as well as extending intracranially through foramina and fissures. The tumors can degenerate into neurofibrosarcomas.

Calvarial lesions

Vascular channels mimicking lytic lesions (see Figure 6.46, page 95)

Large (giant) parietal foramina mimicking lytic lesions (see Figure 6.47, page 95)

Pacchionian granulations (arachnoid granulations) mimicking lytic lesions (see Figure 6.48, page 95)

Metastatic disease and multiple myeloma (see Figures 6.49, 6.50, page 96)

Hemangioma (see Figure 6.51, page 97)

Epidermoid (see Figure 6.52, page 97)

Dermoid

Langerhans cell histiocytosis (eosinophilic granuloma) (see Figure 6.53, page 98)

Fibro-osseous lesions – mixed fibrous (soft tissue density or signal) and osseous (ground glass) tissue (see Figure 6.54, page 99)

Osteoma (see Figure 6.55, page 100)

Paget's disease (see Figure 6.56, page 101)

Vascular channels mimicking lytic lesions

Look for linear, branching channels connecting with each other and with intradiploic vascular lakes (expansions of these luscencies in the skull). Parietal foramina are linear tract-like defects in the parietal bone through which emissary veins travel, are often bilateral, and have sclerotic margins extending from the outer to the inner table.

Large (giant) parietal foramina mimicking lytic lesions

These are developmental defects in ossification often associated with underlying cerebral venous anomalies.

Pacchionian granulations (arachnoid granulations)

These will erode the inner table. Common locations are within 3 cm of the mid-sagittal plane in the frontal and parietal bones and near the torcular herophili (confluence of dural venous sinuses).

Metastatic disease and multiple myeloma

Intradiploic, expansile lesions with or without frank destruction of the inner and/or outer table of the skull. Certain metastatic bone lesions may be blastic (sclerotic) and/or mixed blastic and lytic. Blastic lesions often arise from prostate cancer in men and breast cancer in women.

Hemangioma

These are intradiploic, with expansion of the inner and outer table, and often more pronounced along the outer table. They have a spiculated, honeycomb, spoke-wheel appearance, with non-sclerotic margins.

Epidermoid

These lesions are expansile, intradiploic, with well-defined, sclerotic margins.

Dermoid

Typically associated with suture lines, these lesions are often midline, with fat density/signal characteristics.

Langerhans cell histiocytosis (eosinophilic granuloma)

They are intradiploic with a beveled edge owing to eccentric growth. There is no sclerosis unless healing or healed. Common locations include the mastoid bone, orbit, and bony calvarium.

Fibro-osseous lesions (fibrous dysplasia)

These are found in mixed fibrous (soft tissue density or signal) and osseous (ground glass) tissue, with the temporal bone, maxilla, and mandible commonly involved. You will see expansion of involved bone. On CT look for the characteristic ground glass appearance but you may see varying degrees of focal soft tissue (fibrous tissue) and bony tissue (ground glass). On MRI you will see T1 hypointensity and variable T2 hyperintensity with enhancement of involved bone.

Osteoma

These are benign, focal tumors of dense compact bone usually arising from the outer table, and usually <1 cm in size. There is no soft tissue component and no enhancement. When in the paranasal sinuses, they may expand and erode surrounding bony margins and/or obstruct normal sinus drainage, leading to mucocele formation.

Paget's disease (osteitis deformans)

This is a chronic, metabolic bone disease with variable degrees of bone destruction and/or sclerosis. The early stage in the skull is osteoporosis circumscripta with geographic areas of destruction. There is an intermediate phase of the disease with areas of bone destruction and sclerosis, and a more chronic phase where the sclerotic changes dominate. Look for enlargement of the affected bone, thickening of bony cortices, widening of the diploic space with coarsened, irregular trabeculations and a cotton wool appearance. The differential diagnosis can include metastatic disease and fibrous dysplasia.

Skull base lesions

Chordoma (see Figure 6.57, page 102)
Chondrosarcoma (see Figure 6.58, page 103)
Meningioma (see Figures 6.59, 6.60, pages 103, 104)
Glomus tumor (paraganglioma) (see Figure 6.61, page 104)
Endolymphatic sac tumor (see Figure 6.62, page 105)
Skull base schwannoma (see Figures 6.63, 6.64, page 106)
Rhabdomyosarcoma (see Figure 6.65, page 107)
Multiple myeloma
Metastatic disease
Lymphoma/leukemia
Cholesterol granuloma of petrous apex (see Figure 6.66, page 108)
Congenital epidermoid of petrous apex (see Figure 6.67, page 109)
Petrous apex cephalocele (see Figure 6.68, page 110)

Chordoma

This is a midline notochordal, slow growing tumor. It most often occurs between 30 and 60 years old, peaking in the fifth decade; 50% are found in the sacrum, 35% in the skull base in the spheno-occipital region, and 15% in other spinal segments. The cervical spine (especially C2) and lumbar spine are the most common spinal sites above the sacrum. It is a destructive lesion with a large soft tissue mass. Intratumoral calcification (amorphous) is more common in sacrococcygeal tumors. Sclerosis in spinal lesions above the sacrum is common (~50%). Lesion on MRI shows low to intermediate T1WI and very high, heterogeneous T2 signal (cystic-gelatinous content). In addition, there are low signal septations and a pseudocapsule, it is lobulated, and enhancement is common. It is often hyperdense on CT.

Chondrosarcoma

This tumor has a higher incidence in the second and third decades of life, is almost always low grade, and is thought to arise from the skull base near cartilaginous sites because the skull base arises from endochondral ossification. They are off-the-midline tumors, the petro-occipital fissure region being the most common site. Other sites are sella turcica and the sphenoethmoidal junction region. They are locally invasive tumors and metastases are uncommon. On imaging, note off-midline lytic, destructive/invasive lesions with chondroid matrix (best seen on CT), hemorrhage, variable enhancement and high T2 signal.

Meningioma

This tumor occurs most commonly during middle age, more in females than males. It is a common skull base extra-axial tumor with unusual primarily intra-osseous and extracranial variants, which may arise in soft tissue in adjacent extracranial spaces such as the infratemporal fossa/masticator space. Look for hyperostosis of bone. Tumors may be multiple, especially with NF-2.

Glomus tumor (paraganglioma) of skull base

This lesion occurs more often in the fifth and sixth decades. Sites of origin include the glomus tympanicum (middle ear along cochlear promontory), glomus jugulare (from jugular foramen), or both regions (jugulotympanicum). They are highly vascular soft tissue masses, often with a permeative bony erosive/destructive pattern (best seen on CT). When large, you may see prominent vascular flow voids on MRI or enhancing vascular channels on CT, because of marked vascularity. A salt-and-pepper appearance on MRI is because of the large number of small vascular channels.

Endolymphatic sac tumor

Most of these tumors arise sporadically from endolymphatic sac epithelium, but are rarely associated with Von Hippel–Lindau syndrome. The highest incidence is in the posteromedial temporal bone near the endolymphatic duct/sac. The age range is 20–80 years. It is a slow growing tumor. On CT, note the retrolabyrinthine mass with bony erosion/destruction, bone spicules, and possibly a thin rim of expanded bone around the periphery. On MRI, note a heterogeneous mass with areas of high T1 signal on unenhanced images (blood breakdown products) and prominent enhancement but lacking prominent flow voids (unlike glomus tumors). When small, the tumors do not involve the jugular foramen.

Skull base schwannoma

These arise from the lower cranial nerves, but may arise within the bony apertures of the skull base: within the internal auditory canal (CN 7 and 8), jugular foramen (CN 9 in pars nervosa, and CN 10 and 11 in pars vascularis), and hypoglossal canal (CN 12). Vestibular schwannoma is the most common, with a trigeminal nerve origin being the second most common (but far less so than the vestibular nerve type). There is a nonspecific imaging appearance, with low T1, high T2, but when large often heterogeneous signal, owing to calcification or necrosis/cystic changes. Enhancement is variable from strong to mild. A clue to diagnosis is to identify the growth pattern along the course of the specific nerve.

Rhabdomyosarcoma

This is the most common soft tissue sarcoma in children, usually in the head and neck. The three main histologic types are: (1) embryonal with a botryoid variant, (2) alveolar, and (3) pleomorphic. Embryonal is the most common; it arises in the middle ear near the eustachian tube, orbit, paranasal sinuses, and nasopharynx. Parameningeal sites are the nasopharynx, sinonasal region, and ear, which have the worst prognosis. Often you see extensive bone destruction. The tumor has a nonspecific appearance on MRI with prominent enhancement. The differential diagnosis with Langerhans cell histiocytosis is difficult.

Multiple myeloma

Can be a solitary plasmacytoma versus diffuse myeloma. Imaging shows a nonspecific destructive process in the elderly. Differential diagnosis should always include metastatic disease.

Metastatic disease

This arises from direct invasion of the skull base from an adjacent malignancy or by hematogenous spread. Always include multiple myeloma in the differential diagnosis with metastatic disease.

Lymphoma/leukemia

You can see primary involvement of the osseous skull base versus secondary involvement from adjacent dural disease.

Cholesterol granuloma of the petrous apex

This involves a pneumatized petrous apex with poor ventilation, mucosal edema, recurrent bleeding, and cholesterol formation. It is best diagnosed on MRI with high T1 and T2 signal; with time, it expands the petrous apex. Pneumatization of the contralateral petrous apex supports diagnosis as pneumatization is often symmetric.

Congenital epidermoid of the petrous apex

This arises from trapping of aberrant ectoderm and occurs more in children and young adults. On CT, you see a non-enhancing expansile lesion with variable bone destruction which may be difficult to differentiate from cholesterol granuloma when there is lack of bone destruction. MRI shows low to intermediate T1, high T2 and no enhancement. Look for diffusion restriction.

Petrous apex cephalocele

This is an uncommon, benign expansion of the sub-arachnoid space, extending from the region of Meckel's cave into the petrous apex, with associated smooth, bony expansion of the petrous apex, which is occupied by only fluid-filled, CSF identical density/signal. There is no internal enhancement.

Sinonasal lesions

Sinusitis (see Figure 6.69, page 111)

Fungal sinusitis (see Figure 6.70, page 112)

Mucocele of paranasal sinuses (see Figure 6.71, page 113)

Sinonasal polyp disease (see Figure 6.72, page 113)

Juvenile nasopharyngeal angiofibroma (JNA) (see Figure 6.73, page 114)

Sinonasal malignancy

Nasopharyngeal carcinoma (see Figure 6.74, page 115)

Esthesioneuroblastoma (primary olfactory neuroblastoma) (see Figure 6.75, page 116)

Sinusitis

This is a common finding on both CT and MR studies of the head. It may follow a viral upper respiratory infection, or be triggered by allergens or pollutants. Sinus drainage is impaired by mucosal edema, leading to sinus obstruction and subsequent proliferation of bacteria. See thickening along the mucosal surfaces of involved sinuses. Often you see elevation and enhancement of the mucosal surfaces on MRI (also seen with CT) with thickened, edematous submucosal edema. You may see fluid density/signal layering or complete opacifying of the involved sinus. Complete sinus opacification with air-fluid levels is only seen in about 60% of patients with acute sinusitis. Changes of chronic inflammatory sinus disease include thickening of the bony margins (reactive osteitis), and central increased density/signal on CT/MRI. Differential diagnosis of increased density/signal within the paranasal sinuses on unenhanced CT/MRI includes chronic inspissated secretions, fungal sinus disease, blood, and calcification.

Fungal sinusitis

1. *Invasive fungal sinusitis: acute invasive* – seen in diabetics with ketoacidosis and immunocompromised patients. It is rapidly progressive with a high mortality rate. The nasal cavity is the most common site of infection, with involvement of the middle turbinate in two-thirds of patients. There is fungal invasion of mucosa, submucosa, bone, and blood vessels, with intraorbital, intracranial, and maxillofacial extension. Often unilateral involvement of ethmoids and sphenoid sinuses is seen. An early sign is avascular regions on post-contrast images. There is soft tissue thickening in involved sinuses with aggressive bone destruction. You can see cavernous sinus thrombosis, leptomeningeal enhancement, and cerebritis/cerebral abscess develop.

   Chronic invasive form – seen in immunocompetent people, or in patients with diabetes or an impaired immune system. Patients have a history of rhinosinusitis. It develops over months to years. You see hyperdense material in the sinus on non-enhanced CT, which is hypointense on T1WI and markedly hypointense on T2WI. Associated bone destruction, extension into adjacent compartments including orbits, maxillofacial structures, and intracranially; and increased soft tissue extending beyond the confines of the involved sinuses are also seen. This condition can mimic malignancy.

2. *Noninvasive fungal sinusitis: allergic fungal sinusitis* – most common form of fungal sinusitis; more common in warm, humid climates. It is felt to be a hypersensitivity reaction to inhaled fungal organisms, resulting in a chronic, non-infectious, inflammatory reaction. Imaging shows multiple sinus involvement often with nasal cavity involvement. Often you see near complete opacification and expansion of sinuses with increased density on non-enhanced CT. On MRI, T1WI signal can be variable with high, low, intermediate, or mixed signal intensity. On T2WI, the characteristic low signal or signal void is seen. The signal void is secondary to metals concentrated by the fungal organisms, and from high protein and low free water content of the mucin material. See enhancement of the inflamed mucosal surfaces. You do not see enhancement of the abnormal central contents of the sinus. Bony expansion with erosion can lead to intracranial and intraorbital complications.

3. *Fungus ball or mycetoma* – uncommon form of fungal sinus disease. This is felt to be secondary to impaired mucociliary clearance of the sinus, with persistent accumulation of the fungus. The fungus reproduces and results in an inflammatory

response within the sinus. The fungus ball is a tangle of fungal hyphae. There is no invasion of fungus into the surrounding structures. The most common organism is *Aspergillus fumigates*. On imaging, the fungus ball is usually limited to a single sinus, most commonly the maxillary but occasionally the sphenoid sinus. Note increased density on non-contrast CT owing to the matted hyphae and punctuate calcifications that may be present. Inflamed mucosa appears as decreased density on CT and increased T2 signal on MRI. No enhancement of central fungus ball is seen. Surrounding bony margins show variable thickening or thinning. The fungus ball is hypointense on T1WI and T2WI owing to calcifications, absence of free water, and concentration of metals by fungi.

Mucocele of paranasal sinuses

This is a completely opacified, expanded sinus containing mucoid material secondary to sinus outflow obstruction. See completely opacified, expanded sinus without pathologic contrast enhancement. It occurs in the frontal sinus in about 65% and ethmoids in about 25% of cases, and less frequently in the maxillary sinus and rarely in the sphenoid sinus. This is the most common expansile lesion of the sinuses. Symptoms depend upon location of the mucocele and the direction of expansion. Frontal or ethmoid mucoceles may expand into the orbit, resulting in proptosis and diplopia, or they may expand intracranially. They are often painless. If pain develops and you see enhancement along the peripheral margins of the mucocele, it may represent a mucopyocele. On CT, see a non-enhancing, expanded, completely opacified sinus with smooth remodeling of surrounding bony margins. The contents may be hypodense (if predominantly simple mucus) and/or hyperdense (inspissated secretions and/or colonization with fungus). The lesion is hypointense on T1 and hyperintense on T2 when there is predominantly a water/mucoid signal, or hyperintense on T1 and hypointense on T2 with high protein, inspissated contents.

Sinonasal polyp disease

Sinonasal polyps represent inflammatory thickening and upheaval of the sinonasal mucosa. See nodular, polypoid thickening along the mucosal surfaces of the paranasal sinuses and nasal cavity. They are associated with allergic fungal sinusitis in about 66% of patients. CT reveals multiple, nodular, polypoid densities in multiple sinus cavities and the nasal cavity. They can be mucoid or soft tissue in density or have high density on non-contrast CT owing to increased protein, decreased water, and/or fungal elements. You can see bone expansion and erosion that may be so extensive as to expand into the orbit or intracranial compartment. You may see enhancement along the peripheral margins of the polyps, but no central enhancement. MRI appearance is variable depending upon water content and presence of fungal disease. They can have a bizarre, swirl-like appearance owing to variable contents on T1WI. On T2WI they can also have variable signal based upon content. Peripheral not central enhancement on MRI may be present.

Juvenile nasopharyngeal angiofibroma

This is the most common benign tumor arising in the nasopharynx. These locally aggressive, benign tumors are most often seen in adolescent males, with a history of recurrent epistaxis. They are highly vascular tumors arising in the posterior nasal cavity from the fibrovascular stroma near the sphenopalatine foramen, through which they can gain access into the masticator space, orbit, skull base, and intracranially. Often you see remodeling of adjacent bone with expansion, such as anterior bowing of the posterior wall of the maxillary sinus. See marked enhancement of the tumor on CT and MRI, and marked hypervascularity on angiography. They are often embolized preoperatively. There is a high incidence of recurrence and they are often difficult to completely resect owing to their infiltrative nature.

Sinonasal malignancy

These tumors only account for about 3%–4% of all head and neck cancers; 80% are squamous cell, and 10% are adenoid cystic carcinoma and adenocarcinoma. There is a poor prognosis owing to the advanced stage at presentation. Spread is by direct extension, which may be into the orbit and intracranial compartment.

Nasopharyngeal carcinoma

This may result in direct invasion into the skull base and/or perineural spread. It is important to do fat suppressed post-contrast MRI (because of inherent fatty marrow in the skull base), looking for skull base invasion and perineural spread.

Esthesioneuroblastoma (primary olfactory neuroblastoma)

These tumors arise from olfactory nerve cells in the high nasal cavity (olfactory recesses) or ethmoid vault, and expand and grow intracranially through the cribriform plate into the subfrontal region and inferiorly into the nasal cavity. They are vascular tumors with enhancement and are often associated with cysts along the cranial margin of the tumor. They have a bimodal distribution in the second and sixth decades of life.

Intracranial tumors

Primary intra-axial neoplasms

Neuroepithelial (glial) tumors

Astrocytic origin – diffuse
Astrocytic origin – focal
Brainstem glioma
Non-astrocytic glial tumors
Mixed oligodendroglioma

Astrocytic diffuse

In children infratentorial tumors and in adults supratentorial neoplasms are more common.

Astrocytoma (WHO grade II) (see Figure 6.76, page 117) – found more often in older children and younger adults up to the age of about 45 years. It can appear poorly or well marginated, usually with no enhancement. It has a high tendency to dedifferentiate into WHO grade III and IV tumors with time.

Anaplastic astrocytoma (WHO grade III) (see Figure 6.77, page 117) – can mimic the appearance of a grade II astrocytoma. It may show no or patchy enhancement but you should not see heterogeneous, ring-like enhancement. Its natural history is for transformation into a higher grade (grade IV).

Glioblastoma multiforme (GBM) (WHO grade IV) (see Figure 6.78, page 118) – 15%–20% of all intracranial tumors, about 50% of all cerebral gliomas, and 40% of all primary brain tumors in all ages. It is usually supratentorial and many arise from transformation of less malignant astrocytomas as well as having a de novo appearance. It is more common in the fifth to sixth decades of life. Hallmarks are necrosis and neovascularity. You usually see a solitary, deep heterogeneous mass with irregular enhancement and prominent vasogenic edema. It often extends through the corpus callosum.

Gliomatosis cerebri (WHO grade III) (see Figure 6.79, page 119) – usually supratentorial, found more commonly in the middle adult age group but may occur at any age. It has an extensive multilobar, often bihemispheric infiltration but usually no enhancement, and often presents with minimal symptoms because it infiltrates without destroying neural connections.

Astrocytic focal

Pilocytic astrocytoma (WHO grade I) (see Figures 6.80, 6.81, pages 119, 120) – more common in children and in the posterior fossa. It is cystic, solid, or both; 10%–20% calcify, 60%–70% have cysts.

Subependymal giant cell astrocytoma (WHO grade I) (see Figure 6.82, page 120) – greater incidence in tuberous sclerosis, more common in the lateral ventricle near the foramen of Monroe, usually attached to the caudate nucleus. It is usually greater than 1 cm in size if symptomatic.

Pleomorphic xanthoastrocytoma (PXA) (WHO grade II) (see Figure 6.83, page 121) – found in children and young adults. It is associated with chronic epilepsy, and is often cortical, supratentorial, and most common in the temporal lobe. It is typically a cyst with an enhancing mural nodule along the pial surface, and often attaches to overlying dura. It may remodel/erode the inner table.

Brainstem glioma (see Figure 6.84, page 121)

This tumor accounts for approximately 10%–20% of all pediatric brain tumors and approximately 20%–30% of infratentorial tumors in children, mean age about seven years at the time of diagnosis. It forms a heterogeneous group of tumors ranging from pilocytic astrocytomas to glioblastoma multiforme. Diffuse, infiltrating gliomas of the pons are most common (~80%) and often extend exophytically into the prepontine cistern, surrounding without narrowing the basilar artery. You see diffuse enlargement of the pons. Calcification and hemorrhage are rare with variable enhancement in about 25% of images. Hydrocephalus occurs in only about 10% of cases. There is diffuse hypodensity on CT and decreased T1 and increased T2/FLAIR signal on MRI. Focal tumors account for approximately 5%–10% of brainstem gliomas and are discrete tumors without infiltration or peritumoral edema that may be exophytic. Dorsally, exophytic tumors are more likely to represent pilocytic astrocytoma (WHO grade I). Focal brainstem gliomas most often involve the midbrain or medulla. Patients with focal tectal gliomas do well with shunting. These tumors rarely progress. Focal, well-demarcated medullary gliomas may grow exophytically into the lower fourth ventricle without invasion. Brainstem gliomas have a poor prognosis with an overall two-year survival of about 20%. Their location within the brainstem influences the outcome with the best prognosis with a midbrain location, worst in the pons, and intermediate in the medulla.

Non-astrocytic glial tumors

Oligodendroglioma (see Figure 6.85, page 122) – approximately 5%–10% of all intracranial tumors and 18% of all gliomas. Histologic grading is less refined. Many advocate a two-tiered system of: (1) oligodendroglioma WHO grade II, and (2) anaplastic oligodendroglioma WHO grade III. The peak age is 35–40 years. It is slow growing, often heterogeneous, and arises in deep white matter and grows toward the surface. It occurs more commonly in the frontal lobe and is often cortical and large at presentation. Calcifications are common, which are often in superficial regions. Enhancement is variable (~50%). You may see necrosis and hemorrhage.

Ependymoma (WHO grades II or III) (see Figures 6.86, 6.87, pages 123, 124) – intraventricular most often but may be intra-axial from cell rests, especially when supratentorial. The supratentorial location is found more commonly in adults than infratentorial (70%) which is more common in children. There are two age peaks: one at 5 years and the other at 35 years. Seventy percent are malignant – 50% in the posterior fossa and 85% supratentorial ependymomas. They often recur and 10%–20% metastasize along CSF pathways. They are more often found along the floor of the fourth ventricle when in the posterior fossa, and more being extraventricular (parenchymal) when supratentorial. Large cysts are more common with supratentorial tumors. In the fourth ventricle they are often heterogeneous with calcifications, smaller cysts, and hemorrhage, and often form a cast of the lumen, having plastic type of growth with extension through outlet foramina like toothpaste. They show variable, heterogeneous enhancement. Supratentorial tumors often are calcified with mixed solid and cystic components with heterogeneous enhancement.

Subependymoma (WHO grade I) (see Figure 6.88, page 124) – supra- or infratentorial. Found in middle aged to elderly persons (fifth to sixth decades). This tumor is common in the inferior floor of the fourth ventricle or in the lateral ventricle, attached to the septum pellucidum or lateral wall. It is usually a homogeneous solid mass, may be lobulated, and may have calcification in larger lesions. Most are small but may be large. There is usually no to mild enhancement.

Choroid plexus papilloma (WHO grade I) (see Figure 6.89, page 125) or carcinoma (WHO grade III–IV) – intraventricular, occurring more frequently in the atrium of the lateral ventricles in children, more in the fourth ventricle in adults; 85% are present in children younger than five years old, with about 40% presenting in the first year of life. This tumor may arise in the CP angle cistern near the foramen of Luschka. It is lobulated with papillary fronds, highly vascular, and prominently enhances. It may hemorrhage, and hydrocephalus may be from overproduction of CSF or obstruction of CSF pathways (depending on its location).

Mixed oligodendroglioma

This tumor occurs more frequently in the frontal lobes than temporal lobes. It has slow growth, nonspecific decreased T1 and increased T2 signal with enhancement in 50% of cases. It begins in the WM and often extends into the cortex, which may be expanded. The mean age for its incidence is 35–45 years.
Examples: oligoastrocytoma (WHO grade II, low grade) and anaplastic (malignant) oligoastrocytoma (WHO grade III).

Neuronal and mixed neuronal–glial tumors

Central neurocytoma (see Figure 6.90, page 126)
Ganglioglioma (see Figure 6.91, page 127)
Ganglioneuroma (gangliocytoma) (see Figure 6.92, page 128)
Dysembryoplastic neuroepithelial tumor (DNET) (see Figure 6.93, page 128)

Central neurocytoma (WHO grade II) – occurs in young adults. It is nearly always intraventricular but may be extraventricular. The tumor is classically described as being attached to the septum pellucidum, with greater frequency in the lateral and third ventricles. Calcification is common. It was previously called and can be confused with intraventricular oligodendroglioma.

Ganglioglioma (WHO grade I or II) – found more in the temporal lobe, in the group with a mean age of

20–30 years. It may be cystic (~50%), show calcification (~35%–40%), and have a peripheral location, rarely eroding the inner table, with expansive growth leading to well-defined margins. Peritumoral edema and enhancement (~50%) are mild. It may look like oligodendroglioma (but ganglion cell tumors have a higher incidence in the temporal lobe and younger age).

Ganglioneuroma/gangliocytoma (WHO grade I) – is a well-differentiated ganglion cell tumor. (Includes Lhermitte–Duclos disease in the cerebellum.)

Dysembryoplastic neuroepithelial tumor – intracortical and causes seizures; occurs more commonly in children, in the temporal lobes then frontal lobes, and often has a long history of partial complex seizures. The average age is about 20 years. It is associated with cortical dysplasia, a nonspecific appearance on MRI (hypointense T1 and increased T2 signal), and is focal, well-circumscribed, with no adjacent edema, and minimal to no enhancement. On CT it is hypodense with a cystic appearance. You may see overlying thinning of the inner table and occasional calcification.

Embryonal tumors

Primitive neuroectodermal tumors (PNET) – include cerebral PNET (see Figure 6.94, page 129), medulloblastoma (in the fourth ventricle in children) (see Figures 6.96, 6.97, pages 131, 132), desmoplastic medulloblastoma (in the lateral cerebellum and more common in adolescents and young adults with a mean age of 17 years), pineoblastoma (see Figure 6.104, page 138), retinoblastoma (see Figure 6.95, page 130), ependymoblastoma, neuroblastoma, and ganglioneuroblastoma. They are highly malignant, cellular tumors, composed of over 90% undifferentiated cells. They can develop along a variety of cell lines, are common tumors during childhood, and most are infratentorial. Supratentorial PNETs are rare, occurring most often before five years of age. Typically, you see a large (>5 cm), deep, hemispheric mass with rapid growth and often CSF seeding. Necrosis/cyst formation is seen in 30%–60%, calcification in 50%–70%, and hemorrhage in about 10%, which may occur within a necrotic component.

Atypical teratoid/rhabdoid tumor (WHO grade IV) (see Figure 6.98, pages 132–133) – rare, aggressive tumor, usually seen in children under three years old; 50% are infratentorial (off-the-midline), and may be located in the CP angle. It is usually heterogeneous with cysts, calcification, and hemorrhage, and shows heterogeneous enhancement.

Other primary intra-axial neoplasm

Primary CNS lymphoma – once considered a rare disease; now seen with increasing frequency in both immunocompetent and immunosuppressed patients. The histology most often demonstrates intermediate to high-grade non-Hodgkin's lymphoma of B-cell origin.

Primary CNS lymphoma in immunocompetent patients (see Figures 6.99, 6.100, 6.101, pages 133–135) – most common locations are the deep periventricular WM, corpus callosum, septum pellucidum, and cerebellum. The tumor usually presents with a large, solitary hemispheric mass; it is most often seen as a solitary, homogeneously enhancing mass, usually demonstrating high density (70%) on unenhanced CT in the deep hemispheric WM, often extending to and/or crossing the midline. The high density on unenhanced CT relates to high cellularity, which often results in diffusion restriction on MRI. Calcification is unusual unless previously treated. Hemorrhage is rarely seen. MRI usually demonstrates isointensity or hypointensity of mass relative to GM on T2WI and intermediate to low signal intensity on T1WI. Post-contrast MRI shows dense homogeneous contrast enhancement in most cases. Both CT and MRI demonstrate surrounding edema and associated mass effect.

CNS lymphoma in immunosuppressed patients (includes AIDS lymphoma) – higher incidence in the supratentorial compartment. There is often involvement of the corpus callosum, basal ganglia, and other deep GM nuclei. Variable contrast enhancement is seen, which is often heterogeneous and complex compared with lymphoma in immunocompetent patients. Ring-like peripheral enhancement can be seen. Necrosis is seen in a significant proportion of AIDS related lymphoma. Hemorrhage within the lymphoma is not common but more often seen in lymphoma patients with AIDS. Multiple lesions are evident in up to 50% of patients. It is often difficult to differentiate from toxoplasmosis infection. When periventricular, it often invades and grows along the ependymal surface of the ventricles.

Miscellaneous tumors/tumor-like lesions
Hemangioblastoma (WHO grade I) (see Figures 6.24, 6.102, pages 85, 136–137)

The highest incidence of these tumors is in the posterior fossa (cerebellum most common) and spinal cord; they are rarely supratentorial. Peak incidence is in the fourth decade. These tumors are the most common primary intra-axial type of tumor in the posterior fossa in adults (but still only account for about 10% of neoplasms). They are associated with von Hippel–Lindau syndrome (VHL) in approximately 20% of cases and are usually sporadic and solitary, but in 5% of all or 30%–60% with VHL, these tumors are multiple. Sixty percent have cysts with a mural nodule; 40% are solid. They are very vascular and may look like a high-flow vascular malformation. When there is a cyst with a nodule, the nodule is usually subpial in location. Associated edema is usually mild, unless hemorrhage has occurred. The cyst wall is generally not neoplastic and does not need to be resected.

Lhermitte-Duclos disease (dysplastic gangliocytoma) (WHO grade I) (see Figure 6.92, page 128)

This is a rare cerebellar lesion with features of both a congenital malformation/hamartoma and a neoplasm. It is associated with Cowden's disease, which consists of multisystem hamartomas. It is often asymptomatic in early life, becoming clinically apparent in the third and fourth decades. The characteristic appearance on imaging studies is that of a focal lesion with a striated, lamellated appearance with thickened cerebellar folia and is referred to as having a corduroy or tiger-striped appearance. Calcifications may be present; it may be associated with mass effect but there is no enhancement. There are reports of elevated rCBF and rCBV. It may recur after resection.

Pineal region tumors/masses

Pineal cell origin

    Pineocytoma (see Figure 6.103, page 137)

    Pineoblastoma (see Figure 6.104, page 138)

Germ cell tumors

    Germinoma (see Figure 6.105, page 139)

    Teratoma (see Figure 6.106, page 140)

    Embryonal cell carcinoma, endodermal yolk sac tumor, choriocarcinoma

Gliomas (see Figure 6.107, page 140)

Meningioma (see Figure 6.108, page 141)

Metastasis

Vascular lesions (see Figure 6.109, page 142)

Benign pineal region cyst (see Figure 6.110, page 143)

Pineal cell origin

These tumors are often hyperdense on CT and isointense on T2WI from increased cellularity; about 50% calcify, and about 85% have associated hydrocephalus from obstruction of the aqueduct of Sylvius. Mass effect on the tectal plate results in Parinaud's syndrome. There is no gender predilection.

Pineocytoma – tumors are moderately cellular, and have a variable degree of neuronal differentiation. Prognosis depends on the degree of cellular maturation, and the median age is 36 years, with a 67% five-year survival. The tumor is more well defined, homogeneous, and hyperintense on T2 than pineoblastoma, and has no CSF dissemination.

Pineoblastoma – a form of PNET, with an overall median age of 18 years. The tumor is more heterogeneous, with hemorrhage and necrotic/cystic changes, than pineocytoma, showing CSF spread in approximately 10% of cases. They are termed trilateral retinoblastoma when associated with bilateral retinoblastomas (usually inherited and diagnosed before the age of two years).

Germ cell tumors

These tumors often spread through CSF pathways, and have a peak age near puberty.

Germinoma (most common) – form about 60% of all pineal region tumors with a much higher incidence in males than females (~10:1), and approximately 65% of pineal germ cell tumors with no gender predilection for suprasellar germinomas. The tumor is usually homogeneously hyperdense on CT and isointense on T2WI, well circumscribed, with tumor calcification (frequently engulfs the calcified pineal gland). If you see a suprasellar mass with a pineal mass, then the diagnosis suggests a germ cell tumor (germinoma). These tumors are highly responsive to radiation and chemotherapy.

Non-germinoma pineal germ cell tumors – make up about 25% of pineal germ cell tumors, and include immature and mature teratomas, embryonal cell carcinoma, endodermal sinus yolk sac tumors, and choriocarcinoma. Mature teratoma accounts for about 10% of pineal germ cell tumors. Teratoma has a much higher incidence in males, with a peak age near puberty. Immature teratomas are more common than mature teratomas. These tumors have elements of all three germ layers. They appear as a heterogeneous mass with calcification, fat, bone, cysts, and hemorrhage.

Metastasis

The pineal gland lacks a blood brain barrier and can be seeded by hematogeneous metastases.

Vascular lesions

Vein of Galen aneurysms – these are not true aneurysms but represent dilatation of the embryologic precursor (median prosencephalic vein of Markowski) of or the actual vein of Galen, owing to a high-flow AVM. Both are associated with the persistence of the falcine sinus, which is a normal venous channel in the falx cerebri that involutes after birth. It may persist in cases of outflow obstruction through the straight sinus. Different types are:

1. Vein of Galen aneurysmal malformation (VGAM) is a high-flow AVM, which is classified into choroidal type (choroidal arteries shunt into a common venous pouch before entering the primitive median vein) or mural type (direct AV shunts within the wall of the primitive median vein) depending upon the underlying angioarchitecture. Both demonstrate AV shunting into an enlarged median prosencephalic vein (embryologic precursor of the vein of Galen). The embryonic median vein does not drain normal brain parenchyma, only the AV shunt. This type develops early in gestation, prior to 12 weeks.

2. Vein of Galen aneurysmal dilatation (VGAD) is a subpial (typical parenchymal type) AVM (located supra- or infratentorially) that shunts into the true vein of Galen, which dilates. The dilated vein of Galen also drains normal brain parenchyma. The degree of dilatation of the vein of Galen depends upon the degree of outflow obstruction secondary to stenosis or obstruction where the vein of Galen joins the straight sinus.

3. Vein of Galen varix – this is a dilatation of the vein of Galen without an associated arteriovenous shunt. The vein of Galen in these cases drains the normal brain. There are two varieties. The first develops in association with cardiac failure in the newborn and disappears with improvement in cardiac function. The other is secondary to extensive DVAs, draining much of the cerebral hemisphere into the deep venous system.

4. Dural AVF with vein of Galen dilatation – these are acquired lesions usually secondary to thrombosis of the straight sinus, resulting in AV shunts located within the wall of the vein of Galen, and usually occur in adults.

Benign pineal region cyst

These are generally small, well-circumscribed, intra-pineal non-neoplastic cysts, which are most often smaller than 5–10 mm in size but occasionally can be large. You may see mild flattening of the superior tectum. Most are incidental findings. The cyst may be slightly hyperintense to CSF on T1WI, often hyperintense to CSF on FLAIR images, and isointense to CSF on T2WI on MRI. Typically it is thin walled with thin peripheral enhancement and may slightly enlarge or involute over time. If there is nodular, irregular enhancement, rapid growth, or development of symptoms, be suspicious for neoplasm.

Primary pituitary tumors

Pituitary adenoma – micro- and macroadenoma (see Figures 6.111–114, pages 143–145)
Pituitary carcinoma
Pituicytoma (see Figure 6.115, page 146)

Pituitary adenoma

Pituitary gland height should not exceed 9 mm and it normally has a flat or concave superior margin, although hormonally active females can show glands larger than 9 mm with upward bulging, and be normal. The gland should be symmetric and homogeneous in signal with the infindibulum midline. Occasionally the normal pituitary gland will show asymmetry with sloping of the sella floor and even mild deviation of the infindibulum. Look very closely in these cases for subtle signal alterations, which might indicate an adenoma. Adenoma is the most common tumor of the sella turcica and accounts for about 10%–15% of all intracranial tumors. These are benign epithelial tumors, which arise from cells in the adenohypophysis (anterior lobe). They are termed a microadenoma if ≤1 cm and a macroadenoma if ≥1 cm in size. Approximately 75% present with hormonal dysfunction (secreting prolactin, ACTH, growth hormone) and are usually microadenomas; 25% are non-functioning and usually macroadenomas. A microadenoma is hypointense to isointense on unenhanced T1WI and hypointense (enhances less than normal pituitary tissue) on early post-contrast images. A macroadenoma tends to be isointense on

T1 and hyperintense on T2WI, is often more hetero-geneous in signal and enhancement, with areas of necrosis/cystic change and hemorrhage compared with a microadenoma. These tumors can become locally invasive (but are not considered malignant), extending into surrounding areas including the dura, sphenoid sinus, cavernous sinus, and bony skull base. Adenomas may undergo spontaneous hemorrhage. The patient may present with signs and symptoms of pituitary apoplexy. As the tumor enlarges and extends into the suprasellar cistern, look for upward compression of the optic chiasm/nerves and the anterior floor of the third ventricle.

Pituitary carcinoma

This is rare and is defined by the presence of cranio-spinal and/or systemic metastases.

Pituicytoma

This is a rare tumor of the neurohypophysis. It arises from glial cells (pituicytes) in perivascular zones and is a low-grade astrocytoma. It is histologically benign, very vascular, and homogeneously enhancing. It can be located in the posterior lobe or along the infindi-bulum/suprasellar region.

Tumors/tumor like lesions related to the craniopharyngeal duct

Craniopharyngioma (see Figure 6.116, pages 146–147)
  Adamantinomatous
  Squamous papillary
Rathke's cleft cysts (see Figure 6.117, page 147)

Craniopharyngioma

These are benign but aggressive tumors, most often (>90%) arising in the suprasellar region, but they may arise solely within the sella from remnants of Rathke's pouch (craniopharyngeal duct) and rarely within the third ventricle. They originate from squa-mous epithelium. They account for more than 50% of suprasellar tumors in childhood and more than 50% occur in children and young adults with a smaller second peak in middle-aged adults. There are two main types: (1) adamantinomatous, with a peak age of 10–20 years old, and (2) squamous papillary, with a peak age of 40–50 years old. Adamantinomatous type – 90% are cystic, 90% calcify (nodular or rim), and 90% enhance. Cysts are often hyperintense on unen-hanced T1 images. Squamous papillary type – about

50% are cystic (and usually hypointense on T1) and 50% are solid, often lacking calcification.

Rathke's cleft cyst

Rathke's pouch is an embryonic upward growth of the ectoderm from the primitive oral cavity (stomodeum), and is the precursor of the anterior and intermediate lobes of the pituitary gland. If the intrasellar extension of this embryonic pouch persists, it can develop into a non-neoplastic Rathke's cleft epithelial-lined cyst. This is usually intrasellar but may also extend to the supra-sellar region. It is lined by columnar or cuboidal mucus-secreting epithelium. Most cysts are asymptomatic and have a variable signal on MRI depending upon the serous or mucus content, but may be hyperintense on unenhanced T1WI. Cysts should not enhance and are not associated with calcifications, unlike craniopharyn-giomas. An intracystic nodule with T1 hyperintensity and T2 hypointensity is described in the literature as a potential indicator of these cysts.

Other suprasellar masses/mass-like lesions (SATCHMOE) (if not described below, see discussion elsewhere in Chapter 3)

Suprasellar pituitary adenoma, sarcoid (see Figures 6.119, 6.170, pages 148, 182)
Aneurysm, arachnoid cyst
Teratoma (germ cell tumors) (see Figure 6.118, page 148), tuberculosis (TB) (see Figure 6.168, page 180)
Craniopharygioma, cysticercosis (see Figure 6.172, page 184)
Histiocytosis (see Figure 6.120, page 149), Hypothalamic glioma (see Figure 6.122, page 150), Hypothalamic hamartoma (see Figure 6.142, page 163), Hypophysitis (lymphocytic) (see Figure 6.121, page 149)
Meningioma, metastases
Optic glioma (see Figure 6.20, page 82)
Epidermoid/dermoid cyst (see Figure 6.123, page 151)

Germ cell tumors

Suprasellar germinomas account for 35% of all intra-cranial germinomas. Germinomas in this region may be associated with concurrent pineal region germin-omas. There is equal gender predilection unlike the pineal region germinoma. The tumor is often slightly hyperdense on CT and hypointense on T1 and T2 MR imaging, with prominent contrast enhancement. Seeding of the subarachnoid space is common. Invasion into adjacent brain parenchyma is also common. You may see thickening of the infindibulum, but the tumor is not associated with cysts or calcification. It is very radiosensitive.

Teratoma is a rare suprasellar mass containing elements of all three germ layers; therefore on imaging you see heterogeneous density/signal intensities with variable presence of fat, bone/cartilage, and other elements derived from ectoderm, endoderm, and mesoderm.

Histiocytosis (Langerhans cell histiocytosis)

This is a proliferation of histiocytes, which can involve the calvarium, and mastoid and orbital regions, as well as infiltrate the suprasellar region. It is often present with diabetes insipidus, with loss of normal posterior pituitary bright spot. On MRI you may see a focal enhancing suprasellar mass or an infiltrative enhancing lesion involving the infindibulum and/or hypothalamic region.

Epidermoid cyst

A congenital cholesteatoma, this mass-like lesion is lined by stratified squamous epithelium with its contents consisting of desquamated, keratinized debris and cells. It is a slowly expansile lesion with an infiltrative pattern surrounding and engulfing blood vessels and cranial nerves. Most often it appears hypodense on non-contrast CT, with similar or slightly higher density to CSF, and hypointense on T1 and hypertense on T2, with subtle differences in signal compared with CSF. You may see subtle internal architecture with strands of tissue – often you can accentuate the internal architecture on 3D-CISS images. Generally there is no enhancement or calcification. Rarely, epidermoids may appear hyperdense on CT (non-contrast) and show T1 hyperintensity and T2 hypointensity on MRI. This is the so-called bright epidermoid. Look for diffusion restriction with bright signal on diffusion trace images and dark signal on the ADC map to differentiate this tumor from the arachnoid cyst.

Intraventricular tumors

Choroid plexus papilloma (carcinoma) (see Figure 6.89, page 125) – see discussion elsewhere in Chapter 3 and list in Chapter 4

Ependymoma/subependymoma (see Figure 6.86, 6.88 pages 123, 124) – see discussion in Chapter 3

Medulloblastoma (see Figures 6.96, 6.97, pages 131, 132)

Meningioma (see Figure 6.124, page 152) – similar in appearance to meningiomas in other locations. Most common intraventricular location is the atrium of the lateral ventricle. See discussion in Chapter 3

Central neurocytoma (see Figure 6.90, page 126) – see discussion in Chapter 3

Glioma – see discussion in Chapter 3

Colloid cyst (see Figure 6.125, page 152) (not a true neoplasm, acts as a mass due to location)

Medulloblastoma

This is a posterior fossa PNET seen most often in children, comprising about 30%–40% of posterior fossa tumors in childhood. Most present between the ages of 5 and 15 years, with occasional presentation as a congenital tumor at birth or as tumors later in life. They usually arise from the roof of the fourth ventricle, in the midline (80% in childhood), and grow into the fourth ventricle. Lateral cerebellar medulloblastomas do occur in the older age group and more often as the desmoplastic variant. Approximately 30%–40% have evidence of CSF dissemination and/or solid tumor CNS metastases at the time of presentation. Imaging studies usually show a relatively well-circumscribed, homogeneous to heterogeneous mass in the fourth ventricular roof that may extend into the lumen of the fourth ventricle, and which is often iso- or hyperdense on pre-contrast CT (owing to increased cellularity). Twenty percent show coarse calcification on CT. On MRI the tumor is iso- to hypointense on T1 and iso- to hyperintense on T2 images, with heterogeneous T2 signal common owing to calcification, cysts, necrosis, and hemorrhage. Post-contrast enhancement is seen in about 90% of tumors. More than 90% of cases have hydrocephalus at presentation. The desmoplastic variant usually occurs in the older age group, in adolescents and young adults (mean age of 17 years), and is most often located laterally in the cerebellar hemispheres.

Colloid cyst

These are rare benign lesions, virtually always located in the anterosuperior third ventricular region near the foramen of Monro, and are often associated with intermittent obstruction at the foramen of Monro resulting in headaches, which may be positional. They have been associated with sudden hydrocephalus and death. Cyst contents are variable, including thick gelatinous material secondary to secretions from the epithelial lined wall. Blood products and cholesterol crystals may be present in the cyst. On CT the cysts are usually hyperdense compared to the brain (although they may be iso- or hypodense) on non-contrast images, and may demonstrate minimal enhancement (usually peripheral). On MR they have a variable appearance, which may be homogeneous or heterogeneous. About 50% are hyperintense on T1WI and usually hypointense on T2WI. Calcification is very rare.

Primary extra-axial neoplasm
Tumors of meninges

Meningioma (WHO grade I [typical], II [atypical], and III [anaplastic/malignant]) (see Figures 6.126, 6.127, 6.128, pages 153, 154) – constitute approximately 13%–25% of primary intracranial tumors, more common in adults with a peak in the sixth and seventh decades, and a greater incidence in females than males. Higher grade tumors are more common in men. The majority being WHO grade I (typical). The tumors are known to be induced by ionizing radiation. Multiple tumors occur in NF-2 and in families with a hereditary predisposition. They arise from arachnoid cap cells, and are usually supratentorial (90%) – parasagittal/convexity, sphenoid, parasellar, olfactory groove/planum sphenoidale. In infratentorial (10%) tumors, CP angle is most common. On CT they are hyperdense on pre-contrast images with homogeneous enhancement. Calcification occurs in about 20%; look for hyperostosis/blistering of adjacent bone. On MRI they are often nearly isointense with GM on T1WI and T2WI but this is variable. Look for an enhancing dural tail, but this is not specific. They can be a focal mass-like growth or *en plaque* along the dural surfaces. They are hypervascular with enlargement of the middle meningeal artery and/or other extra-axial vessels and pial supply may be evident. When small, primarily see meningeal (extra-axial) vascular supply, which enters the tumor centrally with a centrifugal/spoke-wheel-like branching pattern. As it enlarges, there is recruitment of pial vessels (along the periphery). Assess the adjacent dural venous sinuses for invasion and/or occlusion. On angiography note the mother-in-law

sign. Tumor stain comes early and stays late. As a general rule of thumb (but remember rules are made to be broken), the higher/more cranial the tumor the greater the edema, with tumors near the skull base often without any significant vasogenic edema. Elevated alanine on MR spectroscopy may be seen.

Non-meningothelial tumors of meninges (rare)
Mesenchymal
Hemopoietic
Primary melanocytic

Mesenchymal tumors (rare) – these include hemangiopericytoma (previously called angioblastic meningioma) (see Figure 6.129, page 155). This is a neoplasm of the capillary pericytes. It is highly vascular with multiple vascular channels, extra-axial, multilobulated with a dural attachment, and associated with bone destruction. There is no calcification, and it is heterogeneous on T1, T2, and contrast images. This tumor has a higher incidence in the fourth to sixth decades, is locally invasive, and has recurrent, extracranial metastases in up to 30% of cases. Other rare mesenchymal tumors of the meninges include osteocartilaginous tumors, rhabdomyosarcoma, lipoma, and fibrous histiocytoma.

Hemopoietic neoplasms of the meninges – include primary malignant lymphoma, granulocytic sarcoma (chloroma), and plasmacytoma. Granulocytic sarcoma is seen in acute myelogenous leukemia. On CT it can look hyperdense (like an extracerebral hematoma or meningioma), enhance homogeneously, and have a variable signal on MRI. Sixty percent are more than 15 years old.

Primary melanocytic lesions of the meninges (see Figure 6.130, page 156) – rare tumors distinct clinically and histologically from melanomas elsewhere in the body. They can be primary parenchymal or leptomeningeal and benign or malignant. They are thought to originate from pigmented cells of the leptomeninges, and arise where there is the highest concentration of melanocytes in the leptomeninges – the pons, cerebellum, cerebral peduncles, medulla, interpeduncular fossa, and inferior surfaces of the frontal, temporal, and occipital lobes. You see hyperdense parenchymal/leptomeningeal foci on unenhanced CT, with variable enhancement depending upon the benign or malignant nature of the tumor. MRI shows increased T1 (on unenhanced images) and decreased T2 signal with variable enhancement. The tumor may be associated with neurocutaneous melanosis.

Cranial nerve sheath tumor

Schwannomas (see Figures 6.131, 6.132, 6.133, pages 156–158) – constitute 5%–8% of all intracranial tumors; 98% arise from cranial nerves, all of which are covered by Schwann cell sheaths except olfactory and optic nerves (these are really parts of the CNS); 1–2% arise intracerebrally (intra-axial). Most cranial nerve schwannomas arise from sensory nerves, and are benign encapsulated nerve sheath tumors. They are hypointense on T1WI and hyperintense on T2WI. When large, their signal can be heterogeneous from necrosis/cystic change. Rarely they may have calcification. Prominent enhancement is often seen but they may show heterogeneous enhancement in a third of cases. A clue to their diagnosis is their location and sometimes the tubular configuration along the course of the nerve. Ninety percent arise from CN VIII – the vestibular schwannoma that is often erroneously called an acoustic schwannoma because it arises from the vestibular division (usually superior division) of the nerve and from Schwann cells. The trigeminal nerve is a distant, second most common cranial nerve schwannoma.

Secondary intracranial neoplasms

Intra-axial metastases (see Figure 6.134, page 159)
Extra-axial metastases
  Leptomeningeal (see Figure 6.135, page 159)
  Dural (see Figure 6.136, page 160)

Intra-axial metastatic disease

This arises from distant primary sites, and accounts for approximately 20% of brain tumors; 40% of metastatic lesions are solitary, 80% are supratentorial (frontal more common than parietal), which parallels the predominant blood flow pattern, and 20% occur in the posterior fossa (cerebellum, 10%–15% and brainstem, 3%–5%). Intra-axial metastases are usually well circumscribed with a distinct peripheral margin. Often extensive vasogenic edema out of proportion to the size of the enhancing lesion is seen. The hallmark of metastatic disease is enhancement. The highest incidence is in the fourth to seventh decades of life, often at the GM–WM junction (possibly owing to change in the caliber of arterioles, causing tumor emboli to lodge here). Hemorrhagic metastases, especially renal, lung, breast, thyroid, and melanoma in 20% of cases may have central necrosis. As a rule of thumb, prostate carcinoma never metastasizes to the brain, only to the dura and skull. Rarely (~1%) a military pattern can be seen with diffuse tiny enhancing nodules without edema.

Extra-axial metastatic disease

Leptomeningeal (leptomeningeal carcinomatosis) – most commonly from breast and melanoma but any primary can cause this. See curvilinear, gyriform, or nodular enhancing lesions along the pial surfaces, within sulci and in the different cisterns, including the internal auditory canals, and along the surfaces of cranial nerves. It is associated with communicating hydrocephalus secondary to involvement of arachnoid granulations.

Dural metastases – spread directly to the dura hematogenously, or by invasion from adjacent skull metastasis or directly from a malignant intracranial tumor (i.e. GBM). Incidence is higher in prostate and breast cancer, lymphoma, and leukemia. Be careful, this may look like a subdural hematoma, meningioma, or extramedullary hematopoesis. See nodular, loculated, or plaque-like enhancing lesions.

Always include multiple myeloma/plasmacytoma in the differential diagnoses along with metastatic disease when you see extra-axial tumor-like lesions.

Non-neoplastic mass-like lesions

These lesions can mimic neoplasms – consider them in the differential diagnosis of intracranial masses.

Hematoma (see Figures 6.137, 6.138, 6.203a–b, pages 160, 161, 206)
Infectious/inflammatory processes (see Figures 6.139, 6.140, 6.169, 6.172, 6.173, pages 161, 184, 185). For example abscess, granuloma, cerebritis
Tumefactive demyelinating lesions (see Figure 6.141, page 162) – focal demyelinating lesions can occasionally present as a focal mass-like lesion with extensive edema, mass effect, and enhancement mimicking a neoplastic process.
Hamartoma – These are disorganized normal tissue elements located in abnormal sites such as hypothalamic hamartoma (see Figure 6.142, page 163).
Mass-like congenital malformations – cortical dysplasia (see Figure 6.9, 6.10, on page 77), polymicrogyria (see Figure 6.7b, page 76).
Arachnoid cyst (see Figures 6.143, 6.144, 6.145, 6.146, pages 163, 164) – This is secondary to splitting of the arachnoid membrane

Neuroepithelial cyst (see Figure 6.147, page 165) – This contains ependymal or epithelial lined fluid collections within the parenchyma of the CNS without an obvious connection to the ventricle or subarachnoid space. The cysts are of unknown etiology with no pathologic enhancement.

Vascular lesions – aneurysms (see Figures 6.204, 6.205, pages 207, 208), varices, AVM's (see Figures 6.149, 6.209, 6.210, 6.211, 6.212, pages 165, 209–211).

Congenital inclusion lesions – epidermoids (see Figures 6.123, 6.150, 6.151, on pages 151, 166, 167), dermoids (see Figure 6.152, page 167), and lipomas (see Figure 6.153, page 168)

Idiopathic hypertrophic pachymeningitis (see Figure 6.154, on page 168) – this rare entity is characterized by marked dural thickening, which may be mass-like, of unknown etiology. Diagnosis by exclusion usually made by biopsy. The affected dura is usually hypointense on T1WI and T2WI and shows contrast enhancement.

Intracranial infectious/inflammatory lesions

Pediatric infectious diseases

The TORCH complex comprises a variety of congenital and neonatal infections seen in the pediatric population. The effects of these diseases depend upon the stage of development of the fetus at the time of infection and the host's immune response. Early infection occurring in the first or second trimester can result in malformations of the CNS, including microcephaly and neuronal migration anomalies ranging from lissencephaly to polymicrogyria/pachygyria. Infections acquired late in uterine development or in the perinatal/neonatal period can result in hydranencephaly, porencephlay, multicystic encephalomalacia, delayed or demyelination, cerebral calcifications, infarction, and hemorrhage. The CNS manifestations of these congenital/neonatal infections may be present at birth, evolve over the first few weeks of life, or develop months to years later.

Toxoplasmosis

Transmission of infection from the mother is transplacental. Approximately 10% of newborns infected with

Toxoplasmosis gondii exhibit clinical manifestations of the disease and most have some degree of CNS involvement. You may see aqueductal stenosis, hydrocephalus, parenchymal calcifications scattered in the periventricular regions, basal ganglia and cerebral WM and areas of parenchymal destruction, and chorioretinitis.

Other infections including HIV infection

Most cases of childhood HIV infections (~78%) are maternally transmitted. This most commonly occurs in utero via the transplacental route. It can also be transmitted through breast milk postpartum and intrapartum during birth. HIV is a lymphotropic and neurotropic virus. Direct invasion of the CNS results in apoptosis and myelin damage that leads to HIV encephalopathy. Infants are usually asymptomatic at birth and develop chronic symptoms slowly over a period of months. You may see microcephaly, ventricular enlargement, cerebral atrophy with patchy areas of parenchymal density/signal abnormality without mass effect, and calcifications (often in the basal ganglia and WM). Basal ganglia calcifications are rare under one year of age. Classically you see bilateral symmetric calcifications of the globus pallidus, putamen, thalamus, and at the GM–WM junction.

Rubella

This is rare because of immunization efforts. Transplacental infection occurs at the time of the primary maternal infection. The time of fetal infection is important in determining the outcome. The earlier in gestation the infection occurs, the greater the incidence of congenital lesions. Imaging findings can include microcephaly, chronic meningoencephalitis, areas of parenchymal necrosis, calcifications in the basal ganglia and cortex, delayed myelination, ventriculitis, and hydrocephalus.

Cytomegalovirus (see Figure 6.155, page 169)

Cytomegalovirus (CMV) belongs to the herpes virus family. It is the most common cause of congenital viral infection in the United States. Transmission to the fetus can occur via the transplacental route, during birth owing to infection of the cervix, via direct contact of maternal secretions with the newborn at the time of delivery, or through breastfeeding. Those infections that occur during or after birth rarely result in CNS manifestations. The most severe effects on the CNS occur with infection early in gestation (first and second trimester). There is a predilection for involvement of subependymal germinal matrix cells. This can explain the preferential periventricular calcifications seen on imaging and neuronal migration abnormalities including lissencephaly, polymicrogyria, pachygyria, and heterotopias. Infections later in gestation may result in hydranencephaly and porencephaly. Periventricular infections are found in more than 50% of cases, but there can also be involvement of the cerebral cortex, deep WM, and cerebellum.

Herpes simplex infection

The majority of congenital herpes infections at birth represent herpes simplex virus (HSV) type 2 (associated with genital lesions) and arise from contact with infected genital secretions at the time of delivery. Thirty percent of these have CNS involvement and 80% of these are fatal. Neonatal herpes infection acquired during birth is a diffuse, generalized process resulting in extensive brain destruction. It may result in microcephaly, ventriculomegaly, and multicystic encephalomalacia. Early CT imaging may show hypodense lesions in the periventricular WM and finger-like areas of increased density within the cortical GM (this may be related to increased blood flow to the cortical infection). With disease progression, you can see focal areas of hemorrhagic necrosis, parenchymal calcifications, and cystic encephalomalacia.

Pyogenic – infratentorial and/or supratentorial infections

- Meningitis (see Figure 6.156, page 169)
- Subdural/epidural empyema (see Figures 6.157, 6.158, pages 170, 171)
- Cerebritis (see Figure 6.159, page 172)
- Abscess (see Figure 6.160, page 173)

Acute bacterial (pyogenic) meningitis

Hemophilus influenzae, Neisseria meningitides and *Streptococcus pneumoniae* account for approximately 80% of cases of acute bacterial (pyogenic) meningitis in the United States. Certain organisms are more common at certain ages. In neonates, *Escherichia coli* and group B streptococci are more common; in infants and children, *H. influenzae* is most common; in adolescents and young adults, *N. meningitides* is most common; and in the elderly population, *S. pneumoniae* and *Listeria monocytogenes* are more common pathogens. Preferential location of exudate is associated with the specific organism. In *H.*

influenzae meningitis, basal predilection of exudates is seen whereas in pneumococcal meningitis, the exudates are more prominent over the cerebral convexities near the superior sagittal sinus. Most common complications of acute bacterial meningitis are: (1) cerebral infarction (~37% of cases) – arterial or venous, (2) diffuse cerebral edema (~34%), (3) hydrocephalus (most often communicating) (~30%), (4) cranial nerve dysfunction (~10%–20%), and (5) subdural effusions and subdural/epidural empyema. Imaging of meningitis is more sensitive when utilizing MR than CT, but abnormal contrast enhancement on MRI has been reported to occur in only 55%–70% of patients with clinically proven infectious meningitis. Two patterns of meningeal enhancement can be seen: (1) leptomeningeal (seen as a thin layer of continuous enhancement along the surface of the brain, which extends into the depths of the sulci), and (2) dural (thicker and follows the inner margin of the calvarium). While the leptomeningeal pattern is more common in inflammatory disease and dural enhancement is more common in neoplastic disease, there is some overlap. Also favoring neoplastic meningeal enhancement is nodular irregular enhancement of meninges. Imaging findings in early meningitis are often normal. On CT, there may be loss of visualization of the basal cisterns and other subarachnoid spaces from the presence of high protein exudates. Post-contrast CT images may show enhancement of the high protein exudates in the cisterns/subarachnoid spaces and meninges (more often leptomeningeal). Pathologic enhancement of the meninges is usually more conspicuous on MRI. FLAIR sequence is the most sensitive unenhanced sequence to detect leptomeningeal disease.

Subdural effusion and subdural/epidural empyema

This can represent a complication of meningitis, be related to calvarial or paranasal sinus/mastoid/middle ear inflammatory disease, or arise as a consequence of penetrating trauma or surgery. Frontal sinusitis is the most common cause of subdural/epidural empyema. On imaging, you see a subdural or epidural fluid collection, which is usually of higher density/signal intensity than simple CSF, with peripheral enhancement of the collection of varying thickness. MR better depicts both the inner and outer enhancing layers of the extracerebral collections. Subdural effusions are sterile, non-infected, subdural fluid collections that can result as a reactive phenomenon of meningitis.

These non-infected collections generally show fluid density/signal similar to CSF and may or may not demonstrate peripheral enhancement. DWI will not show diffusion restriction with sterile subdural effusions (but will with empyema), and will generally resolve with curative treatment of the meningitis. This condition is often seen in association with *H. influenzae* meningitis in infants/children.

Cerebritis/abscess

This occurs secondary to local abnormalities such as sinusitis, otomastoiditis, or trauma, is iatrogenic from neurosurgical procedures, or can result from hematogenous dissemination of infection. Hematogenous origin is often secondary to lung infections, in IV drug abusers and immunodeficient patients such as diabetics. Focal cerebritis goes through various stages of evolution toward the development of a cerebral abscess. There is early and late cerebritis leading to early and late capsule stages in abscess formation. The most common location is the frontal lobes but it can occur anywhere. Look for a local source of infection such as sinus disease, otomastoiditis, or calvarial/scalp infection. Early cerebritis is a localized area of brain inflammation without enhancement, which is poorly demarcated and seen as hypodensity on CT and increased T2/FLAIR signal with localized mass effect. In late cerebritis, look for patchy, irregular enhancement. With continued progression of the disease, the process becomes more localized with an area of liquefactive necrosis that develops a peripheral collagen capsule, which evolves and becomes more mature with time. The capsular wall is usually thinner on the medial/ventricular side of the abscess because of the greater vascularity along the lateral (cortical side). In addition, the capsule of an abscess is usually thin and of uniform thickness. These characteristics help to distinguish an abscess from a tumor, which usually has a thicker, more nodular, irregular wall and does not show relative thinning along the medial/ventricular side of the lesion. Hematogenous abscess formation usually occurs at the GM–WM junction owing to change in caliber of the arteries in this region. MRI of an abscess shows a peripheral rim, which is iso- to mildly hyperintense to brain on T1WI and hypointense on T2WI. Central increased T2/FLAIR signal related to the liquefactive necrosis is seen. There is usually surrounding increased T2/FLAIR signal from edema. The hypointensity within the capsule on T2WI is felt to be secondary to the presence of collagen, hemorrhage, and/or paramagnetic free radicals within phagocytic macrophages. Successful treatment of an abscess results in the resolution of the T2 hypointense rim and may be a better indicator of the treatment response, as persistent, residual peripheral enhancement may be present despite successful treatment. Imaging of an abscess on CT also shows a peripheral ring enhancing lesion with similar morphologic characteristics as seen on MRI. Owing to the thinner medial/ventricular wall of an abscess, it may rupture into the ventricle resulting in ependymitis, ventriculitis, and choroid plexitis (which can also occur from hematogenous spread because of a lack of a blood brain barrier in the choroid plexus).

Viral – infratentorial and/or supratentorial infections

Meningitis

Encephalitis (see Figure 6.162, page 175)

Viral meningitis

This is often referred to as acute aseptic meningitis, characterized by relatively mild illness with fever, meningeal irritation, and CSF pleocytosis with lymphocyte predominance. Enteroviruses (echovirus, coxsackievirus, and non-paralytic poliovirus) are the most common cause and responsible for 80% of cases where a pathogen is identified. Mumps is a common cause in unimmunized populations. Arboviruses also cause meningitis, and St. Louis encephalitis virus is the most common cause of aseptic meningitis from this group in the United States. CT and MR imaging are usually normal in the absence of encephalitis. When meningoencephalitis occurs, you may see associated meningeal enhancement.

Viral encephalitis

This can be a focal or generalized viral infection of the brain. Some have associated meningitis (meningoencephalitis). A wide variety of viral organisms are responsible for encephalitis. Imaging of viral encephalitis shows greater involvement of GM compared to WM in immunocompetent people. Patients showing greater WM involvement have a higher likelihood of having an impaired immune system. Different cell types in the CNS have varying sensitivities to certain viruses, which results in differing patterns of disease. For example, the poliomyelitis virus has the propensity to infect motor neurons; the rabies virus mainly infects neurons and to a lesser degree oligo-dendrocytes; the herpes virus infects neurons and glial cells in the limbic system; the JC virus only infects oligodendrocytes; and West Nile viral encephalitis involves the deep thalamic regions. These predilections may be related to specific viral receptors on the host target cells. Therefore, the pattern on imaging studies depends upon the specific virus involved.

Acute infective encephalitis

1. Herpes type 1 (see Figure 6.161, page 174–175) accounts for 95% of herpetic encephalitis and 10%–20% of viral encephalitis in the United States. It is the most common cause of sporadic encephalitis. It has a predilection for the limbic system with involvement of the temporal lobes, orbital frontal gyri, insular cortex, and cingulate gyrus, with the tendency to spare the putamen. Bilateral involvement is typical and may be symmetric or asymmetric. Often hemorrhagic encephalitis occurs. Early identification with CT may be difficult owing to the beam hardening artifact through the temporal lobes, but you may see hypodensity and possible hemorrhagic changes and enhancement (which may be gyriform) as the disease progresses. MRI is much more sensitive in delineating the disease process.

2. Neonatal herpes encephalitis is most often secondary to HSV type 2. Eighty-five percent of cases occur during the peripartum period, 10% postnatally, and 5% in utero. There is a more diffuse pattern of involvement compared with HSV type 1 infection, with inclusion of cerebral WM and sometimes the cerebellum. Imaging studies show patchy WM involvement with possible stippled areas of hemorrhage. You may see rapid progression to brain necrosis and hemorrhage.

3. Arboviruses may also result in acute encephalitis and have an arthropod vector (mosquitoes). Different types include: (1) eastern equine encephalitis, (2) western equine encephalitis, (3) St. Louis encephalitis – the most common arboviral encephalitis – MR may show abnormal signal in the substantia nigra but it is not specific, (4) La Crosse encephalitis, and (5) West Nile encephalitis.

4. Rabies virus shows predominant involvement of the GM of the brain and spinal cord.

5. Polio virus (an enterovirus). The polio virus receptors are found in the motor cortex, cerebellum, and spinal motor neurons.

6. Japanese encephalitis (JE) is the most common form of focal encephalitis in Asia, showing areas of signal abnormality in the thalami (more commonly in the posterior medial thalami), basal ganglia, brainstem, cerebellum, and cortical areas. It may involve the posterior part of the medial temporal lobe/hippocampus, and may be associated with hemorrhage.

Subacute encephalitis

This type is associated with a more insidious onset and includes subacute sclerosing panencephalitis (SSPE) secondary to the measles virus, progressive rubella panencephalitis, progressive multifocal leukoencephalopathy (discussed in Chapter 1) secondary to infection with the JC virus, HIV encephalitis, CMV encephalitis (discussed in Chapter 3), kuru, and Creutzfeldt–Jakob disease (prion disease: caused by a proteinaceous infectious particle that contains little or no nucleic acid and does not evoke an immune response. Prions propagate by altering the shape/folding of normal cellular prion protein into abnormal prion protein, which accumulates within and destroys brain tissue – discussed elsewhere in Chapter 3).

HIV encephalitis

The most common imaging findings are cerebral atrophy, which can be predominantly central, peripheral, or mixed. WM lesions may be diffuse, patchy, focal, or punctuate. They do not enhance or show mass effect.

Rhomboencephalitis

This is the term used when a viral encephalitic process primarily involves the brainstem and cerebellum. It is seen with *Listeria monocytogenes*, adenovirus, and enterovirus infections.

Non-infectious encephalitis

Acute disseminated encephalomyelitis (ADEM) (see Figure 6.166, pages 178–179) – usually occurs five days to two weeks after a viral illness (usually upper respiratory tract infection) or vaccination (especially measles, mumps, and rubella). It is probably immune mediated, with perivenular demyelination similar to that found with multiple sclerosis. This is a monophasic illness. It involves the brain and spinal cord (30% of patients have cord lesions). Cord lesions can involve GM, WM, or both. Spinal lesions usually do not enhance and segmental lesions usually involve two to three vertebral bodies. Intracranially you see scattered, poorly marginated T2 hyperintense lesions in WM in the posterior fossa and the cerebral hemispheres. Greater involvement of the subcortical and deep WM compared to periventricular areas occurs. WM lesions are typically asymmetric whereas involvement of the basal ganglia and thalami often is symmetric. The cerebral cortex is involved in about 30% of cases and occasionally you may only see cortical involvement. There is posterior fossa involvement in more than 50% of patients. No mass effect is evident, although brainstem lesions may have considerable swelling. There is variable contrast enhancement and you may see diffusion restriction early in the disease. Differential considerations favoring ADEM over MS include GM involvement, a greater predilection to involve more peripheral WM, more prominent involvement of the posterior fossa in children with ADEM, and a monophasic course. ADEM lesions usually resolve or remain unchanged at six months following the onset of the illness. MS should be considered if new lesions appear at or after this time.

Rasmussen's encephalitis (see Figure 6.167, page 179) – this is the childhood form of chronic encephalitis, possibly viral or autoimmune in origin, resulting in an intractable seizure disorder resistant to medical therapy that may require hemispherectomy for treatment. It usually involves only one cerebral hemisphere. On MRI, you see focal involvement initially with swelling/edema (increased T2/FLAIR signal) in involved region(s) early in the disease, with subsequent spread of the lesion across the ipsilateral hemisphere or parts of it, with progressive hemispheric atrophy.

Granulomatous infections/inflammatory lesions

These lesions may be meningial (more commonly basal) or parenchymal (infratentorial and/or supratentorial).

TB (see Figures 6.168, 6.169, pages 180, 181)
Sarcoid (see Figures 6.119, 6.170, pages 148, 182)
Fungal (see Figure 6.171, page 183)

Tuberculosis

The incidence of CNS TB has been increasing since the mid 1980s since the rise of HIV/AIDS. The most common pattern of CNS disease is a diffuse meningoencephalitis. TB meningitis results in thick,

gelatinous infiltration of the basal meninges. Basal vascular structures are often affected with spasm and arteritis, which may result in infarction. Imaging studies show an enhancing meningitic process, most severely affecting the basilar cisterns, often with associated ring or solid nodular enhancing parenchymal tuberculomas and hydrocephalus (usually communicating). TB exudates in the cisterns and sulci often are hyperintense on T1WI and demonstrate intense enhancement. Post-inflammatory calcification in the basal cisterns can be seen with or without treatment.

Sarcoidosis

This is a systemic, non-infectious granulomatous process characterized by the presence of non-caseating granulomas. About 5% of cases with sarcoid develop CNS involvement. CNS manifestations reflect dural/leptomeningeal and vascular involvement by the granulomatous process with a predilection for the basilar cisterns. Sarcoid can gain access into the parenchyma of the brain via the perivascular spaces (Virchow-Robin spaces). You may see dural, leptomeningeal, and parenchymal lesions in neurosarcoid. Nodular dural/leptomeningeal and parenchymal enhancement can also be seen. In addition, there may be cranial nerve involvement. Dural lesions appear isointense to GM on T1WI and hypointense on T2WI with relatively uniform enhancement. Enhancing parenchymal lesions often follow the course of perivascular spaces. Non-enhancing periventricular WM lesions simulating MS may also be seen. Leptomeningeal and pachymeningeal involvement is the most common form and is the most frequent cause of chronic meningitis.

Fungal

There has been a steady rise in CNS involvement by fungi over the last 30 years with the advent of transplant immunosuppression and the rise of HIV/AIDS. Different genera of fungi exist in various forms; they may exist as a single cell referred to as the yeast form, or in colonies that may have a branched appearance called the hyphal form. If these two different forms coalesce they can become mycelia. As a result of the smaller size of the single yeast cell form, they commonly spread hematogenously through the meningeal microcirculation resulting in a leptomeningitis or granuloma formation. The hyphal forms, which are larger, more likely involve the brain parenchyma

49

producing a cerebritis or encephalitis. Large mycelia forms can result in vasculitis, leading to septic infarction and mycotic aneurysms. Besides hematogenous spread, fungal disease can gain access via direct communication secondary to trauma, surgery, or fungal infection involving the sinonasal region. Immunosuppressed patients are more prone to develop these infections. Different fungal infections include aspergillosis, mucormycosis, candidiasis, histoplasmosis, *Coccidioides immitis*, *Blastomyces dermatitidis*, and cryptococcus.

Parasitic infections

These infections are more commonly supratentorial than infratentorial.

Cysticercosis (see Figure 6.172, page 184)

Cysticercosis

This is the most common parasitic CNS disease and involves the larval pork tapeworm (*Taenia solium*) from contaminated water or food. CNS involvement is parenchymal, leptomeningeal, or intraventricular. The parasite becomes lodged within the brain parenchyma or meninges and develops a cystic covering around the scolex. Parenchymal cysts are usually 10 mm or less in size, and because of increased blood flow may be preferentially located near the cortex and in the basal ganglia. Subarachnoid/basal cistern cysts may become large owing to lack of restricted growth of surrounding structures. Intraventricular cysts (in only 7%–20% of cases with neurocysticercosis) may be single (more common) or multiple, and may be attached to the ventricular wall or free floating. The fourth ventricle is the most common location for intraventricular cysts, most of which are not associated with cysticercosis in other locations. MRI is more sensitive in most cases except where the predominant findings are small calcifications. Parenchymal cysts have different stages. Stage 1 is the vesicular stage when there is a small marginal nodule (scolex) projecting into a small cyst containing clear fluid. These are viable organisms and do not elicit an inflammatory response and therefore no contrast enhancement of the cyst wall. Stage 2 occurs with the host immune response leading to the colloidal vesicular stage. The larva begins to degenerate with gradual shrinkage of the scolex. Cyst fluid becomes more turbid and you see surrounding WM edema and contrast enhancement of the cyst wall. Stage 3 is the granular nodular

stage when the cyst wall thickens and the scolex becomes a coarse mineralized granule. The surrounding edema begins to regress. You may see a thick, small, ring-like enhancement pattern of the cyst as it shrinks. Stage 4 is the nodular calcified stage when the lesion shrinks and becomes completely mineralized/ calcified. No surrounding inflammatory edema is evident. Rarely you may see minimal enhancement surrounding the calcified lesion. Identification of the scolex (mural nodule) is nearly pathognomonic of this infection. Leptomeningeal/subarachnoid cysticercosis can produce the racemose form where multilocular cysts are seen in the subarachnoid cisterns (more often basal cisterns) with the absence of the scolex within these cystic conglomerations. They may show contrast enhancement when degenerating, and may result in communicating hydrocephalus, cranial nerve dysfunction, and vasculitis.

Infections in immunocompromised patients

These infections are more commonly supratentorial than infratentorial.

HIV – see previous discussion under viral encephalitis (see Figure 6.165, page 177)

PML – see discussion in Chapter 1 (see Figure 6.163, page 176)

CMV

Toxoplasmosis (see Figures 6.140, 6.173, pages 161, 185)

Cryptococcal (see Figure 6.171, page 183)

Cytomegalovirus infection

Adults: most adults are infected by CMV but CNS disease develops only in immunosuppressed patients. This is the most common opportunistic infection in AIDS. The effect of CMV on the CNS can mimic infection by HIV and other viruses. It causes a ventriculoencephalitis, and can lead to necrotizing encephalitis and ventriculitis. Encephalitis is seen as increased T2 signal without enhancement in the WM (there is more propensity to involve deeper periventricular WM than in HIV encephalitis). Ventriculitis/periventriculitis with diffuse increased T2 signal occurs in the periventricular/ subependymal regions with thin, linear enhancement along the ventricular walls. CMV polyradiculopathy can demonstrate thickened, clumped, enhancing nerve roots of the cauda equina.

Neonatal: this is secondary to an in utero infection. The risk of acquiring a primary maternal infection in utero is 40%–50%. There are a wide range of CNS manifestations, which can lead to death. Surviving infants may show porencephaly, polymicrogyria, periventricular calcifications, hydrocephalus, and cerebellar hypoplasia.

Toxoplasmosis

This is a parasitic infection secondary to an intracellular protozoan, *Toxoplasma gondii*. Twenty to seventy percent of adults in the United States are seropositive. In AIDS, toxoplasmosis causes a necrotizing encephalitis. Imaging studies show multiple lesions with solid nodular or peripheral ring enhancing lesions, with associated vasogenic edema and mass effect. The most common location is the basal ganglia, and GM–WM junction. Lesions may show variable T2 signal – iso-, hypo-, or hyperintensity. Usually there is a response to anti-toxoplasma drugs about 10 days after beginning treatment but full resolution may take up to six months, and patients are kept on lifelong therapy. You may see calcifications of treated lesions. It is not possible to differentiate the appearance of toxoplasmosis from lymphoma in AIDS patients with conventional MRI. Lymphomas are usually necrotic in AIDS patients. MR spectroscopy may help suggest lymphoma by elevated choline and elevated lactate peak.

Cryptococcus infection

The yeast-like fungus *Cryptococcus neoformans* is the most common fungal disease in AIDS patients, with approximately 5%–10% of cases developing CNS cryptococcus disease and 80%–90% of all patients being AIDS related. The most common CNS manifestation is meningitis. The subarachnoid spaces are filled with thick, gelatinous material containing organisms. Meningeal enhancement is usually not seen on CT but may be evident with contrast MRI; however, this is not typical. If you see prominent meningeal enhancement, consider causes other than cryptococcus first. Look for enlarged perivascular spaces with slightly higher signal than CSF on T1WI. There is a notable lack of an inflammatory response and therefore enhancement. With progression and confluence of perivascular spaces, you will see gelatinous pseudocysts within the expected regions of the perivascular spaces, including the dentate nuclei regions. If the organism invades the brain, a granuloma called a cryptococcoma may form. This has an appearance similar to other granulomas with low T1 and high T2 signal and solid,

nodular, or ring-like enhancement and surrounding edema (high T2 signal).

Intraventricular infection – infratentorial/supratentorial

> Ependymitis/ventriculitis (see Figures 6.174a–b, 6.175, pages 186, 187)
> Choroid plexitis (see Figure 6.174c, page 186)
> Intraventricular exudate (see Figure 6.174a–b, page 186)

Ependymitis/ventriculitis

This can be seen in association with meningitis, secondary to rupture of a parenchymal abscess, or be secondary to the placement of an intraventricular catheter (iatrogenic). Note subtle hypodensity (CT) and T1 hypointensity and T2 hyperintensity in the immediate periventricular regions (in the ependymal/subependymal regions) with linear enhancement along the wall of the ventricles on post-contrast CT and MRI. You may see areas of increased density (CT) and areas of signal abnormality on MRI, representing exudates layering within the occipital horns of the lateral ventricles.

Choroid plexitis

Infection of the choroid plexus may accompany a ventriculitis or be secondary to hematogenous seeding directly as the choroid plexus lacks a blood brain barrier. A normal choroid plexus enhances, therefore look for enlargement of the choroid plexus in cases of plexitis.

Intraventricular exudate

This usually accompanies ventriculitis. You will see exudative debris, which layers in the dependent portions of the ventricular system.

Demyelinating disorders

> Acute disseminated encephalomyelitis (see Figure 6.166, page 178) – see previous discussion in non-infectious encephalitis
> Multiple sclerosis (MS) (see Figures 6.176–180, pages 188–191)
> > Variants:
> > Balo's concentric sclerosis (see Figure 6.181, page 191)
> > Marburg's variant (see Figure 6.182, page 192)

Devic's disease (neuromyelitis optica) (see Figure
6.183, page 193)

Marchiafava–Bignami disease – toxic
demyelination of the corpus callosum (see
Figure 6.184, page 194)

Osmotic demyelination (central pontine/extrapontine
myelinolysis) (see Figure 6.185, page 195)

Multiple sclerosis (see discussion in Chapter 1)

Balo's concentric sclerosis variant of multiple sclerosis

This rare variant of MS is characterized pathologically
by alternating rings of myelin preservation (remyelin-
ation) and myelin loss (demyelination). It was initially
thought to have a fulminant clinical course similar
to Marburg's variant leading to death, but there is
now evidence that there may be self limiting cases.
Typical MR features are concentric rings on T2WI.

Marburg's variant of multiple sclerosis

This is a rare, acute, fulminant, monophasic variant of
MS without remissions, with rapidly progressive
demyelination leading to severe disability and death.
MRI usually shows multiple lesions typical for MS but
occurring simultaneously with a more destructive
pattern and more prominent inflammatory infiltrates.

Devic's disease (neuromyelitis optica)

This condition was initially thought to represent a
variant of MS but may represent a distinct entity of
its own. This is characterized by a demyelinating
disease involving the optic nerves and spinal cord,
which can lead to blindness and permanent spinal
cord injury. There is a greater incidence in young
adults but it may occur in any age from infancy to
the elderly, and is more common in females than
males. MRI imaging shows findings of optic neuritis
(enlargement and enhancement of the optic nerves) in
addition to swelling, abnormal spinal cord signal, and
enhancement, often involving long segments of the
spinal cord as opposed to MS where shorter segments
are typically seen.

Marchiafava–Bignami disease

This is toxic demyelination of the corpus callosum
usually seen in chronic alcoholism, owing to deficiency
in the vitamin B complex. It typically affects the body of
the corpus callosum followed by the genu and then the
splenium. The corpus callosal degeneration/necrosis
progresses and splits into three layers with the middle
layer the most severely involved. On MR in the
acute stage, there may be decreased T1 and increased
T2/FLAIR signal in the body of the corpus callosum,
which may extend to involve the genu. No mass effect
is seen, but there may be peripheral contrast enhancement and diffusion restriction in the acute stage.
Lesions eventually cavitate and are well demarcated.

Osmotic demyelination (central pontine/extrapontine myelinolysis)

Acute demyelination in this disease is caused by rapid
correction of hyponatremia. Imaging shows abnormal
density (CT) or signal intensity within the central pons
sparing the periphery. When this is extrapontine, it may
involve the basal ganglia and cerebral WM. Typically
there is no enhancement although this may occasionally
occur. You may see restricted diffusion on DWI.

Traumatic lesions

These can occur anywhere. Traumatic head injury is a
major cause of death and disability in today's society
and a frequent indication for brain imaging. In the
setting of acute head injury, CT is the imaging modality of choice. In the setting of remote/chronic traumatic head injury, MRI can be a useful adjunct.

Scalp hematoma (see Figure 6.186, page 196) –
cephalohematoma, subgaleal hematoma
(see discussion in Chapter 3)

Parenchymal contusions (see Figures 6.188, 6.189,
page 197)

Diffuse axonal injury (DAI)/shear injury (see
Figure 6.190, page 197)

Subarachnoid hemorrhage (SAH) (see Figure 6.191,
page 198)

Subdural (SDH)/epidural hematoma (EDH) (see
Figures 6.191–195, pages 198–201)

Duret hemorrhage

Intraventricular hemorrhage (IVH) (see Figure
6.191, page 198)

Post-traumatic cytotoxic edema (see Figure 6.191,
page 198)

Non-accidental trauma (child abuse) (see Figures
6.196–198, pages 202, 203)

Post-traumatic encephalomalacia (see Figure 6.199,
page 204)

Parenchymal contusions

The brain is held in a rigid shell, which is our skull. There are many regions of naturally occurring bony irregularities along the inner table of the skull and skull base, which create natural sites where focal mechanical injury to the brain may occur in the setting of trauma. The orbital plates of the frontal bone, the floor and anterior bony walls of the middle cranial fossa, the region of the pterion, and along the superior margin of the petrous portion of the temporal bone are some of these areas of bony irregularity and common sites of contusions. You can easily feel these by running your hand along these surfaces on a skull specimen. Contact of the brain against the inner table and skull base can result in hemorrhagic contusions (superficial bruises of the brain), which represent focal areas of brain injury with bleeding. These can occur beneath the site of direct injury and are referred to as *coup* contusions, or on the opposite side of the brain along the major vector force and are called *contre-coup* contusions. These often expand/bloom in the first 24–48 hours after the initial head injury. Imaging demonstrates areas of blood density (~50–90 HU) with associated edema in the cortical and juxtacortical regions, with associated mass effect.

Diffuse axonal injury/shear injury

Axonal injury results from rapid angular/rotational acceleration and deceleration of the brain. Brain tissue in the cortex and underlying WM have different compositions so that the differential movement of these structures during this type of trauma has a shearing or tearing effect upon the axons. Favored sites of DAI are the corpus callosum (greater in the posterior part), GM–WM junction in the frontal and temporal lobes, and the WM in the superior frontal gyrus, superior cerebellar peduncles, and dorsal midbrain. DAI lesions have traditionally been considered small (between 1 mm and 5 mm in size), non-hemorrhagic foci of increased T2 signal on MRI. Reports now indicate that there is a high percentage of hemorrhagic DAI lesions, especially when utilizing 3T magnets and gradient echo T2/susceptibility weighted MR sequences, even when standard MRI pulse sequences are normal.

Subarachnoid hemorrhage

Trauma is the most common cause of subarachnoid hemorrhage. The appearance is similar to SAH from other causes. It can be focal or diffuse. CT is more sensitive than MRI in detecting SAH; however, FLAIR sequences appear to be most sensitive in detecting SAH with MRI.

Subdural/epidural hematoma

Traumatic injury can result in subdural and/or epidural hematomas. Often there is a combination of both types of extracerebral hemorrhage. EDHs often occur after fracture of the temporal squamosal bone with injury to the middle meningeal artery, although venous EDHs also occur. These hematomas are also found in the parietal and frontal regions and less commonly in the posterior fossa (where venous EDHs are more common). Acute EDHs are classically described as biconvex, lenticular shaped, hyperdense extra-axial collections on non-contrast CT. Areas of hypodensity within an acute EDH may represent sites of active bleeding with non-retracted, unclotted blood. When patients are anemic or have low hematocrit, acute SDH and EDH may be lower in density than you would typically expect. Acute SDHs are biconcave, hyperdense, extra-axial collections of blood that spread more diffusely and along the margins of the inner table and surface of the brain. They are less frequently associated with skull fracture than EDHs. EDHs which can extend across the margin of a dural venous sinus (can cross the midline) but generally do not cross sutures and do not extend into the interhemispheric fissure. SDHs may extend into the interhemispheric fissure but are limited by the dural venous sinuses (they do not cross the sinus/midline).

Duret hemorrhage

This refers to post-traumatic brainstem hemorrhages, which occur as a result of stretching and tearing of perforating vascular structures within the brainstem. When there is significant supratentorial mass effect with downward transtentorial herniation, the brainstem is displaced caudally. This results in traction and stretching upon the vertebrobasilar system and subsequent tearing of perforating vessels within the brainstem.

Intraventricular hemorrhage

Trauma related IVH appears similar to IVH from other causes. You will see hyperdense material that may layer within the dependent portions of the ventricular system, such as in the occipital horns of the lateral ventricles and in the dorsal aspect of the fourth ventricle. Intraventricular blood may occur within the choroid plexus of the ventricular system and therefore not act as free-floating material.

Cytotoxic edema

Post-traumatic edema can be vasogenic and cytotoxic and represents secondary injury caused by a cascade of mechanisms triggered at the moment of injury. Cytotoxic edema results in the accumulation of water inside the neurons, which swell reducing the intercellular space and limiting movement of free water. This is identified on MRI by increased T2 signal and diffusion restriction (high signal on diffusion trace sequence images and decreased signal on the ADC map). You tend to see loss of GM–WM differentiation on CT.

Non-accidental trauma (child abuse)

In this type of trauma, you often find multiple post-traumatic changes of varying ages; for example, subdural hematomas in varying stages of evolution. Look for subarachnoid and intraparenchymal hemorrhages/contusions and evidence of DAI. You may see cytotoxic edema with loss of GM–WM differentiation and the CT reversal sign, with relative sparing/hyperdensity of the basal ganglia and posterior fossa structures relative to the hypodense cerebral hemispheres. Search for skull fractures, which are often better detected with plain x-rays.

Post-traumatic encephalomalacia

Areas of macrocystic (seen as density on CT and signal intensity on MRI, similar to CSF) and microcystic (tissue injury without frank cavitation, which shows increased signal intensity on FLAIR MR images) encephalomalacia are found in areas prone to traumatic brain injury, such as the anteroinferior frontal lobes, anterior temporal lobes, and in the mid-temporal lobes just above the petrous temporal bone.

Vascular lesions

Most vascular lesions can occur anywhere.

Hemorrhage – subarachnoid, intraparenchymal, intraventricular, and epidural/subdural
Aneurysms (see Figures 6.204–208, pages 207–209)

Vascular malformations (see Figures 6.149, 6.209–223, pages 165, 209–217)
Microvascular ischemic disease/small vessel disease (see discussion in Chapter 1 and Figure 6.224, page 218)
Cerebral infarction (stroke) (see Figures 6.226–245, pages 219–229)
Non-atherosclerotic vasculopathies/vasculitis, CADASIL, moyamoya disease (see Figures 6.246–248, pages 229–231)
Cortical venous/dural sinus thrombosis (see Figures 6.249–253, pages 232–237)
Vasospasm (see Figures 6.254, 6.255, page 238)
Vascular dissection (see Figure 6.256, page 239)
Fibromuscular dysplasia (FMD) (see Figure 6.257, page 239)
Vascular injury (see Figures 6.258, 6.259, page 240)
Posterior reversible encephalopathy (PRES, hypertensive encephalopathy) (see Figure 6.260, page 241)

Hemorrhage

Hemorrhage can occur into any intracranial compartment in the posterior fossa or in supratentorial compartments. Patients on anticoagulants and those with coagulopathy are at increased risk of spontaneous intracranial hemorrhage without or with underlying lesions and with minor trauma.

Subarachnoid hemorrhage

The most common cause is trauma.

1. Benign non-aneurysmal perimesencephalic hemorrhage (see Figure 6.200, page 205) – an entity characterized by spontaneous SAH, with the blood centered anterior to the midbrain or pons with or without extension around the brainstem, and which can extend into the suprasellar cistern and medial horizontal Sylvian cisterns without extending into the lateral Sylvian or interhemispheric fissures. Blood is typically anterior to the brainstem. This condition is usually not associated with an identifiable intracranial aneurysm on angiography, and patients have a good outcome. The precise cause is unknown but may be a result of a venous bleed. About 5% of cases, however, are related to rupture

of basilar tip aneurysms. The pattern of subarachnoid blood may suggest this diagnosis but cannot completely exclude aneurysmal SAH.

2. Aneurysmal subarachnoid hemorrhage (see Figure 6.201, page 205) – distribution of blood may provide a clue as to the location of the ruptured aneurysm. Look for a localized clot.

3. Superficial siderosis (see Figure 6.202, page 205) – characterized by repetitive episodes of SAH resulting in staining of the surface of the brain with hemosiderin (toxic to the brain). It is best identified on gradient echo T2 images because of the magnetic susceptibility of hemosiderin with blooming. It is often present with bilateral sensorineural hearing loss and ataxia. Imaging shows linear/curvilinear hypointensity on gradient echo T2 images conforming to the surface of the brain.

Intraparenchymal hemorrhage

1. Hypertensive hemorrhage (see Figures 6.137a, 6.203a,c, pages 160, 206) – common locations are the putamen, thalamus, pons, and cerebellum. This type of hemorrhage is often associated with intraventricular extension of blood. You may see a pattern of multiple microbleeds best seen on gradient echo T2 or susceptibility weighted images.

2. Hemorrhage from amyloid angiopathy (see Figures 6.137b, 6.203b, pages 160, 206) – you may see multiple lobar hemorrhages of differing ages, which often extend superficially, and/or scattered microbleeds throughout the cerebral hemispheres, best demonstrated on gradient echo T2 or susceptibility weighted images.

3. Hemorrhage secondary to other causes including AVM, vasculitis, septic emboli, and intra-axial tumors.

Intraventricular hemorrhage – causes

1. Trauma
2. Tumor
3. AVM, aneurysm

Epidural/subdural hematoma

1. Most often traumatic
2. Dural AVF and pial AVM may rupture into the subdural and subarachnoid spaces

Aneurysms

Current opinion regarding pathogenesis is that aneurysms result from a combination of hemodynamic stress and acquired degenerative changes within the vessel wall, even if inherited diseases may predispose their formation by weakening the vessel wall. The prevalence is approximately 3%–5%, with multiple aneurysms in 15%–45% of cases. The peak age at presentation is in the fourth decade. There is a higher incidence in smokers and females, in patients with polycystic kidney disease, connective tissue disorders (Marfan's disease and Ehlers–Danlos Syndrome), moyamoya disease, aortic coarctation, neurofibromatosis, fibromuscular dysplasia, and in patients with AVMs (flow related and dysplastic). Giant aneurysms are diagnosed if they are more than 25 mm in size. 90% arise from the anterior circulation. The anterior communicating artery complex is the most common site (~30%–35%), about 30% originate from the internal carotid artery (includes the posterior communicating artery, internal carotid artery bifurcation, ophthalmic segment, superior hypophyseal artery), and about 30% from the middle cerebral artery bifurcation/trifurcation. Approximately 10% arise from the posterior circulation with the basilar artery apex the most common site followed by the origin of the posterior inferior cerebellar artery. The annual rate of rupture is about 1.4% with increased risk associated with aneurysm size, posterior circulation location, and history of previous SAH. When multiple aneurysms are present and there is SAH, the question is which one ruptured? The prediction of which bled includes the following factors: the largest, most irregular (has blebs or "Murphy's tit"), focal vasospasm, and location of SAH/clot. Treatment of ruptured aneurysms includes open neurosurgical clipping, endovascular coiling, or occasionally combined endovascular and open clipping.

Saccular (berry type) aneurysms

These are thin-walled sacs connected to the parent vessel by an orifice of variable size called the neck. True aneurysms contain at least some layers normally found in arteries; however, the wall is very thin with deficiencies in the internal elastic lamina and tunica media, which typically occur at the bifurcations of vessels.

Non-saccular aneurysms

These arise at non-branching sites and are less common.
Traumatic aneurysms – 1% of cases, often distal, and
mostly from penetrating trauma, an adjacent fracture,
or impact on the falx or tentorium.
Mycotic aneurysms – often distal and secondary to direct
invasion and destruction of the vessel wall; associated
with endocarditis, meningitis, and thrombophlebitis.
Neoplastic aneurysms – often distal and most are
from atrial myxoma and metastatic choriocarcinoma
secondary to direct invasion and destruction of the
arterial wall.
Dissecting aneurysms – these contain components of the
native vessel wall but result from intimal disruption;
associated commonly with fibromuscular dysplasia, connective tissue disorders, polyarteritis nodosa, and syphilis.

Other rare aneurysms

Serpentine aneurysms are partially thrombosed giant
aneurysms with separate inflow and outflow channels
composed of a residual lumen made up of channels
formed within the thrombus, not the true lumen of the
parent artery. More than 50% arise from the middle
cerebral artery. They can mimic a neoplasm on cross-
sectional imaging, with heterogeneous enhancing mass
and symptoms that may be related to mass effect.

Vascular malformations

The main types are:

1. High flow (pial) AVM – account for about 85% of
    high-flow vascular malformations intracranially,
    more commonly occurring in the supratentorial
    than infratentorial regions. This is a congenital
    abnormality in the development of the capillary
    bed. The lack of a normal capillary bed results in
    arterial venous shunting. The three components
    include: (1) arterial feeders, (2) AVM nidus, and
    (3) draining veins. Complications related to
    AVMs include hemorrhage (50%), seizures (25%),
    headache, and progressive focal neurologic deficit.
    They make up less than 10% of the incidence of
    intracranial aneurysms. These malformations
    generally become symptomatic between the ages
    of 20 and 40 years, with a rate of hemorrhage of
    2%–4% per year, which is cumulative. The brain
    adjacent to the AVM may be gliotic and atrophic
    with increased T2 signal secondary to vascular
    steal of flow through the AVM, which is a
    high-flow, low-resistance sump. Imaging studies

show enlarged arteries representing arterial
feeders, a cluster of pathologic vessels representing
the nidus, and enlarged draining veins. Unless there
is a hemorrhage or infarction in or around the
AVM, there is usually little associated mass effect.
You may see calcifications in/around the AVM.
Morphologic characteristics that increase risk of
hemorrhage are intranidal/perinidal aneurysms; a
posterior fossa, basal ganglia/thalamic, or
intraventricular/periventricular location; a single
draining vein or stricture of the draining vein,
central/deep venous drainage, or small AVM size
(have higher pressures).

2. Dural AVF – can be a high-flow or slow-flow type
    and account for 10%–15% of high-flow vascular
    malformations. They are felt to be acquired
    lesions (unlike AVMs), which may be related to
    dural sinus thrombosis with or without
    subsequent recanalization. There are normal AV
    shunts within the dura, which may enlarge when
    dural sinus thrombosis occurs. Unlike an AVM,
    there is no nidus. The arterial supply is from
    dural/meningeal branches. The venous drainage
    pattern is variable with drainage into dural
    sinuses, cortical veins, or both. The pattern of
    venous drainage determines the aggressiveness
    (whether there is a high risk of hemorrhage) of the
    malformation. Direct cortical venous drainage is
    associated with a higher risk of hemorrhage. The
    peak age at diagnosis is the fifth to sixth decade,
    but this AVF may occur in children where they
    can be more complex, higher flow, and aggressive.
    Symptoms are determined by their location.
    Pulsatile tinnitus is found with a transverse
    sigmoid sinus location, and visual symptoms with
    a carotid cavernous sinus location. Imaging
    studies including MRA may be completely normal
    and the gold standard for diagnosis is catheter
    angiography with injection of the external carotid,
    internal carotid, and vertebral arteries. On CT/
    MRI, look for dural sinus thrombosis, tiny
    vascular channels (flow voids) within or adjacent
    to a dural sinus (on MRI), enlarged cortical veins,
    cavernous sinus, or ophthalmic veins, and
    vasogenic edema (from venous congestion). They
    can result in hemorrhage into the subarachnoid,
    subdural, and/or intraparenchymal regions.

3. DVA – these are not true vascular malformations.
    They represent primitive/extreme variations in
    normal venous drainage. These cannot be resected

because they drain normal brain parenchyma and therefore would result in venous infarction if removed. The typical appearance is that of numerous small venous branches converging on and draining through a single, large venous trunk. They can drain either superficially toward cortical veins or deeply into subependymal veins and the deep venous system. Their appearance has been described as a *caput medusa* or like a large tree with multiple small branches converging on the main trunk of the tree. Cavernous malformations may develop in close proximity to the DVA, with the theory being that increased venous pressure (venous restriction) through the single common draining vein may result in hemorrhages of the smaller venous radicals of the DVA. Imaging studies show multiple small vascular channels converging on a single, common draining vein, which is directed either superficially or deeply. Look for associated cavernous malformations with susceptibility sensitive MR sequences. You may see edema in the parenchyma surrounding a DVA if there is venous congestion.

4. Cavernous malformations (cavernomas, cavernous angiomas) – they have a supratentorial/infratentorial location, and are slow flow vascular malformations that consist of a dilated capillary bed without normal intervening brain parenchyma. In the era of cerebral angiography they were included in the term occult vascular malformation because they were generally not identified on angiography owing to their slow flow. They can be solitary or multiple. Familial cohorts where individuals have multiple lesions have been described with an increased occurrence in Hispanic families. The classic imaging appearance is of a popcorn-like, round, lobulated lesion with heterogeneous signal on T1WI and T2WI with a complete peripheral rim of hemosiderin. However, when small and seen in familial cohorts, they may only be evident as regions of hypointensity best demonstrated on gradient echo T2 imaging. See the blood products of varying ages within these lesions. They tend to ooze and expand along the periphery and usually do not present with acute catastrophic hemorrhages. On CT, you may see stippled calcification related to a subtly hyperdense lesion, and little if any mass effect

unless there has been a recent bleed. No surrounding vasogenic edema occurs except with a recent bleed. MRI is much more sensitive in detecting these lesions, especially when using gradient echo T2/susceptibility weighted sequences owing to detection of magnetic susceptibility of the blood breakdown products.

5. Capillary telangiectasia – these are slow flow vascular malformations also included in the occult vascular malformation category, characterized by dilated capillary channels with normal intervening brain parenchyma. They are most common in the pons but may occur in the cerebral cortex, WM, and rarely in the spinal cord. They are usually solitary but may occasionally be multiple, are generally asymptomatic, and are incidental findings on imaging studies. They do not hemorrhage. On MRI, they usually demonstrate iso- to slight hypointensity on T1WI and isointensity to slight hyperintensity on T2WI, but are more conspicuous on gradient echo T2/susceptibility weighted sequences secondary to the presence of deoxyhemoglobin within the lesion (from the slow flow). Post-contrast images show a brush-like or stippled pattern of enhancement, sometimes with a small dominant vascular channel within the lesion. Unenhanced CT and MRI (T1 and FSE T2) may be completely normal and you may only see the lesions on post-contrast images.

6. Mixed transitional vascular malformations – this term is used when lesions do not fit precisely into one category and demonstrate morphologic characteristics of more than a single vascular type lesion. Included in this category are DVAs with arteriovenous shunting and capillary telangiectasias with DVAs.

Microvascular ischemic disease/small vessel disease

Risk factors include hyperlipidemia, diabetes, and hypertension. There is patchy and/or confluent decreased T1 and increased T2/FLAIR signal in periventricular, deep WM and deep GM nuclei, but no diffusion restriction, enhancement, or mass effect. You may see other evidence of small vessel disease such as lacunar infarcts (deep perforating artery territory infarcts, smaller than 10 mm in size).

Cerebral infarction (stroke)

The third most common cause of death after myocardial infarction and cancer and the leading cause of disability is stroke. It is one of the most common indications for CT/MR imaging of the brain. Non-contrast CT of the brain is the current imaging standard for acute stroke because of its wide availability and high sensitivity in detecting acute intracranial hemorrhage. In the setting of acute stroke, this excludes the patient from receiving anticoagulation and fibrinolytic agents. MRI with diffusion imaging is exquisitely sensitive in the detection of early stroke and, along with perfusion imaging, can help define the ischemic penumbra (area of at-risk, ischemic, but not yet infarcted brain tissue). The ischemic penumbra is defined by the diffusion–perfusion mismatch. Areas that demonstrate diffusion restriction are considered regions of irreversible injury. An ischemic penumbra exists if the perfusion defect (CBF, MTT) is larger than the diffusion defect. These imaging techniques can aid in the planning of stroke therapy. Areas of abnormal density (on CT) and signal intensity (on MRI) of acute stroke (infarction) should conform to the distribution of known vascular territories. Diffusion restriction is usually present for approximately 7–10 days after acute stroke. The signal abnormality on the diffusion trace image can persist for some time secondary to T2 shine despite normalization of signal on the ADC map. Enhancement of subacute stroke occurs as described in Chapter 1.

Watershed ischemia

This refers to areas of ischemic injury/infarction at the border zones between different vascular territories. These are common types of ischemic injury seen in patients with low flow states such as carotid stenosis and hypotensive episodes. A common finding with significant carotid artery stenosis (in the neck) is hypodensity (CT) and T1 hypointensity and T2 hyperintensity within the frontal and frontoparietal centrum semiovale. This represents the watershed zone between the distal anterior and middle cerebral artery vascular territories.

Severe acute ischemia

Because of abrupt and dense ischemia, the regions of highest metabolic demand are at risk for infarction, which includes the cortical GM as well as the deep GM nuclei. There is no time for re-routing of blood to these areas of highest demand. The pattern can be seen with near drowning or cardiac arrest with resuscitation.

Hypoxic-ischemic encephalopathy in infants

The pattern of brain injury is dependent upon the degree of brain maturation and the severity of ischemia. The most sensitive and specific imaging technique is MRI.

The watershed zones in the premature infant (<36 weeks) differ from those in the full-term infant (>36 weeks). During the first two trimesters the primary blood supply arises from peripheral blood vessels that flow centrally toward the ventricles (ventriculopetal flow), resulting in the watershed zones being located in the periventricular regions. In the full-term infant ventriculofugal blood flow develops from the intraventricular and periventricular regions in addition to the already developed blood supply extending centrally from the surface of the brain. As a result the watershed zones move more peripherally to the parasagittal intervascular watershed regions between the anterior cerebral artery and middle cerebral artery, and the middle cerebral artery and posterior cerebral artery vascular territories.

There are four patterns of hypoxic-ischemic encephalopathy of infants.

1. In mild to moderate ischemia in preterm infants, you most often see periventricular WM injury resulting in periventricular leukomalacia. Imaging findings include loss of the WM volume with increased T2/FLAIR signal in the periventricular regions, particularly lateral to the trigones of the lateral ventricles. The ventricles are enlarged and demonstrate an irregular, wavy contour. Associated thinning of the corpus callosum (most commonly the posterior body and splenium) is seen secondary to the WM volume loss. Differentiating so-called terminal zones of myelination, which demonstrate increased T2/FLAIR signal in the peritrigonal regions, may be confusing. Look for a normal layer of myelinated WM between the ventricular margin and the high T2 signal, absence of ventricular enlargement, and a normal volume of the corpus callosum in these terminal zones.

2. In severe ischemia in preterm infants, the most metabolically active regions are most susceptible to injury, which include the amygdala, basal ganglia, thalami, brainstem, and cerebellum.

3. Mild to moderate ischemic injury in full-term infants results in injury to the parasagittal watershed zones between the anterior and middle cerebral arteries and between the middle and posterior cerebral arteries. This involves both the cortex and subcortical WM regions.

4. Severe ischemia in full-term infants involves the most metabolically active regions at this stage in development, which include the lateral thalami, posterior putamen, hippocampi, brainstem, corticospinal tracts, and the sensorimotor cortex.

Non-atherosclerotic vasculopathies/ vasculitis/CADASIL

Non-atherosclerotic vasculopathy

This refers to a variety of disorders unrelated to atherosclerosis or vasculitis that can result in cerebral infarction. Some entities included in this category are connective tissue disorders such as neurofibromatosis (mesodermal dysplasia), sickle cell disease, moyamoya disease, anticardiolipin antibody syndrome, radiation, and fibromuscular dysplasia.

Vasculitis

This is an infectious/inflammatory process involving the vascular wall that can result in vascular stenosis or occlusion with subsequent cerebral infarction and/or hemorrhage. It can be a process primarily involving the CNS or be part of a more systemic process. Etiologies include: (1) primary angiitis of the CNS; (2) CNS angiitis secondary to contiguous infection, such as meningitis (bacterial, tuberculous, fungal, or syphilitic), septic embolic disease, and sarcoid; (3) primary systemic angiitis with CNS involvement, such as polyarteritis nodosa, temporal arteritis, Takayasu's arteritis, and Wegener's granulomatosis; and (4) CNS angiitis secondary to systemic disease, such as rheumatoid disease, SLE, or Lyme disease. Cross-sectional imaging studies can show areas of ischemic change within the WM, or if medium and large vessel involvement occurs both GM and WM infarction. Hemorrhage may also result from vasculitic changes. Angiographic imaging studies in vasculitis may show multiple, segmental areas of vessel narrowing, sometimes alternating with areas of vessel dilatation resulting in a beaded appearance; focal areas of vascular occlusion may also be evident. Be aware that this appearance, while suggestive of vasculitis, is not specific. Severe atherosclerotic vascular disease can mimic this appearance at times.

Moyamoya ("puff-of-smoke") disease

This is a non-atherosclerotic vasculopathy of unknown etiology, first described by and most common in the Japanese, but now known to occur in other populations including those in the United States. It is characterized by progressive stenosis, leading to occlusion of the supraclinoid internal carotid artery and progressing to involve the adjacent M1 and A1 segments of the middle and anterior cerebral arteries. This leads to enlargement of the basal perforating arteries, which on angiography gives a puff-of-smoke appearance. It can be idiopathic or associated with sickle cell disease (or other hematologic disorders), congenital syndromes, and radiation. Severe atherosclerotic disease may mimic its appearance. It is usually bilateral, associated with transdural collateral vessels, more often involves children than adults, and may present with stroke or TIA and/or hemorrhage.

Cerebral autosomal dominant arteriopathy with subcortical infarcts and leukoencephalopathy

This is a familial small vessel arteriopathy secondary to a mutation in the Notch3 gene on chromosome 19, leading to dementia in the 30–60 year-old range in patients without known risk factors for cerebrovascular disease. Imaging studies reveal extensive and symmetric increased T2 signal in the cerebral WM including the external capsules. Increased T2 signal in the anterior temporal lobe WM is highly sensitive and specific for CADASIL. Clinically, patients present with migraine attacks and transient ischemic attacks (TIAs), which lead to dementia later in the course of the disease.

Cortical venous/dural sinus thrombosis

The diagnosis of cortical/venous sinus thrombosis is often underdiagnosed because of nonspecific clinical and imaging findings. Imaging studies may show areas of parenchymal edema with or without hemorrhage. Venous infarcts are commonly hemorrhagic. Superficial cortical venous thrombosis/dural sinus thrombosis may result in parasagittal, flame-shaped regions of hemorrhage in the subcortical areas. Thrombosis of the deep venous system involving the internal cerebral veins may result in bilateral thalamic edema. Cortical venous thrombosis involving the vein of Labbé often results in venous infarction of the temporal lobe, which initially may be non-hemorrhagic. On non-contrast CT scans, look for hyperdensity of the involved dural venous sinus or cortical vein. The hyperdensity has been referred to as the delta sign or cord sign. Following contrast there is enhancement of the dural surfaces surrounding the thrombosed sinus, giving the open delta sign. On post-contrast images an increased number of enhancing vascular channels, some of which extend through the deep WM (dilated medullary veins), may be seen representing venous collaterals. CT venography and MR venography are easily performed studies providing direct imaging of the venous structures.

Vasospasm

Cerebral vasospasm is often a consequence of aneurysmal subarachnoid hemorrhage. Angiographic vasospasm occurs in at least two-thirds of patients following a subarachnoid bleed, but only about one-third of patients with vasospasm develop clinically significant deficits related to the spasm. If left untreated, vasospasm may lead to cerebral infarction and even death. Management of aneurysmal cerebral vasospasm includes medical management with triple H-therapy, which includes hypertension, hemodilution, and hypervolemia. Patients who do not respond to medical therapy may require endovascular treatment, which can include selective intra-arterial infusion of a vasodilator such as papaverine, or balloon angioplasty. Treatment with papaverine is usually transient and can have deleterious effects such as elevation of ICP and seizures. Vessel dilatation from angioplasty has a lasting effect but can only be used in the proximal vessels of the Circle of Willis. Transcranial Doppler ultrasound is often used to evaluate vasospasm indirectly by assessing cerebral blood flow velocities. As vessels become narrowed, the velocities rise. MR and CT perfusion studies can be used in the assessment of cerebral vasospasm.

Vascular dissection

Vascular dissection can involve the internal carotid or vertebral arteries. A variety of etiologies can result in dissection such as trauma, connective tissue disorders, and underlying vasculopathy such as fibromuscular dysplasia as well as atherosclerosis. Extracranial dissections of the internal carotid artery generally begin above the common carotid bifurcation and often

extend to the skull base, although they may extend into the carotid canal. This can result in narrowing or occlusion of the internal carotid artery. You often see a tapered appearance to the internal carotid artery as it ascends into the dissection on MRA or catheter angiography. Vertebral artery dissections can involve both its extracranial and intracranial segments. Involvement of the intracranial segment often results in aneurysmal dilatation of the vessel and is associated with subarachnoid hemorrhage. There may also be a steno-occlusive pattern of dissection, which can involve all four segments of the vertebral artery. On MRI, look for an intramural hematoma with an eccentric crescent of increased T1 signal (methemoglobin) within the arterial wall, which is best seen on fat suppressed T1 images.

Fibromuscular dysplasia

There are three forms of FMD:

1. Medial FMD – most common, accounting for about 90%–95% of cases. Rings of fibrous proliferation and smooth muscle hyperplasia occur, with destruction of the internal elastic lamina producing the classic string-of-beads appearance. The areas of dilatation are wider than the normal lumen.
2. Intimal FMD – accounts for about 5% of cases. Intimal thickening and destruction of the internal elastic lamina occurs and results in a web-like linear defect in the vessel lumen.
3. Adventitial FMD – the least common form. Fibrosis of adventitia and periarterial tissue occurs, resulting in long tubular narrowing of the vessel lumen.

Arteries involved in FMD can develop dissections, aneurysms, and AVFs. Patients may present with TIAs secondary to emboli or vascular narrowing. The internal carotid arteries are most often involved (95%), usually extracranially; there is a 60%–85% bilateral involvement, affecting the ICA above the bifurcation, which generally does not extend into the carotid canal. It may also involve the vertebral arteries (12%–43%), and in these cases there is usually evidence of involvement of the carotid arteries. FMD of the vertebral arteries is usually seen at the C2 vertebral level and in most cases does not extend intracranially. FMD is associated with an increased incidence of intracranial saccular aneurysms.

Vascular injury

Injury to the cervical and intracranial vessels can be a result of direct/penetrating injuries including gunshot or stabbing types of wounds or from blunt trauma. Look for dissection/intimal flaps, focal vessel cutoffs, vascular wall injury with adjacent hematoma/pseudoaneurysm, active extravasation if contrast is given in the presence of vessel wall disruption, as well as vascular spasm.

Posterior reversible encephalopathy, hypertensive encephalopathy

These conditions include a loss of vascular autoregulation associated with numerous clinical entities with the common denominator being the presence of hypertension. This results in a disturbance of the blood brain barrier with vasogenic edema. The posterior circulation (vertebrobasilar circulation) has less capacity for autoregulation and is therefore more susceptible. Associated with uncontrolled hypertension, pre-eclampsia/eclampsia, renal disease, lupus, and certain drug toxicities including cyclosporine. Most often they show patchy, cortical and subcortical hypodensity (CT), and T2 hyperintensity (MR) in the parietal and occipital lobes. This is usually bilateral and often symmetric. Diffusion weighted images are usually normal. You may see variable, patchy enhancement. Most cases resolve with normalization of blood pressure.

Neurodegenerative disorders (specific locations)

Alzheimer's dementia (AD) (see Figure 6.261, page 242)

Parkinson's disease

Parkinson plus disorders (see Figures 6.262a,b for multisystem atrophy, page 242)

Dementia with Lewy bodies (DLB)

Wernicke–Korsakoff syndrome (see Figure 6.263, page 243)

Frontotemporal dementia (see Figure 6.264, page 243)

Creutzfeld-Jakob disease (see Figures 6.164, 6.265, pages 177, 244)

Amyotrophic lateral sclerosis (ALS) (see Figure 6.266, page 244–245)

Alzheimer's dementia

This progressive neurodegenerative disease is characterized by the deposition of amyloid and tau protein, associated with the APOE-4 allele on chromosome 19. APOE-4 will increase the susceptibility of patients who have head trauma to develop AD. This is the most common form of dementia, accounting for 50%–56% of cases in clinical studies and at autopsy. It increases with age, and leads to death in three to nine years after diagnosis. There is generalized CNS atrophy, which is accentuated in the medial temporal lobes (hippocampal formations) and in the parietal lobes. The main role of imaging is to exclude treatable causes of dementia and, in the early stages, for possible new therapies that may develop. At autopsy you see neurofibrillary tangles and senile plaques. AD is associated with Down syndrome; the majority of patients with Down syndrome will develop AD by the age of 40 years.

Parkinson's disease

This common disorder affects 1% of the population over 50 years old. It is an extrapyramidal disorder secondary to the loss of dopaminergic cells in the pars compacta of the substantia nigra, locus ceruleus, and dorsal vagal nucleus. Note a decreased width of the pars compacta (the area of relative increased signal intensity between the more hypointense pars reticulata and red nucleus) on T2WI, with blurring of the margins between the hypointense red nuclei and the pars reticulata of the substantia nigra. Increased iron accumulation in the putamen, resulting in hypointensity on T2WI in the putamen is seen in Parkinson plus disorders, but not with idiopathic levo-dopa responsive Parkinson's disease. See nonspecific generalized cortical atrophy and ventricular enlargement.

Parkinson plus disorders

This is a group of heterogeneous degenerative neurological disorders that share but have additional clinical manifestations as PD, are not responsive to treatment with L-dopa, and have a poor outcome. This group includes progressive supranuclear palsy (Steele–Richardson–Olszewski syndrome or PSP), and multisystem atrophy (MSA).

PSP features include atrophy of the dorsal midbrain/tectum, especially the superior colliculi, with enlargement of the aqueduct of Sylvius and increased T2 signal in the periaqueductal region. Clinical features are Parkinsonian features, with supranuclear ophthalmoplegia, pseudobulbar palsy, and dementia.

MSA is a neurodegenerative disorder with cerebellar, pyramidal, extrapyramidal, and autonomic dysfunction. MSA includes Shy–Drager syndrome when autonomic dysfunction predominates, striatonigral degeneration when Parkinsonian features predominate, and olivopontocerebellar atrophy when cerebellar ataxia predominates in the clinical picture. MRI features in MSA overlap, but in olivopontocerebellar atrophy note the cruciform T2 hyperintensity in the pons (hot-cross-bun sign) and brainstem/cerebellar atrophy; in striatonigral degeneration you can see hypointensity in the dorsolateral putamen owing to increased iron deposition.

Dementia with Lewy bodies

This is one of the most frequent types of progressive dementia characterized by progressive cognitive decline, and is associated with the following three features: (1) fluctuations in alertness and attention, (2) visual hallucinations, and (3) Parkinsonian motor symptoms. This is caused by the accumulation of Lewy bodies (alpha-synuclein protein within the nuclei of neurons) in parts of the brain that are involved with motor control and memory. This protein is also found in patients with Alzheimer's disease, PD, and MSA. The average survival after the time of diagnosis is approximately 8 years, similar to Alzheimer's disease. The description of an imaging pattern suggestive of DLB versus Alzheimer's disease includes relatively focused atrophy of the midbrain, hypothalamus, and substantia innominata, with relative sparing of the hippocampus and temporoparietal cortex.

Wernicke–Korsakoff syndrome

This syndrome is characterized by the clinical triad of ophthalmoplegia, ataxia, and confusion, all being present only in 10%–33% of cases. It is secondary to thiamine deficiency, and is a medical emergency treated by thiamine administration. Imaging may show increased T2 signal in the para-third ventricular/medial thalami, floor of the third and fourth ventricles, periaqueductal GM, and mammillary bodies. You may also see atrophy of the mammillary bodies. Contrast enhancement around the third ventricle, aqueduct, and in the mammillary bodies may be evident. Changes

may reverse with treatment. In the chronic phase, you can see enlargement of the third ventricle and mammillary body atrophy.

Frontotemporal dementia

This neurodegenerative process is characterized by focal/regional atrophy involving the frontal and temporal lobes. It is usually asymmetric. Pick's disease, for example, is a type of frontotemporal dementia with Pick bodies seen on pathology. Different varieties of frontotemporal dementia:

1. Frontal variant – characterized by personality and behavior changes with compulsions a prominent feature. Imaging studies show frontal cortical atrophy, increased T2 signal in frontal WM and enlargement of frontal horns.
2. Temporal variant – subtypes, depending on specific location, are in the right or left hemisphere with localization in the temporal lobe.

Left temporal lobe involvement

Semantic dementia involves the loss of long-term memory, language comprehension, and object recognition. Imaging shows atrophy of the anterior temporal lobes, particularly anterolaterally.

Primary progressive aphasia involves preservation of verbal comprehension but disruption of conversational speech and speech fluency. It may progress to mutism. Imaging shows the most severe atrophy in the anterior portion of the superior temporal gyrus/peri-Sylvian region (with enlargement of the Sylvian fissure).

Right temporal lobe involvement

This is characterized by prominent emotional and behavioral changes, and progressive prosopagnosia, which is the progressive and selective inability to recognize and identify faces of familiar people. Imaging shows atrophy in the anterior right temporal lobe, which most severely involves the fusiform (occipital temporal) gyrus.

Creutzfeld–Jakob disease

This is rare with a worldwide prevalence of one person in every million and an annual incidence of one person in two million. It is the most common form of human prion disease and primarily affects GM. About 90% of cases consist of the sporadic form where there is no known source or origin of infection (sCJD). Less common is the familial form of CJD, iatrogenic CJD, the new variant form (vCJD). In vCJD you see bilateral increased T2/FLAIR signal in the posterior and medial thalamic regions, referred to as the pulvinar sign, but this is not specific for vCJD and is also seen in the sporadic form. Most patients die within one year of onset of the disease. Imaging findings in CJD include abnormal increased T2/FLAIR signal in cortical GM and in the basal ganglia, and rapidly progressive atrophy. In one study, cortical GM and deep GM was involved in about 68%, the cortex alone in approximately 24%, and deep GM alone in 5% of cases. FLAIR and DWI appear to be the most sensitive and specific for diagnosing this disorder.

Amyotrophic lateral sclerosis

ALS is the most common type of motor neuron disease and the diagnosis is based upon clinical and EMG criteria, with imaging utilized to exclude other causes such as degenerative cervical canal stenosis, Chiari malformations, or MS. The etiology is unknown and it results in a slowly progressive upper and lower motor neuron degeneration. Typical findings on MRI are increased T2 and FLAIR (more sensitive) signal within the corticospinal tracts, extending from the corona radiata through the posterior limbs of the internal capsule into the ventral brainstem.

Miscellaneous disorders of the brain

Hypertrophic olivary degeneration (see Figures 6.267, 6.268, pages 245, 246)
Wallerian degeneration (see Figure 6.269, page 246)
Mesial temporal sclerosis (see Figures 6.270, 6.271, pages 247, 248)
Intracranial hypotension (see Figure 6.272, page 248)

Hypertrophic olivary degeneration

This occurs secondary to a lesion (such as infarction or hemorrhage) involving the Guillain–Mollaret triangle, which includes the inferior olivary nucleus, contralateral cerebellar dentate nucleus, ipsilateral red nucleus, and connecting tracts. It is associated with palatal myoclonus. MRI may show increased T2 signal and enlargement of the inferior olivary nucleus. When you see this combination of findings, look for a lesion involving the Guillain–Mollaret triangle.

Wallerian degeneration (distal axonal degeneration)

Anterograde degeneration of the axons occurs and is secondary to injury/lesion involving cortical/subcortical regions of the ipsilateral cerebral hemisphere. Look for increased T2 signal extending along the expected course of the corticospinal tracts (within the internal capsule and brainstem) and atrophy of the ipsilateral ventral brainstem. This can occur secondary to supratentorial infarct, hemorrhage, or other injury.

Mesial temporal sclerosis (hippocampal sclerosis)

This is the most common cause of partial complex epilepsy. It is bilateral in about 10%–15% of patients, and is characterized by neuronal loss and gliosis, which is most severe in the CA1 portion of cornu ammonis (part of the hippocampus), also referred to as Sommer's sector (vulnerable sector), followed by similar changes in CA3 and the hilus of the dentate gyrus (CA4), with relative sparing of CA2. The most common findings in this entity are hippocampal atrophy seen in 90%–95%, increased T2 signal in 80%–85%, and loss of internal architecture in 60%–95% of cases. Secondary findings that may be seen are atrophy of the ipsilateral fornix and mamillary body, and dilatation of the ipsilateral temporal horn. Dual pathology that represents the coexistence of another etiology for seizures occurs in 8%–22% of patients and is most commonly cortical dysgenesis.

Intracranial hypotension

This clinical syndrome occurs in patients following postoperative, traumatic, or spontaneous dural tears, resulting in postural headaches and variable additional symptoms including blurred vision, diplopia, photophobia, nausea, vomiting, dizziness, hearing impairment, and neck pain. Clinical and imaging findings are a result of low CSF pressure and follow the Monro–Kellie doctrine, which states an inverse relationship between CSF volume and intracranial blood volume. Imaging studies reveal descent of the brain in the intracranial compartment, in addition to dural thickening and enhancement and enlargement of the pituitary gland secondary to increased intracranial venous volume. The dural sinuses become distended and there may be associated subdural fluid collections.

Within the spinal canal you may also find engorgement of epidural veins and extradural fluid collections.

Hydrocephalus (see Figures 6.273–278, pages 249–252)

Obstructive

Intraventricular (non-communicating)

1. Aqueductal stenosis – benign origin such as web, adhesion, inflammatory debris, or blood, or malignant from neoplasm. Look for enlargement of the third and lateral ventricles with a normal to small fourth ventricle.
2. Intraventricular mass – benign or malignant.
3. Outlet obstruction of the fourth ventricle – can mimic communicating hydrocephalus. The dilated inferior fourth ventricle may herniate (pulsion type diverticulum) through the foramen of Luschka into the low CP angle cisterns.

Extraventricular (communicating)

1. Normal pressure hydrocephalus is a form of communicating hydrocephalus. The characteristic clinical triad (Hakim–Adams triad) is gait apraxia, urinary incontinence, and dementia.
2. Three of the most common etiologies for communicating hydrocephalus are blood (trauma, SAH), inflammatory exudate (meningitis), and tumor (carcinomatous meningitis). The underlying common origin is dysfunction of the arachnoid granulations with impaired resorption of CSF.
3. Look for enlargement of the entire ventricular system but be aware that the fourth ventricle is normal in size in about 25%–30% of cases.
4. In equivocal cases consider provocative removal of about 20–30 mL of CSF via lumbar puncture and see if the patient's symptoms such as gait apraxia transiently improve. Also consider further evaluation with a nuclear medicine cisternogram (Indium-111 DTPA) via lumbar puncture and look for characteristic findings, which include early ventricular reflux with persistent ventricular activity over 24–48 hours and persistent activity over the convexities over the same period without clearing.

Non-obstructive

This shows an increased production of CSF such as seen in choroid plexus papillomas (carcinoma).

Chapter

4 Differential diagnosis by lesion location – refer to their discussions in Chapter 3

Posterior fossa neoplasms in the child

Fourth ventricle

Medulloblastoma (midline, fourth ventricle roof, or vermis)

Ependymoma (usually arises from the ventral aspect of the fourth ventricle/floor)

Choroid plexus papilloma (ca) – in children, more frequently supratentorial, more in the atria of the lateral ventricles but may be in the fourth ventricle

Cerebellum

Astrocytoma, with juvenile pilocytic astrocytoma (JPA) #1 – JPA comprises about a quarter to a third of posterior fossa masses in children and is a close second to medulloblastoma

Atypical teratoid/rhaboid tumor (AT/RT) – very rare

Lhermitte-Duclos disease (dysplastic gangliocytoma) – usually asymptomatic in early life and becomes clinically apparent in the third and fourth decades

Brainstem

Brainstem glioma

Posterior fossa mass-like lesions in the child

Intra-axial

Demyelinating – tumefactive MS – rare in the child

Infection – viral (rhomboencephalitis), granulomatous, i.e. TB, bacterial (abscess), parasitic (cysticercosis)

Hematoma

Vascular malformation

Infarction (stroke)

Extra-axial

Dandy Walker complex

Mega cistern magna

Epidermoid cyst/dermoid cyst

Arachnoid cyst

Aneurysm, vascular malformation

Subdural/epidural hematoma

Posterior fossa neoplasms in the adult

Intra-axial

Metastasis – most common intra-axial tumor in the adult posterior fossa (PF)

Hemangioblastoma – second most common intra-axial PF mass and most common primary intra-axial PF mass in the adult

Astrocytoma

Desmoplastic medulloblastoma – adolescents and young adults, lateral cerebellum

Lhermitte disease (dysplastic gangliocytoma)

Posterior fossa intra-axial mass-like lesions in the adult

Demyelinating – tumefactive MS

Infection – viral (rhomboencephalitis), PML, granulomatous, i.e. TB, bacterial (abscess), parasitic (cysticercosis)

Hematoma

Vascular malformation

Infarction (stroke)

Most common extra-axial cerebellopontine angle mass lesions – most in adults

Vestibular schwannoma – about 80%

Meningioma – about 10%

Epidermoid inclusion cyst

Arachnoid cyst

Vascular lesion, i.e. dolichoectasia of vertebral basilar system, AVM, aneurysm

Other extra-axial posterior fossa masses – vast majority in adults

Chordoma

Chondrosarcoma

Cranial nerve schwannomas (other than vestibular schwannoma)

Intracranial extension of skull base paragangliomas (glomus tumors)

Endolymphatic sac tumors

Metastasis – hematogenous or direct spread (such as nasopharyngeal carcinoma)

Plasmacytoma

Dural-based neoplasms (other than meningioma) – hemangiopericytoma, lymphoma, leukemic infiltrates (chloroma in AML), dural metastasis (particularly breast and prostate)

Differential diagnosis of cerebellar atrophy

Drugs: alcohol (superior vermian most severe)

Dilantin (cerebellar hemispheres)

Chemotherapy

Vascular ischemic disease (infarction)

Paraneoplastic syndrome – ovary, lung, breast, lymphoma

Autoimmune cerebellar ataxia and atrophy – seen in hyperthyroidism, diabetes

Olivopontocerebellar atrophy (OPCA)

Trauma

Intraventricular masses (in all age groups)

Choroid plexus papilloma – most often found in the atrium of the lateral ventricles in children and in the fourth ventricle in adults

Medulloblastoma – from the roof of the fourth ventricle or vermis in children

Ependymoma – most often arises from the floor of the fourth ventricle in children, or less commonly supratentorially, usually in a periventricular (not intraventricular) location in adults

Subependymoma – more often in adults, seen in the inferior fourth ventricle or in the third and lateral ventricle attached to septum pellucidum or the lateral ventricular wall

Astrocytoma – adults and children. Giant cell astrocytomas in particular are seen in patients with tuberous sclerosis

Meningioma – most common in the atrium of the lateral ventricle in adults

Colloid cyst (mass-like benign cyst, not neoplastic) – virtually always located in the anterior-superior third ventricular region. Most often found in early middle age, rarely in children

Metastasis – hematogenous seeding of the choroid plexus (no blood brain barrier) or subependymal/intraventricular spread of a malignant brain tumor, i.e. GBM, medulloblastoma, ependymoma, choroid plexus carcinoma

Lymphoma – can infiltrate the periventricular/subependymal regions and extend into the ventricular system in addition to an extension from infiltration of the corpus callosum and septum pellucidum. More often seen in adults

Cysticercosis (mass-like) – may be freely mobile or attached to the margins of the ventricular walls or choroid plexus. Most often found in adults

Neoplastic involvement of clivus

Chordoma

Chondrosarcoma

Metastasis/myeloma

Meningioma

Hemangiopericytoma

Lymphoma

Invasion from adjacent malignancies

    Nasopharyngeal

    Pituitary mass

    Craniopharyngioma

Pineal region masses

Tumors of pineal cell origin (15%–30%)

    Pineocytoma

    Pineoblastoma

Germ cell tumors (60%)

    Germinoma (same as seminoma) -most common (About 40%–50%)

    Teratoma

    Embryonal cell, choriocarcinoma and yolk sac tumor

Glioma (12%), i.e. tectal

Meningioma

Metastasis

Vein of Galen malformation

Miscellaneous – benign pineal cysts, arachnoid cysts, lipoma, epidermoid/dermoid

Intrasellar lesions

Pituitary adenoma – micro and macro from the anterior lobe – most common

Pituicytoma – posterior lobe

Pituitary carcinoma

Pituitary abscess

Pituitary apoplexy

Craniopharyngioma

Rathke's cleft cysts

Metastatic disease

Sarcoid

Lymphocytic adenohypophysitis

Arachnoid cyst/epidermoid

Extension into the sella from adjacent lesions, i.e. aneurysm, meningioma, suprasellar tumors, etc.

Parasellar lesions

Meningioma

Lateral growth of a pituitary macroadenoma

Aneurysm

Lymphoma

Sarcoid

Arachnoid cyst

Epidermoid/dermoid

Medial temporal lobe lesion

Nerve sheath tumor

Tolasa–Hunt syndrome

Suprasellar lesions – SATCHMOE

Suprasellar pituitary adenoma

Sarcoid

Aneurysm

Arachnoid cyst

Teratoma/germ cell tumor

TB

Craniopharyngioma

Cysticercosis

Hypothalamic glioma/hamartoma

Histiocytosis

Hypophysitis (lymphocytic adenohypophysitis)

Meningioma

Metastasis

Optico-chiasmatic tumor

Epidermoid/dermoid

Ectopic neurohypophysis

Lesions of the infindibulum (pituitary stalk)

Pituitary adenoma along the stalk

Pituicytoma

Lymphocytic adenohypophysitis

Ectopic neurohypophysis

Metastasis

Sarcoid/TB

Histiocytosis

Germinoma

Intracranial extra-axial tumors

Meningioma

Hemangiopericytoma

Lymphomatous/leukemic infiltration of the meninges

Carcinomatous meningitis

Cranial nerve schwannomas

Extension from a calvarial or skull base lesion

Additional extra-axial lesions

Arachnoid cyst

Vascular – dolichoectasia, aneurysm, AVM

SAH, subdural/epidural hematoma

Lepto/pachymeningitis

Subdural/epidural empyema

Sarcoid – nodular, mass-like thickening of the dura

Extramedullary hematopoesis

Supratentorial tumors

Glioma (30%–40%)

> GBM (grade IV astrocytoma) – most common primary CNS neoplasm; 40% of all primary brain tumors considering all ages

> Astrocytomas – grade I (localized), grade II (low-grade infiltrative), grade III (anaplastic)

> Oligodendroglioma

> Ependymoma

> Choroid plexus papilloma

Metastasis (20%–30%) – 40% are solitary; usually at GM–WM junction

Meningioma (16%)

Pineal gland tumors

Pituitary/sella masses

Lymphoma

Tumors associated with chronic seizures/often intracortical

Ganglioglioma
Pleomorphic xanthoastrocytoma (PXA)
Dysembryoplastic neuroepithelial tumor (DNET)
Oligodendroglioma

White matter lesions

Neoplasm
Multiple sclerosis
Acute disseminated encephalomyelitis (ADEM) – WM and GM
Congenital dysmyelinating disorders
  Metachromatic leukodystrophy
  Adrenoleukodystrophy
  Pelizeus–Merzbacher
  Alexander disease
  Canavan's disease
  Vanishing WM disease
Microvascular ischemic disease
  Atrophic demyelination
  Diabetes, hypertension
Toxic effects
  Marchiafava–Bignami disease – toxic demyelination of corpus callosum
  Radiation/chemotherapy effects
Trauma
Infection/inflammatory – viral encephalitis, HIV, PML, Lyme, SLE, sarcoid
Vasculitis
Chronic migraines
Metabolic

Lesions of the corpus callosum

Demyelinating
  MS/ADEM
  Marchiafava–Bignami – owing to chronic and massive alcohol use. Involves the central layers with sparing of dorsal and ventral layers (sandwich sign). Acute form found more often in the genu and splenium, chronic form more common in the body. It often enhances
  PML
Tumors
  High-grade glioma, i.e. GBM
  Lymphoma
Drugs
  Chemotherapy
  Anti-epileptic medication – found more often in the splenium
Post-radiation therapy – seen more commonly in the splenium
Infarction
  Often occurs in association with involvement of the cingulate gyrus, indicating infarction of a larger territory
Trauma
Malnutrition
Lipomas
AVMs

Foramen magnum lesions
Extra-axial

Meningioma/hemangiopericytoma
Paraganglioma
Chordoma (more medial)/chondrosarcoma (more lateral)
Metastasis/myeloma (plasmacytoma)
Nasopharyngeal cancer – direct extension
Nerve sheath tumor
Dural/leptomeningeal disease
  Leptomeningeal – infection
  Dural – tumor, i.e. metastasis, lymphoma, leukemia
Aneurysm/AVM/dolichoectasia
Basilar invagination

Intra-axial (beneath the pia)

Astrocytoma
Ependymoma
Hemangioblastoma
Metastatic disease
Tonsillar herniation

5 Morphologic characterization of lesion appearance

Enhancement patterns

Intra-axial tumors

Primary cerebral neoplasms – variable patterns that include ring, nodular, or irregular enhancement. These are generally thicker and more nodular than inflammatory/abscess cavities

Metastatic tumors to the brain – regular or irregular peripheral ring (thick or thin) and/or solid nodular enhancement

Lymphoma – more often ring-like enhancement in immunosuppressed and solid enhancement in immunocompetent patients

Intra-axial infectious/inflammatory lesions

Bacterial abscess

    Smooth and regular ring

    Clue – medial side is usually thinner with a thicker cortical side owing to greater vascularity laterally. This thinning of the medial wall can lead to intraventricular rupture of the abscess

Parasitic infection – cysticercosis, toxoplasmosis. It usually shows peripheral ring enhancement but may be solid

Granuloma, i.e. TB, sarcoid – peripheral ring enhancement and/or solid

MS/ADEM – may enhance in the acute phase, which may be peripheral, ring-like, and/or solid nodular

Vascular

Resolving hematoma – about 10 days to 3 weeks following hemorrhage. It usually shows ring enhancement and surrounding hypodensity on CT imaging or decreased T1/increased T2 signal on MRI, representing edema

Patent aneurysm/AVM – nodular solid, tubular/serpiginous

Thrombosed aneurysm or AVM – peripheral ring/curvilinear enhancement

Subacute infarct – if small and deep, it may appear solid but subacute cortical/subcortical infarcts usually show gyriform enhancement

Miscellaneous

Radiation necrosis – peripheral ring enhancement, often thick and nodular – it may mimic active tumor. There is a delayed effect of radiation occurring after 6 months to 3 years

Post-surgical cavities – peripheral ring enhancement

Multiple enhancing lesions

Metastatic lesions (hematogenous) – peripheral, near GM–WM junction more often than central

Lymphoma – more often multiple in immunosuppressed patients in the basal ganglia and other deep cerebral nuclei, and corpus callosum where enhancement is more often peripheral, ring, or heterogeneous/complex pattern

Multiple meningiomas

Multicentric glioma

Infectious

    Pyogenic, granulomatous, parasitic, fungal

Demyelinating – indicates active inflammation/demyelination – in WM more than GM

Septic emboli – consider endocarditis

Multiple subacute infarcts

Multiple vascular malformations

Syndromes

    NF-1 and NF-2

    Von Hippel Lindau

    Tuberous sclerosis

Gyral enhancement

Subacute infarct – Rule of 3's. It begins at around day 3 after the infarct, peaks at 3 weeks, and is generally gone by 3 months.

Cerebritis/encephalitis
Leptomeningitis
Seizures – in peri-ictal periods
Carcinomatous meningitis
Lymphomatous meningitis
AVM – enlarged vessels

Meningeal enhancement

Normal postoperative
TB, sarcoid (more basilar), pyogenic infection
    (more often along brain convexity)
Fungal/parasitic infection
Carcinomatous meningitis
Lymphomatous meningitis
Idiopathic hypertrophic pachymeningitis

Ependymal/subependymal enhancement

Ventriculitis
Lymphoma
CSF spread of CNS malignancy – i.e.
    medulloblastoma, GBM, choroid plexus
    carcinoma
Metastases from non-CNS malignancy
Tuberous sclerosis

Hyperdense lesions on non-contrast computed tomography

Acute/subacute hemorrhage
Hemorrhagic neoplasms – metastases from primary
    renal, breast, lung, and thyroid lesions,
    choriocarcinoma, and melanoma
Colloid cyst
Hypercellular neoplasms
    Lymphoma
    High-grade glioma
    Germinoma
    PNET – including medulloblastoma
    Ependymoma
    Metastatic small round blue cell tumors
Meningioma
Calcified/ossified tumors (rare) – i.e. metastatic
    mucinous adenocarcinoma, osteogenic sarcoma
Thrombosed vessels
    Aneurysms
    Dural sinus/cortical vein thrombosis

Radiopaque foreign objects
    Aneurysm clips or other surgical metallic materials
    Pantopaque – retained from remote myelogram

Hyperintense lesions on non-contrast T1 weighted magnetic resonance images

Hemorrhage (subacute – methehemoglobin)
Cortical laminar necrosis – in subacute stages,
owing to deposition of lipid-laden macrophages
Non-Wilsonian chronic hepatic dysfunction –
symmetric increased signal in the globus pallidus. It
is possibly related to the deposition of paramagnetic
substances
Total parenteral nutrition (TPN) – may be from the
deposition of paramagnetic trace elements in the
basal ganglia such as manganese. Increased T1
signal can resolve with the cessation of TPN
Calcifications – usually hypointense on T1 images
but, depending on the crystalline structure, they may
show T1 shortening owing to a greater surface area
Lesions containing fat – lipoma, dermoid
Hamartomas – in NF-1. There is a greater
occurrence in the globus pallidus and internal
capsule. They usually resolve by adulthood. There is
no enhancement or mass effect
Tuberous sclerosis – subcortical WM hamartomas
in infants with immature myelin
Chorea–Ballism associated with hyperglycemia.
This is found in the putamen, caudate nucleus, or
both and may be related to the abundant
gemistocytes (swollen, reactive astrocytes) seen in
acute injury
Craniopharyngioma
Mucinous material
Lesions with hyperproteinaceous fluids
Melanoma – paramagnetic effect of melanin
Colloid cysts
Slow vascular flow

Things that are hypointense on T2 weighted magnetic resonance images

Vascular flow – TOF effect
Calcification, bone
Iron
Hemorrhage (acute owing to intracellular
    deoxyhemoglobin, early subacute because of

intracellular methemoglobin, and chronic
hemorrhage with hemosiderin deposition)
Melanin
Tumors with a high nuclear/cytoplasmic ratio such
as lymphoma, high-grade glioma, PNET tumors
Myelinated WM
Fibrosis
Fungus – calcification or manganese
Air

Lesions demonstrating diffusion restriction

Acute stroke
Pyogenic abscess/infection
Hypercellular neoplasms, i.e. lymphoma,
high-grade gliomas, malignant meningiomas
Epidermoid cysts/cholesteatoma

Traumatic brain lesions
Postoperative brain along the postsurgical bed
Creutzfeld–Jakob disease
Acute demyelinating lesions including central
pontine myelinolysis
Wernicke's encephalopathy
Early, after sustained seizure activity
PRES

Causes of increased signal in sulci on FLAIR images

Meningitis
Any cause of increased protein in CSF including
leptomeningeal spread of malignancy
Subarachnoid hemorrhage
Supplemental oxygen therapy
Drug-related propofil anesthesia

Image gallery

The order in which images are presented will mirror the order of their discussion in Chapter 3.

Congenital lesions/malformations
Disorders of organogenesis

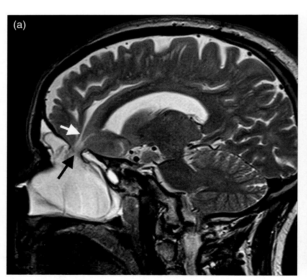 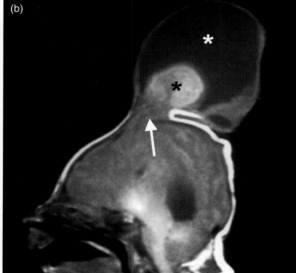

Figure 6.1 **Meningoencephaloceles:** sagittal T2WI (a) shows a large bony defect (black arrow) in the roof of the ethmoid complex (fovea ethmoidalis) with dysplastic, gliotic brain tissue herniating into the nasoethmoidal region (nasoethmoidal encephalocele). Note the tethering of the cingulate sulcus (white arrow) toward the bony defect. Sagittal T1WI (b) shows a rare parietal meningoencephalocele through a large bony defect (white arrow) in the parietal bone. Note the herniated brain tissue (black asterisk) within the CSF-filled meningocele sac (white asterisk).

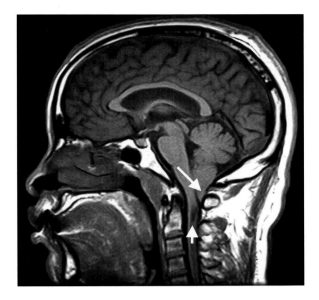

Figure 6.2 Chiari I malformation: sagittal T1WI shows inferiorly displaced, peg-like appearance of the cerebellar tonsil (long white arrow) extending to the posterior arch of C1 and a small upper cervical syrinx (short white arrow).

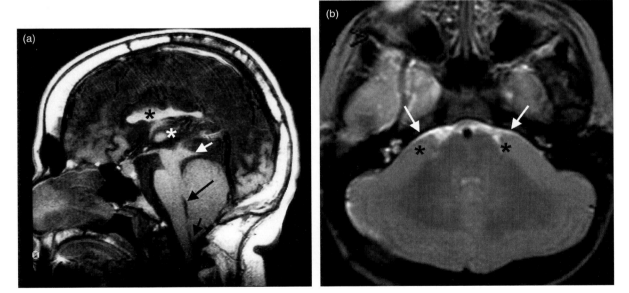

Figure 6.3 Chiari II malformation: sagittal T1WI (a) shows an inferiorly displaced cerebellar tonsil (small black arrow), elongated and inferiorly stretched small fourth ventricle (long black arrow), tectal beaking (white arrow), enlarged massa intermedia (white asterisk), and a dysplastic corpus callosum (black asterisk). Axial T2WI (b) shows scalloping of the posterior petrous ridges (arrows) and wrapping of the cerebellum (asterisks) anteriorly around the brainstem.

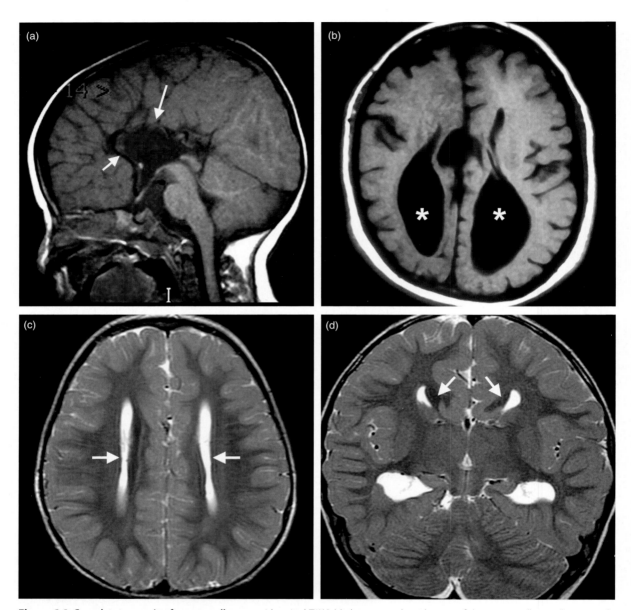

Figure 6.4 Complete agenesis of corpus callosum: mid-sagittal T1WI (a) shows complete absence of the corpus callosum (long arrow). Note the vertical ascending appearance of the A2 segment of the anterior cerebral artery (short white arrow). Axial T1WI (b) shows preferential enlargement of the atria/occipital horns of the lateral ventricles (colpocephaly) (asterisks). Axial T2WI (c) shows the typical widely separated, parallel orientation of the lateral ventricles (arrows). Coronal T2WI. (d) shows the longitudinal bundles of Probst indenting the medial margins of the lateral ventricles (arrows). *Source:* Figure 6.4c,d used with permission from Barrow Neurological Institute.

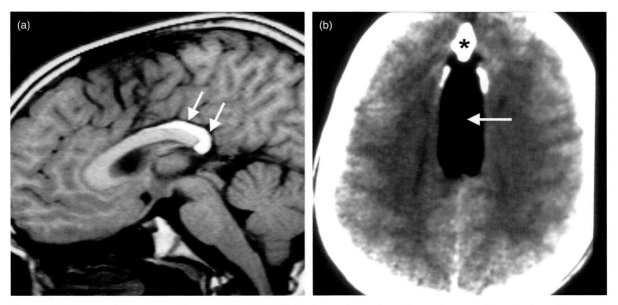

Figure 6.5 Lipomas of the corpus callosum: mid-sagittal T1WI (a) shows a lipoma (arrows) wrapping around the splenium of the corpus callosum. Axial non-contrast CT image (b) of a different patient showing a large lipoma (arrow) in the midline, dorsal to the corpus callosum, associated with calcifications (asterisk).

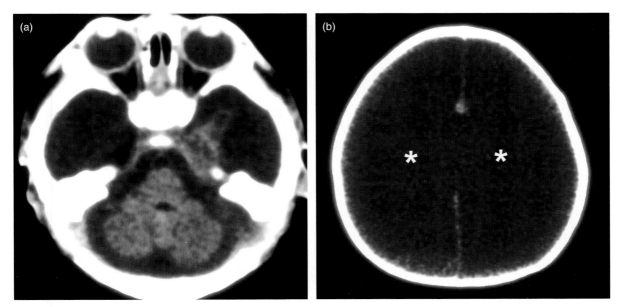

Figure 6.6 Hydranencephaly: non-contrast axial CT image (a) of an infant showing an atrophic brainstem and cerebellum with CSF density replacing the temporal lobes. (b) More superiorly it shows complete replacement of the cerebral hemispheres with CSF fluid (asterisks). Note there is no mantle of cortical tissue to suggest severe hydrocephalus.

Disorders of neuronal migration and sulcation

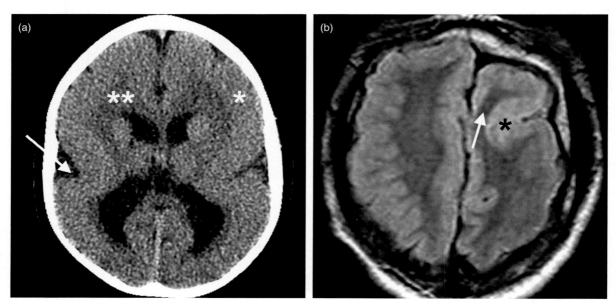

Figure 6.7 Lissencephaly and pachygyria: non-contrast axial CT image (a) shows complete lissencephaly with complete lack of sulcation, thickening of the cortical mantle (single asterisk) with associated thinning of the underlying white matter (double asterisk). Note the immature, shallow/open Sylvian fissure (arrow). Axial FLAIR image (b) shows focal thickening and lack of sulcation of the left frontal cortex/pachygyria (asterisk) with thinning of the underlying white matter (arrow).

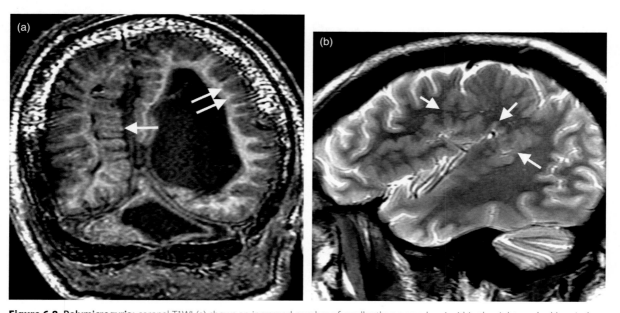

Figure 6.8 Polymicrogyria: coronal T1WI (a) shows an increased number of smaller than normal gyri within the right cerebral hemisphere (single arrow) and a more normal gyral appearance in the left cerebral hemisphere (double arrows). Sagittal T2WI (b) showing an increased number of smaller than normal cortical gyri (arrows) in the peri-Sylvian region.
Source: Figure 6.8b Used with permission from Barrow Neurological Institute.

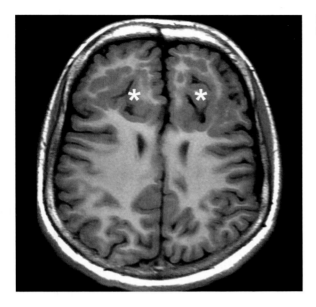

Figure 6.9 Cortical dysplasia: axial T1WI shows thickening and disorganization of the frontal lobe gyri (asterisks).

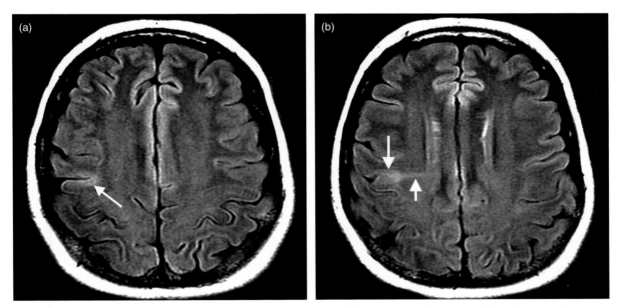

Figure 6.10 Balloon cell cortical dysplasia: axial FLAIR image (a) shows subtle increased signal intensity of the right precentral gyrus (arrow). (b) Demonstrates the comet-like linear tract of increased signal (short white arrow) extending from the cortical surface (long white arrow) toward the superior aspect of the right lateral ventricle.

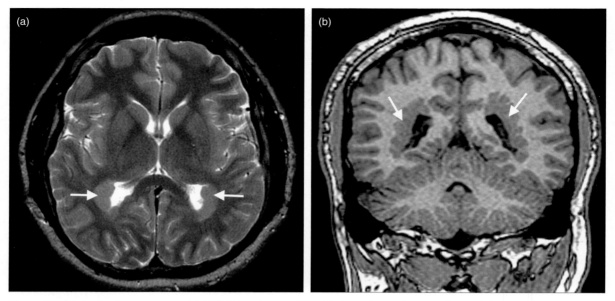

Figure 6.11 Heterotopic gray matter: axial T2WI (a) and coronal T1WI (b) show abnormal tissue with signal identical to the gray matter (arrows) surrounding the atria of both lateral ventricles.

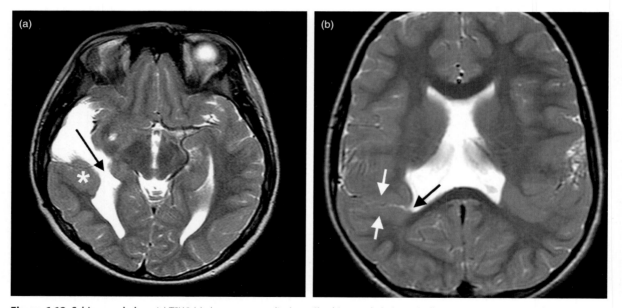

Figure 6.12 Schizencephaly: axial T2WI (a) shows an open-lip (type 2) schizencephaly (arrow), allowing communication of the subarachnoid space with the temporal horn of the right lateral ventricle. Note the thickened, dysplastic appearing gray matter (asterisk) lining the cleft. Axial T2WI (b) shows a closed-lip (type I) schizencephaly with dysplastic, thickened cortex (white arrows) lining the cleft and the pial–ependymal seam (black arrow). Also note the absence of a septum pellucidum. *Source:* Figure 6.12b used with permission from Barrow Neurological Institute.

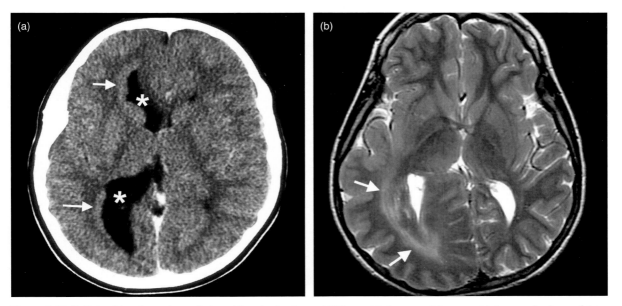

Figure 6.13 Unilateral hemimegalencephaly: axial contrast enhanced CT image (a) shows a mild asymmetric increased volume of the right cerebral hemisphere, with asymmetric enlargement of the right lateral ventricle (asterisks) and periventricular heterotopic gray matter (arrows). Axial T2WI (b) in another patient shows increased volume of the right cerebral hemisphere and abnormal, gliotic appearing white matter (arrows). *Source:* Figure 6.13b used with permission from Barrow Neurological Institute.

Disorders of diverticulation and cleavage

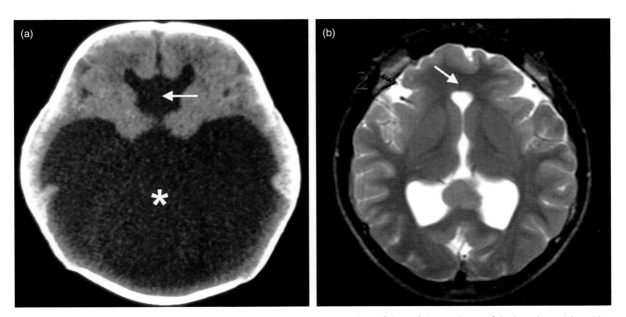

Figure 6.14 Semilobar holoprosencephaly: axial non-contrast CT image (a) shows failure of diverticulation of the lateral ventricles with a mono-ventricle (asterisk) and absence of the septum pellucidum between the frontal horns (arrow). An anterior interhemispheric fissure is present. Axial T2WI (b) shows absence of the anterior interhemispheric fissure/falx (arrow) and fusion of the frontal horns.

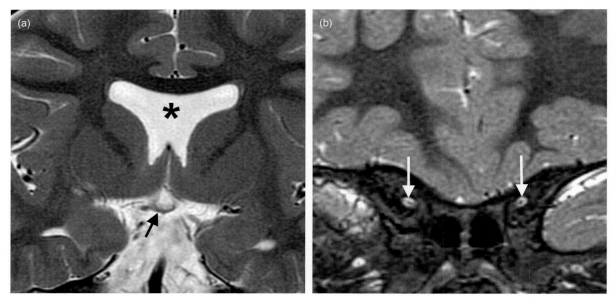

Figure 6.15 Septo-optic dysplasia: coronal T2WI (a) demonstrates absence of the septum pellucidum (asterisk) and hypoplasia of the optic chiasm (arrow). Coronal T2WI (b) shows marked hypoplasia of the optic nerves (arrows) within the posterior orbital regions. *Source:* used with permission from Barrow Neurological Institute.

Posterior fossa cystic malformations

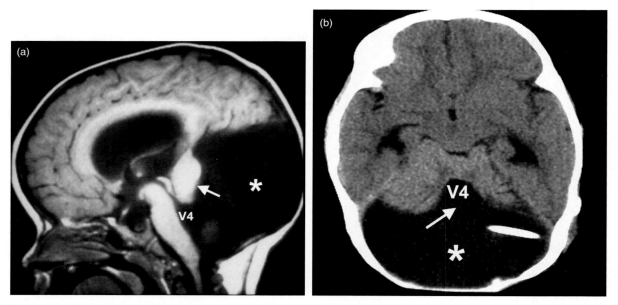

Figure 6.16 Dandy-Walker malformation: sagittal T1WI (a) shows marked hypogenesis of the inferior vermis (arrow) with a large retrocerebellar fluid collection (asterisk), which communicates with the fourth ventricle (V4) through the absent inferior vermis. Axial non-contrast CT image (b) shows the retrocerebellar fluid collection (asterisk) in continuity with the fourth ventricle (V4) through an absent vermis (arrow). A shunt tube is seen within the retrocerebellar fluid collection.

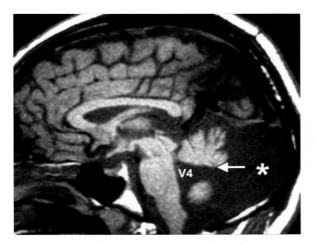

Figure 6.17 **Dandy-Walker variant:** sagittal T1WI shows a hypogenetic inferior vermis (arrow) with a retrocerebellar fluid collection (asterisk) in continuity with the fourth ventricle (V4). Note that there is only mild enlargement of the posterior fossa compared with image 6.16.

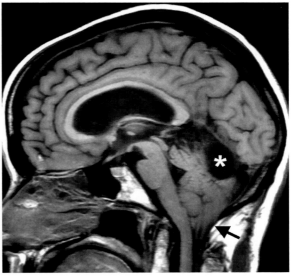

Figure 6.19 **Arachnoid cyst:** sagittal T1WI shows a focal extra-axial CSF-identical fluid collection (asterisk) posterior to the vermis, with mass effect with compression of the underlying vermis and inferior tonsillar herniation (arrow).

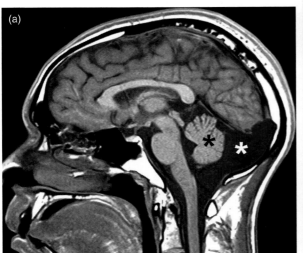

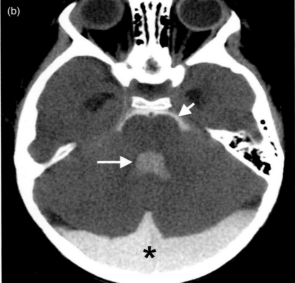

Figure 6.18 **Mega cisterna magna:** sagittal T1WI (a) shows a normally formed vermis (black asterisk) with an enlarged cisterna magna, which protrudes superiorly through a defect in the tentorium cerebelli (white asterisk). (b) Axial CT image following a cisternogram. Contrast freely enters the retrocerebellar fluid collection (asterisk), which confirms a mega cisterna magna. Arrows indicate both subarachnoid and fourth ventricular contrast. Had this been an arachnoid cyst, contrast should not be seen in the fluid collection (early after instillation). *Source:* Figure 6.18b used with permission from Barrow Neurological Institute.

Disorders of histogenesis – phakomatoses (neurocutaneous syndromes)

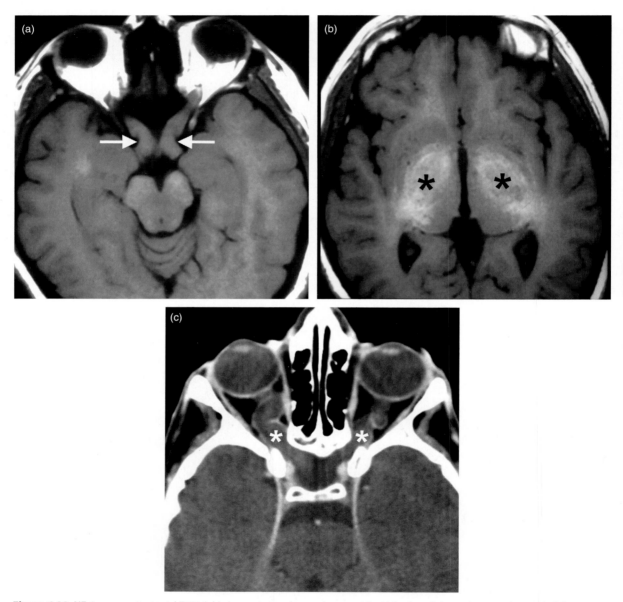

Figure 6.20 NF-1: non-contrast axial T1WI (a,b) demonstrates abnormal, symmetric thickening of the optic nerves (arrows in [a]) representing low-grade gliomas and regions of increased signal intensity within the basal ganglia regions bilaterally (asterisks in [b]) in a patient with NF-1. (c) Demonstrates bilateral optic gliomas (asterisks) in another NF-1 patient.

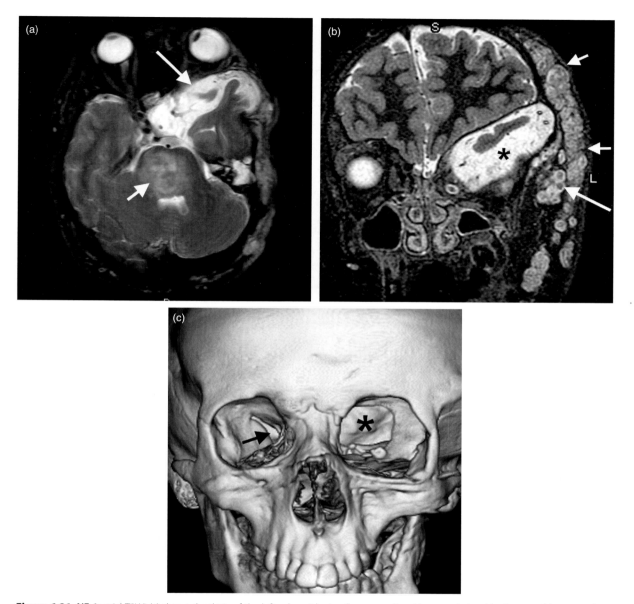

Figure 6.21 NF-1: axial T2WI (a) shows dysplasia of the left sphenoid wing (long arrow) and increased signal in the pons (short arrow), which represents a glioma in this patient with NF-1. Coronal T2WI (b) shows the dysmorphic appearance of the anterior left middle cranial fossa from the sphenoid wing dysplasia (asterisk) in addition to an extensive plexiform neurofibroma (arrows) along the left facial nerve/scalp with the target sign. 3D volume rendered CT reconstruction of the skull (c) shows the dysplastic left sphenoid wing (asterisk) compared with the normal right side, which shows a normal superior orbital CT reconstruction fissure (arrow).
Source: used with permission from Barrow Neurological Institute.

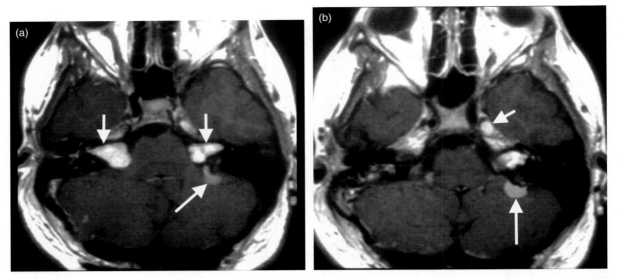

Figure 6.22 NF-2: contrast enhanced axial T1WI (a,b) shows bilateral vestibular schwannomas (short arrows in [a]) and a small meningioma along the left petrous ridge (long arrow in [a] and [b]). (b) Also shows a small schwannoma of the trigeminal nerve in the left Meckel's cave (short arrow).

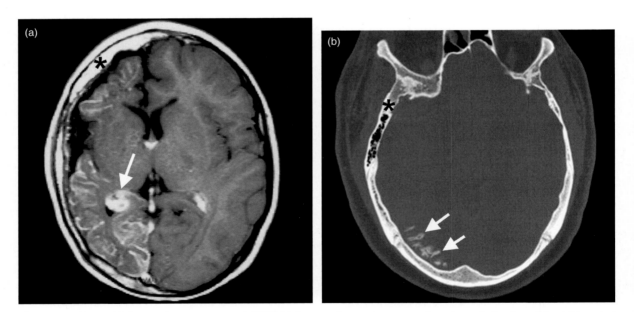

Figure 6.23 Sturge–Weber syndrome: contrast axial T1WI (a) shows gyriform enhancement along the cortical surface of the right cerebral hemisphere and asymmetric enlargement and enhancement of the choroid plexus in the right lateral ventricle (arrow). Bone window CT image (b) shows the gyriform/tram track calcification along the cortical surface in the temporo-occipital region (arrows in [b]). Note the hemiatrophy of the right hemisphere and thickening of the right hemicranium (asterisks in [a] and [b]).

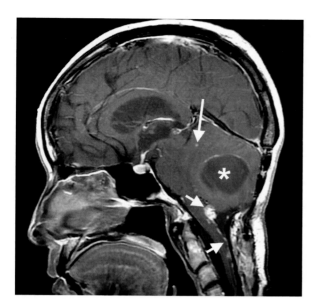

Figure 6.24 Von Hippel–Lindau disease: contrast enhanced mid-sagittal T1WI shows multiple hemangioblastomas in the cerebellum (asterisk is a predominantly cystic form and long arrow is a tiny solid nodular form), and along the dorsal surface of the cervicomedullary junction and dorsal pial surface of the upper cervical spinal cord (short white arrows). *Source:* Used with permission from Barrow Neurological Institute.

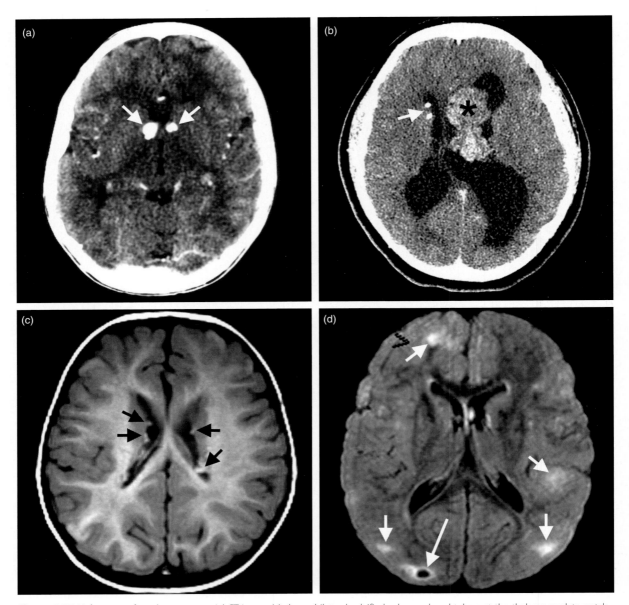

Figure 6.25 Tuberous sclerosis: contrast axial CT image (a) shows bilateral calcified subependymal tubers at the thalamocaudate notch (arrows). Non-contrast axial CT image (b) in another patient shows calcified subependymal tubers (arrow) and a large intraventricular mass (asterisk) representing a giant cell astrocytoma. Non-contrast axial T1WI (c) shows numerous small subependymal tubers (arrows). Axial FLAIR image (d) shows multiple subcortical tubers (short arrows) and a calcified tuber (long arrow).

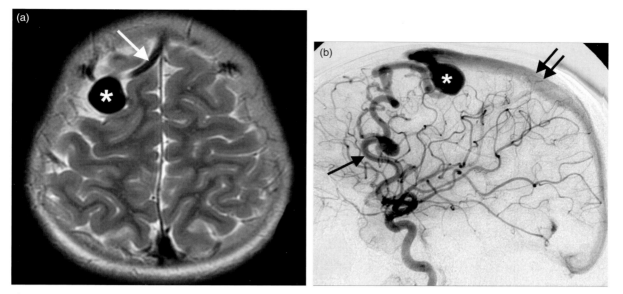

Figure 6.26 **Osler–Weber–Rendu syndrome:** axial T2WI (a) shows a large venous ectasia/varix (asterisk) along the right frontal cortex with an associated enlarged linear vessel (arrow). Lateral digital subtraction angiogram (b) in the same patient shows a pial atriovenous fistula supplied by an ascending frontal middle cerebral artery branch (single arrow), the varix (asterisk), and the drainage into the superior sagittal sinus (double arrows).

Craniosynostosis and head shape

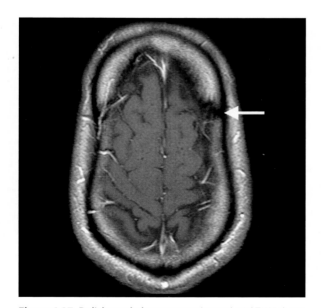

Figure 6.27 **Dolichocephaly:** contrast enhanced axial T1WI shows an elongated, narrow configuration to the calvarium called dolichocephaly or scaphocephaly, owing to premature closure of the sagittal suture. Note the coronal suture which appears normal (arrow).

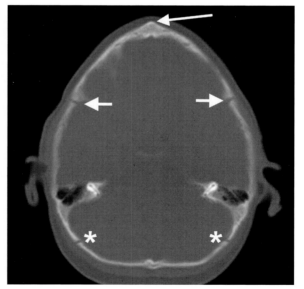

Figure 6.28 **Trigonocephaly:** axial CT bone window shows bony ridging along the anterior midline of the frontal bone (long arrow), secondary to premature closure of the metopic suture. The open coronal suture (short arrows) and lambdoid sutures (asterisks) are noted.

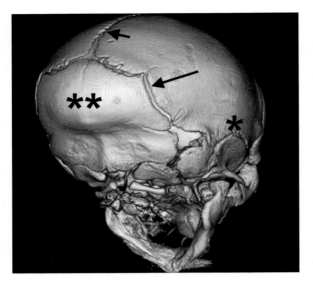

Figure 6.29 Bathrocephaly: 3D volume rendered CT reconstruction demonstrates this normal variant. There is posterior bulging of the interparietal part of the occipital bone (double asterisk). Note the open sagittal suture (short arrow), the lambdoid suture (long arrow), and the temporal squamosal suture (single asterisk).

Metabolic disorders
White matter disorders

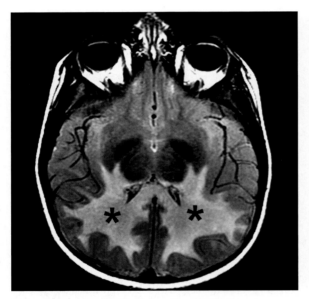

Figure 6.30 Adrenal leukodystrophy: axial FLAIR image demonstrates the dysmyelinating regions as increased signal intensity in the periatrial regions (asterisks), with involvement of the splenium of the corpus callosum and extending anteriorly into the internal and external capsules.

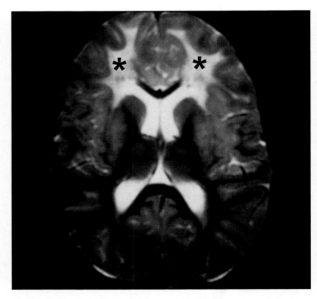

Figure 6.31 Alexander's disease: axial T2WI shows the regions of dysmyelination in the frontal white matter (asterisks).

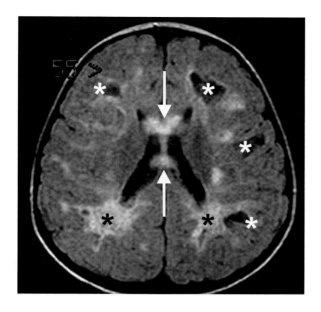

Figure 6.32 Vanishing white matter disease: axial FLAIR image demonstrates multifocal areas of abnormal increased signal (black asterisks) in the white matter, including the arcuate fibers and corpus callosum (arrows). White asterisks indicate areas of CSF signal intensity replacing focal areas of white matter.

Gray matter disorders

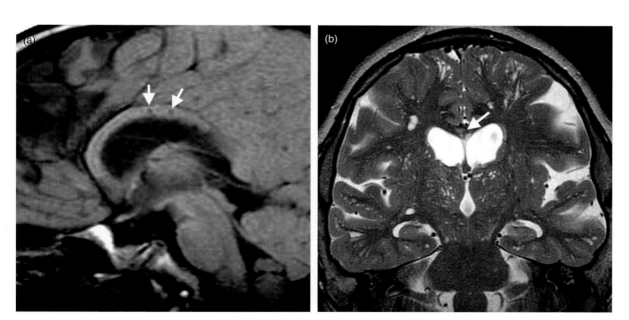

Figure 6.33 Hurler's disease: axial T1WI (a) demonstrates enlarged perivascular spaces within the corpus callosum (arrows). Coronal T2WI (b) shows multiple dilated perivascular spaces within both cerebral hemispheres, including the corpus callosum (arrow).
Source: Used with permission from Barrow Neurological Institute.

Disorders affecting gray and white matter

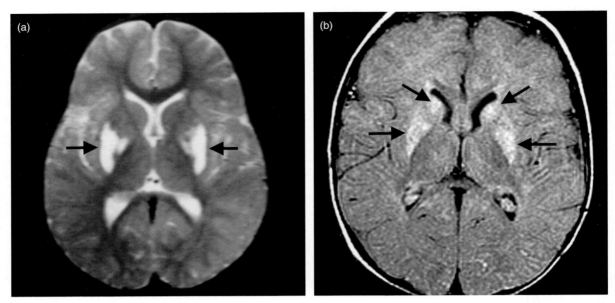

Figure 6.34 Leigh's disease: abnormal increased T2 signal is noted in the lentiform nuclei bilaterally (a,b) as well as within the heads of the caudate nuclei (b) (arrows). *Source:* Figure 6.34b used with permission from Barrow Neurological Institute.

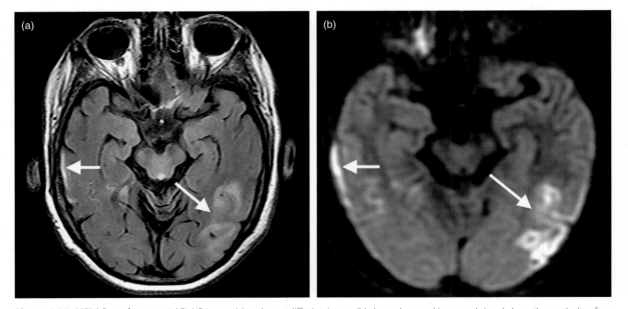

Figure 6.35 MELAS syndrome: axial FLAIR image (a) and trace diffusion image (b) show abnormal increased signal along the cortical surface in the right mid-temporal lobe and in the subcortical white matter in the posterior left temporal lobe (arrows). *Source:* used with permission from Barrow Neurological Institute.

Disorders involving the basal ganglia

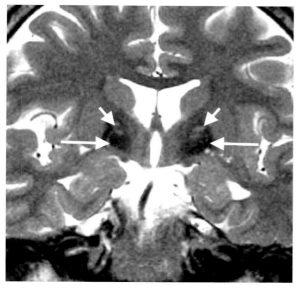

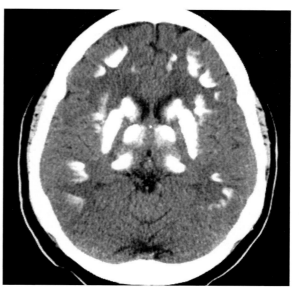

Figure 6.36 Hallervorden–Spatz disease: coronal T2WI demonstrates the eye-of-the-tiger sign with prominent hypointensity (long arrows) surrounding areas of increased T2 signal (short arrows) in the globus pallidi.

Figure 6.37 Fahr's disease: note the extensive bilateral calcifications involving subcortical white matter and the deep gray matter nuclei.

Extracranial lesions
Primary scalp
Skin lesions

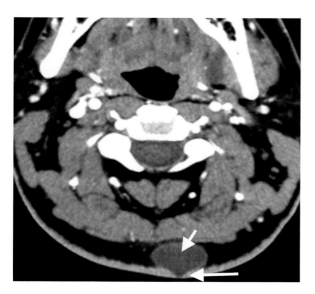

Figure 6.38 Sebaceous cyst: axial contrast enhanced CT image of the upper neck shows the typical appearance of a sebaceous cyst (short arrow) in the subcutaneous fat with attachment to the skin (long arrow).

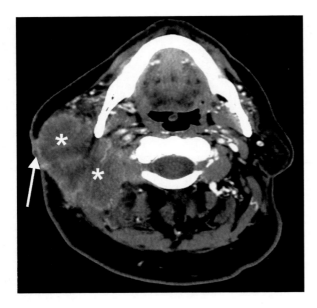

Figure 6.39 Squamous cell carcinoma: axial contrast enhanced CT image of the upper neck shows a large infiltrative neoplasm (asterisks) extending from the skin (arrow) and invading the underlying fascial tissue planes. The parotid gland is involved.

Subcutaneous layer lesions

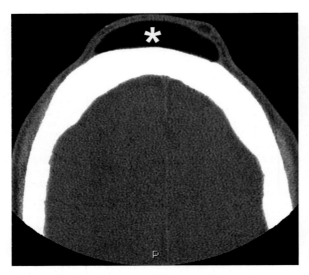

Figure 6.40 Scalp lipoma: axial CT image of the head shows a well-circumscribed mass in the deep frontal scalp (asterisk) representing a benign lipoma.

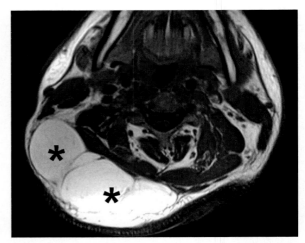

Figure 6.41 Lipoma of the posterior cervical soft tissues: axial non-contrast T1WI shows a large multilobulated mass (asterisks) in the subcutaneous fat of the posterior upper right neck, with septations and signal identical to fat elsewhere, representing a large, benign lipoma.

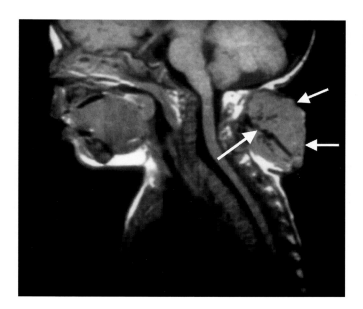

Figure 6.42 **Infantile hemangioma:** sagittal T1WI shows a large suboccipital mass (short arrows) of intermediate signal intensity with large vascular flow voids (long arrow).

Galea/subgaleal/periosteal lesions

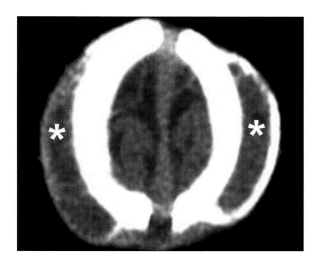

Figure 6.43 **Calcified cephalohematoma:** axial non-contrast CT image of the head shows chronic bilateral frontoparietal subperiosteal hematomas (asterisks) with peripheral calcification.

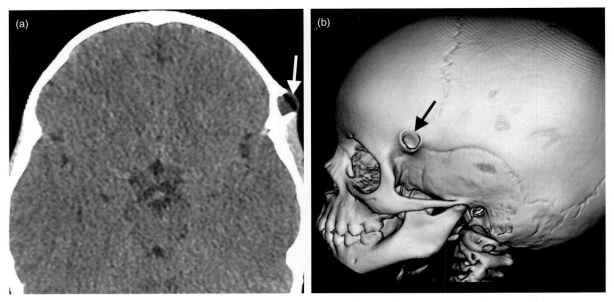

Figure 6.44 Calvarial dermoid: axial CT image of the head (a) shows a mixed density lesion in the left posterior frontal calvarium, just anterior to the pterion, which contains both fat density (arrow) and soft tissue density, surrounded by a partial osseous rim. 3D volume rendered CT reconstruction (b) demonstrates the localized calvarial dermoid at the junction of the coronal, temporal squamosal, and sphenoid sutures.

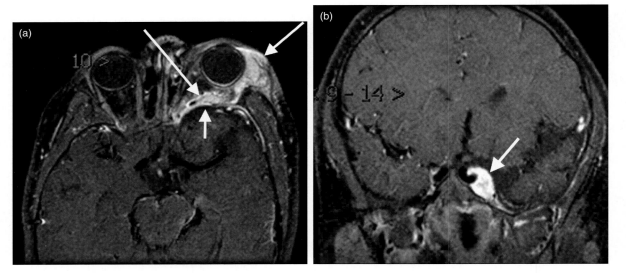

Figure 6.45 Plexiform neurofibroma in NF-1: fat suppressed post-contrast axial and coronal T1WI (a,b) shows an infiltrative enhancing plexiform neurofibroma (long arrows in [a]) in the left periorbital region, extending posteriorly along the lateral wall of the orbit to the orbital apex. Sphenoid wing dysplasia is indicated by the short arrow. (b) Shows the extension reaching the left cavernous sinus, which is enlarged with increased enhancement.

Calvarial lesions

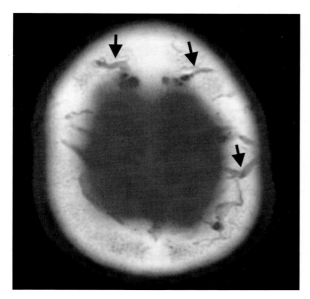

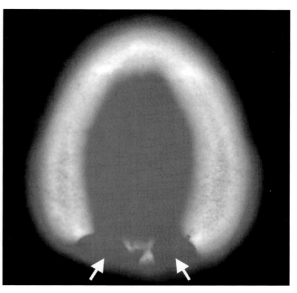

Figure 6.46 **Vascular channels mimicking skull lesions:** axial CT bone window near the vertex shows multiple linear intradiploic lucencies (arrows) representing prominent but normal vascular channels.

Figure 6.47 **Giant parietal foramina:** arrows indicate the markedly enlarged parietal foramina felt to represent a developmental anomaly of parietal bone ossification. These may be associated with anomalies of cerebral venous development. *Source:* Used with permission from Barrow Neurological Institute.

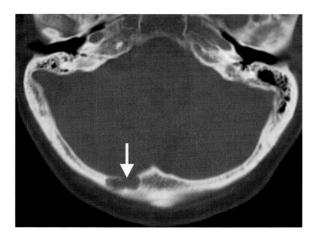

Figure 6.48 **Arachnoid granulation erosions:** axial CT bone window demonstrates scalloped erosion (arrow) along the inner table, extending into the diploic space from a prominent arachnoid granulation. Occipital bones are a common location.

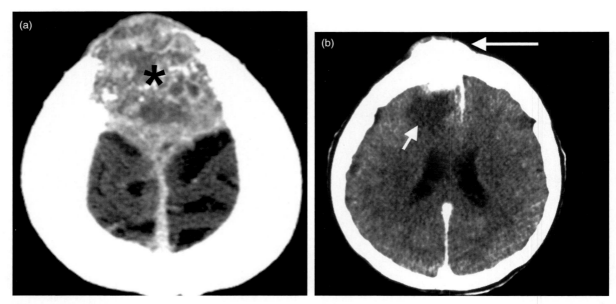

Figure 6.49 Metastatic disease to the skull: axial contrast enhanced CT images (a,b) show a large metastatic lesion from breast cancer destroying the frontal bone and involving the dura of the anterior falx (asterisk in [a]), and (b) a blastic metastatic lesion from prostate cancer growing into the scalp (long arrow) and intracranial compartment, with vasogenic edema (short arrow).

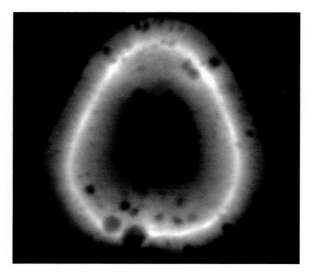

Figure 6.50 Multiple myeloma: CT bone window shows the typical appearance of multiple myeloma involving the skull.

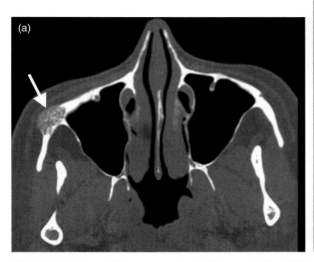

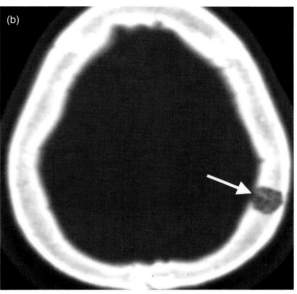

Figure 6.51 Osseous hemangiomas: axial CT bone window (a) shows an expansile lesion within the right zygomatic bone with internal spiculations. Axial CT bone window (b) shows a round, nonexpansile intradiploic lesion with internal spiculations, without surrounding sclerotic margins.

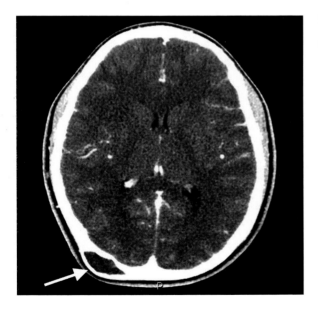

Figure 6.52 Epidermoid of the skull: axial contrast enhanced CT image shows an expansile intradiploic parietal skull lesion with surrounding sclerotic margins (arrow).

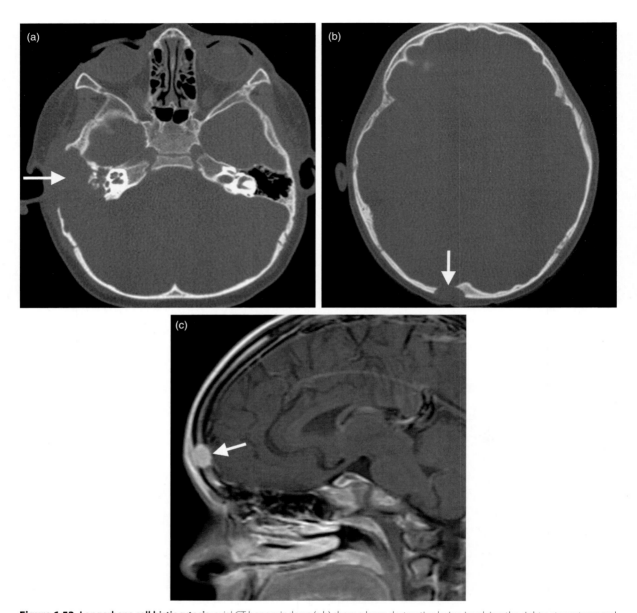

Figure 6.53 **Langerhans cell histiocytosis:** axial CT bone windows (a,b) show a large destructive lesion involving the right petrous temporal bone/mastoid region (arrow in [a]) and a localized expansile intradiploic lesion within the right occipital bone (arrow in [b]). Post-contrast sagittal T1WI (c) shows an enhancing intradiploic frontal bone lesion (arrow). *Source:* Figure 6.53c used with permission from Barrow Neurological Institute.

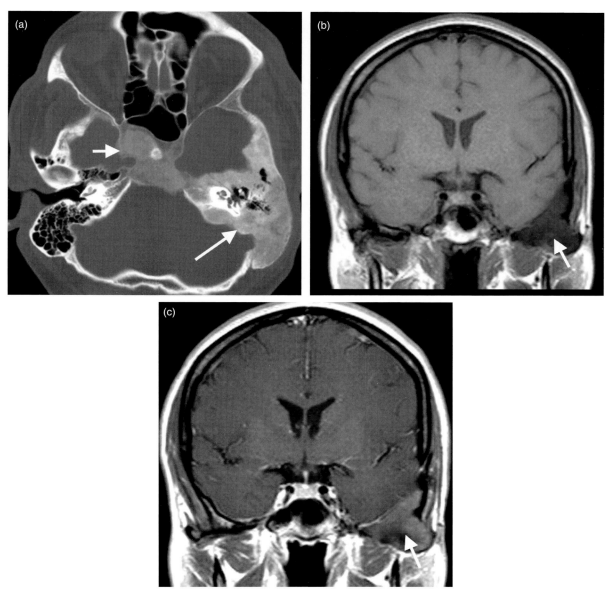

Figure 6.54 **Fibrous dysplasia:** axial CT bone window (a) shows expansion of the sphenoid body (short arrow) and the left temporal bone (long arrow) with a ground glass appearance. Non-contrast coronal T1WI (b) shows the region of osseous abnormality to be expanded with low signal (arrow in [b]), which on post-contrast coronal T1WI (c) shows diffuse enhancement.

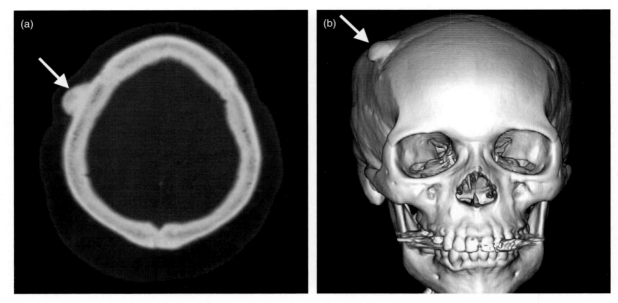

Figure 6.55 Osteoma of the calvarium: axial CT bone window (a) shows a focal mass-like region of dense compact bone arising from the outer table (arrow). 3D volume rendered CT reconstruction (b) clearly shows the osteoma (arrow) protruding from the outer table of the anterior parietal bone.

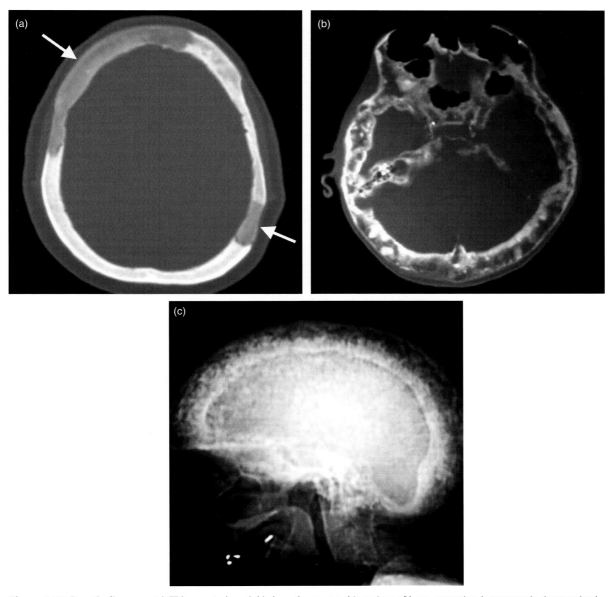

Figure 6.56 Paget's disease: axial CT bone windows (a,b) show the geographic regions of bony resorption (osteoporosis circumscripta), the lytic phase of Paget's disease, indicated by arrows in (a). The mixed lytic/blastic phase is shown in (b), and the scout film from a CT study in (c) shows extensive irregular bony trabeculations, with coarsening and bony thickening diffusely, in advanced Paget's disease.

Skull base lesions

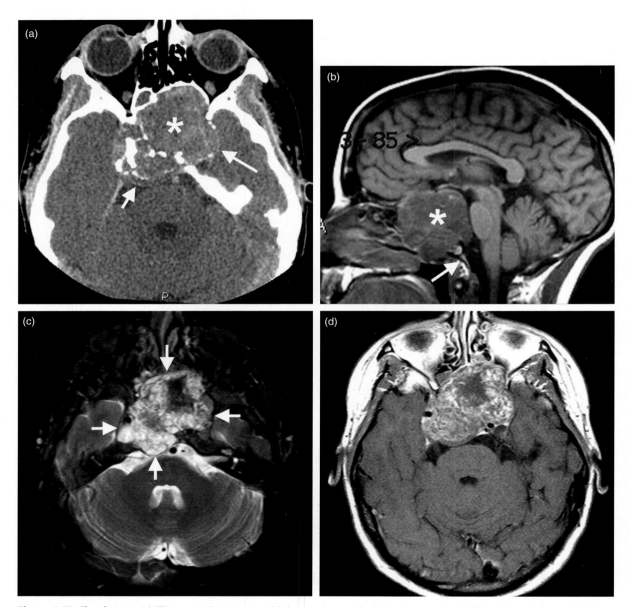

Figure 6.57 Chordoma: axial CT image without contrast (a) shows an expansile, destructive mass (asterisk) involving the central skull base and clivus, with irregular areas of residual/destroyed bone. There is expansion into the prepontine cistern (short arrow) and left middle cranial fossa (long arrow). Sagittal non-contrast T1WI (b) shows the mass (asterisk) and the residual uninvolved inferior clivus (arrow). Axial T2WI (c) shows the heterogeneous high signal (arrows), and there is irregular enhancement on a T1WI in (d).

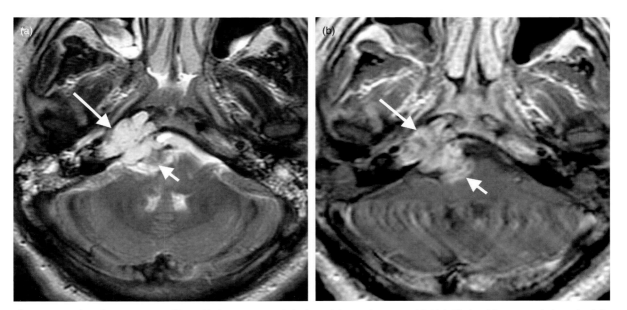

Figure 6.58 **Chondrosarcoma:** axial T2WI (a) shows an irregularly shaped destructive mass with high T2 signal (long arrow) along the right side of the clivus, projecting into the inferior right prepontine cistern (short arrow). Contrast enhanced T1WI (b) shows diffuse, mildly heterogeneous enhancement (arrows). *Source:* Used with permission from Barrow Neurological Institute.

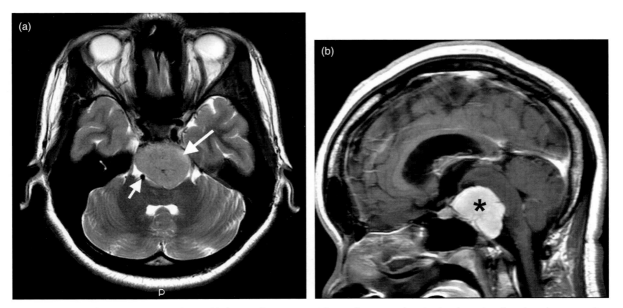

Figure 6.59 **Clival meningioma:** axial T2WI (a) shows a large extra-axial mass (long arrow) projecting from the clivus into the prepontine cistern, with compression of the pons and displacement of the basilar artery posteriorly and to the right (short arrow). The mass demonstrates signal similar to gray matter. Post-contrast sagittal T1WI (b) shows the broad dural base against the clivus and diffuse enhancement (asterisk).

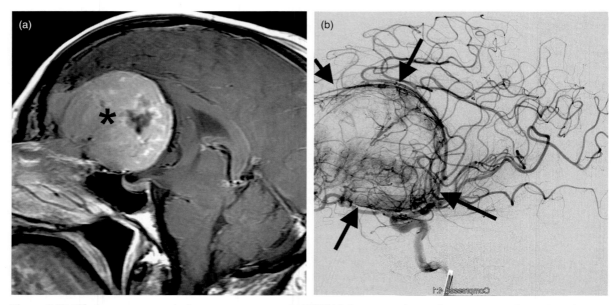

Figure 6.60 Olfactory groove meningioma: post-contrast sagittal T1WI (a) shows a very large enhancing extra-axial mass (asterisk) arising in the subfrontal region. Lateral digital subtraction angiogram (internal carotid injection) (b) shows displacement of surrounding pial vessels and mild tumor stain from the pial vasculature (arrows). *Source:* Used with permission from Barrow Neurological Institute.

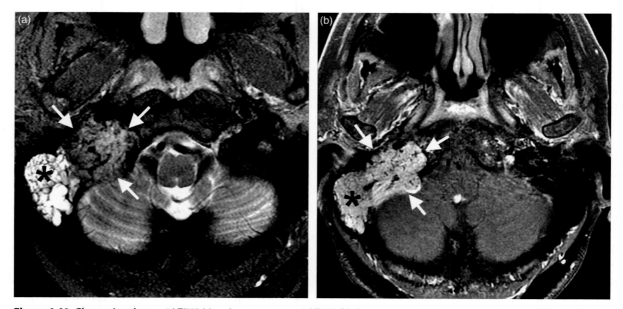

Figure 6.61 Glomus jugulare: axial T2WI (a) and post-contrast axial T1WI (b) show a mass with heterogeneous increased T2 signal and enhancement (arrows in [a,b]) within the jugular foramen, with multiple flow voids. Post-obstructive opacified mastoid air cells are noted (asterisk). *Source:* Used with permission from Barrow Neurological Institute.

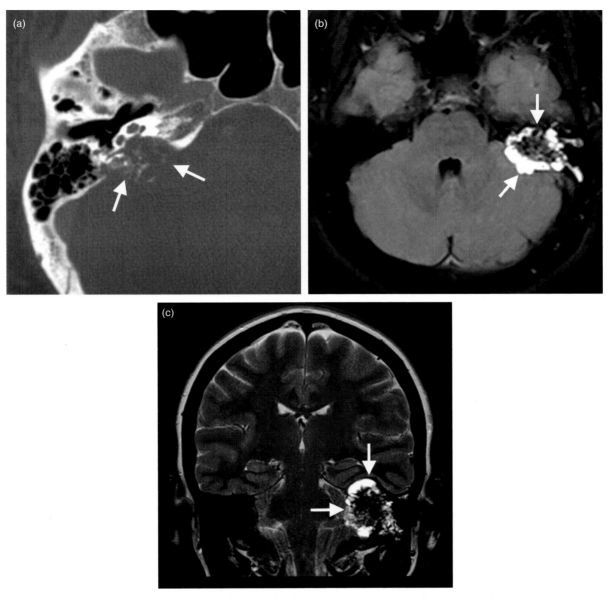

Figure 6.62 Endolymphatic sac tumors: axial CT bone window (a) shows a destructive lesion (arrows) along the posterior aspect of the petrous bone near the endolymphatic duct and involving the internal auditory canal, with bony spicules. Axial T1WI with fat suppression (b) and coronal T2WI (c) in a second patient show an expansile mass in the petrous temporal bone, with a peripheral rim of high signal and heterogeneous central low signal (arrows).

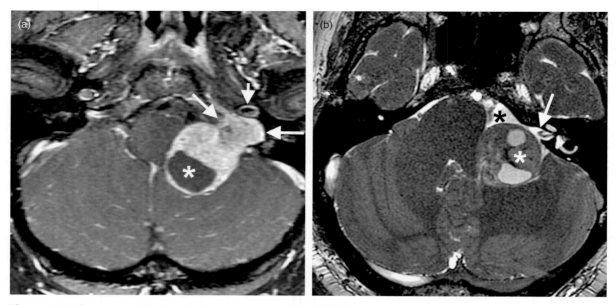

Figure 6.63 Schwannoma of the jugular foramen: post-contrast axial T1WI (a) shows a large, enhancing mass (long arrows), with a cystic component (asterisk) extending from the left jugular foramen (long arrows) into the perimedullary cistern, with associated mass effect. The short arrow indicates the carotid canal. Axial T2WI (b) shows the mass extending into the CP angle cistern (white asterisk) but not extending into the internal auditory canal (arrow). The black asterisk shows the widening of the CP angle cistern adjacent to the mass, a sign of an extra-axial lesion. *Source:* used with permission from Barrow Neurological Institute.

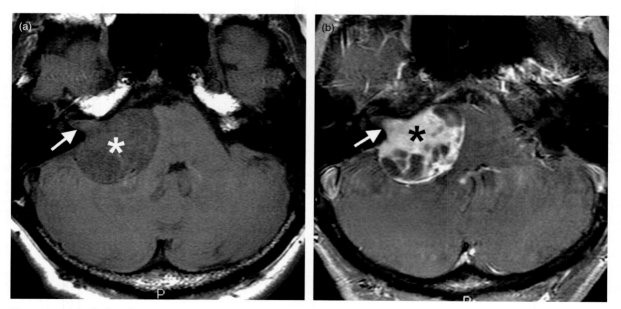

Figure 6.64 Vestibular schwannoma: pre- (a) and post-contrast (b) axial T1WI show a mass (asterisk) widening the internal auditory canal (arrow) and extending into the CP angle cistern, with cystic, non-enhancing regions (in [b]). Associated mass effect with compression of the pons and cerebellum is noted.

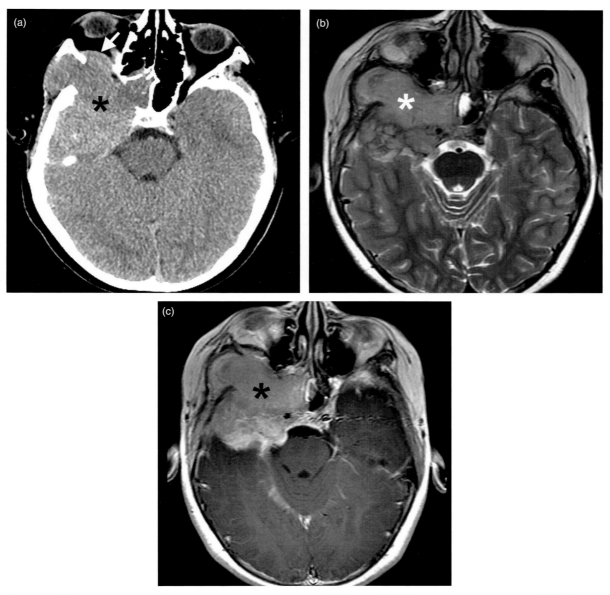

Figure 6.65 Rhabdomyosarcoma (embryonal type): non-contrast axial CT (a), axial T2WI (b), and contrast enhanced axial T1WI (c) show a large, destructive enhancing mass (asterisks) in the region of the sphenoid buttress, with intracranial, epidural extension into the middle cranial fossa, and into the suprazygomatic masticator space as well as the orbit (arrow in [a]) and the sphenoid sinus.

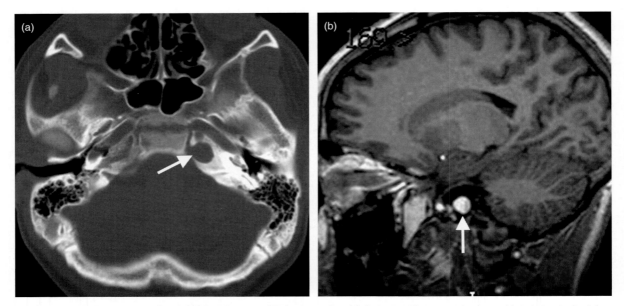

Figure 6.66 Cholesterol granuloma petrous apex: axial CT bone window (a) shows a well circumscribed round lytic lesion in the left petrous apex (arrow). Non-contrast sagittal T1WI (b) demonstrates the high signal intensity characteristic of this lesion (arrow).

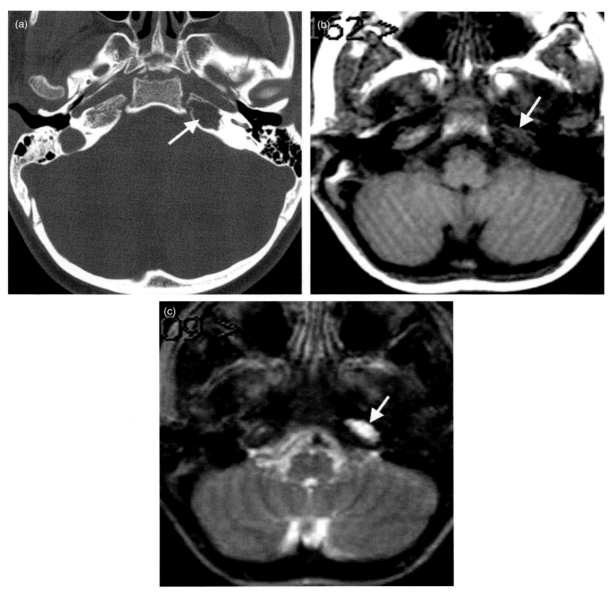

Figure 6.67 **Congenital epidermoid petrous apex:** axial CT bone window (a) shows a mildly expansile lytic lesion at the petrous apex (arrow). Non-contrast axial T1WI (b) shows that the lesion is of intermediate signal intensity, and of increased signal intensity on the axial T2WI (c). Diffusion restriction (not shown) was noted.

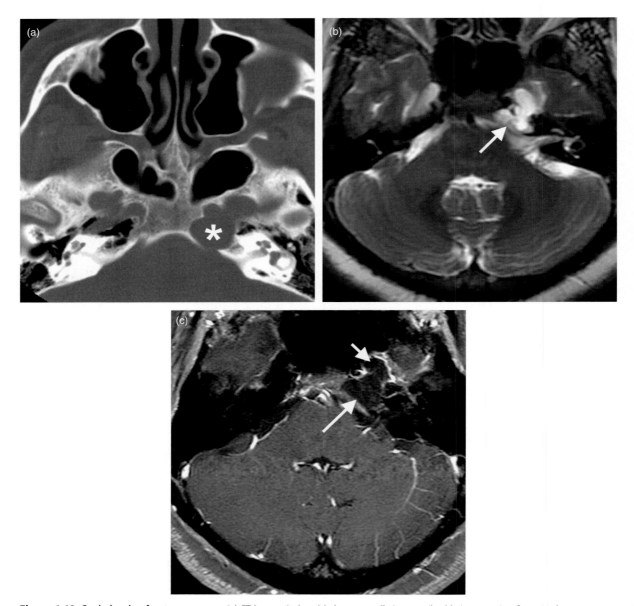

Figure 6.68 Cephalocele of petrous apex: axial CT bone window (a) shows a well-circumscribed lytic appearing focus in the petrous apex (asterisk). Axial T2WI (b) and contrast enhanced axial T1WI (c) show that the region of abnormality has signal identical to CSF and is continuous with Meckel's cave (short arrow in [c]), without pathologic enhancement.

Sinonasal lesions

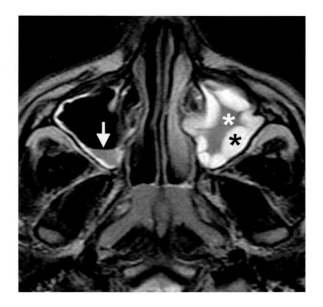

Figure 6.69 **Sinusitis:** axial T2WI shows typical findings with mucosal thickening/edema (black asterisk), with central fluid (white asterisk) opacifying the left maxillary sinus. A small air-fluid level is seen in the right maxillary sinus (arrow), with minimal associated mucosal thickening.

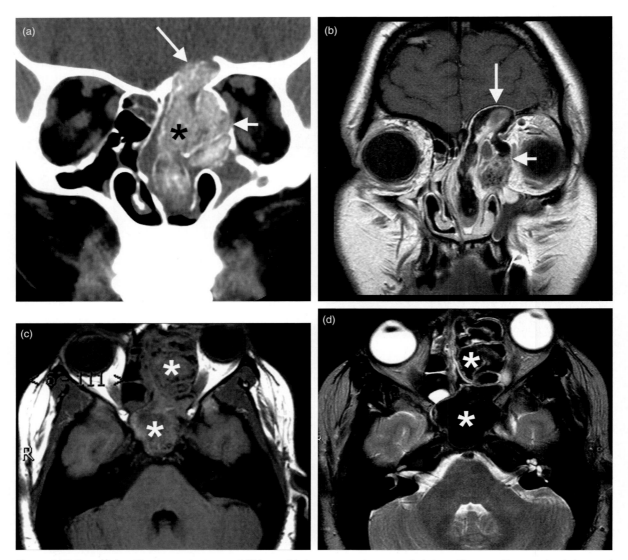

Figure 6.70 Fungal sinusitis: non-contrast coronal CT image (a) shows a complex, expansile lesion with areas of increased and decreased density in the left ethmoid (short arrow) and maxillary sinus and nasal cavity (asterisk), with superior extension into the subfrontal region (long arrow) via destruction of the roof of the ethmoid complex. Post-contrast coronal T1WI (b) shows variable enhancement with prominent areas of hypointensity. Axial non-contrast T1WI (c) shows that the abnormality demonstrates mildly heterogeneous intermediate signal (asterisks), and on the axial T2WI (d) these areas are markedly hypointense (asterisks) and may be mistaken for aerated sinuses.

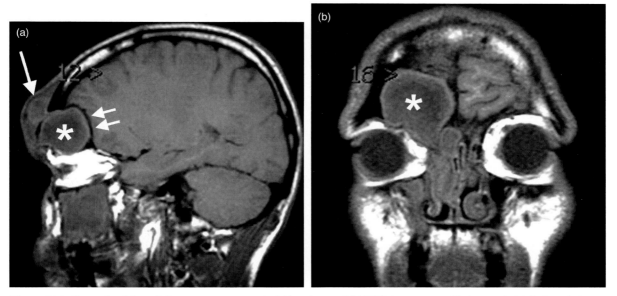

Figure 6.71 Mucocele of frontal sinus: non-contrast sagittal (a) and coronal (b) T1WI shows an opacified, expanded right frontal sinus (asterisk), with expansion into the anterior cranial fossa (short double arrows) and anterior extension into the frontal scalp/Pott's puffy tumor (long arrow).

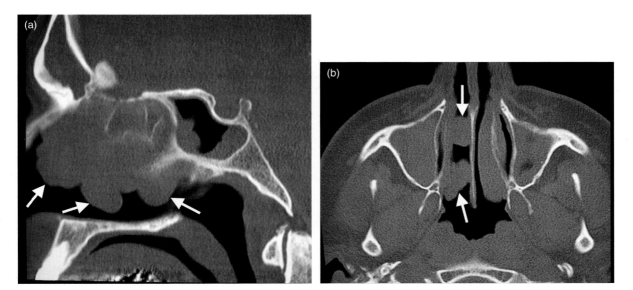

Figure 6.72 Sinonasal polyps: mid sagittal (a) and axial (b) CT bone windows show multiple nodular, polypoid soft tissue densities (arrows) projecting into the nasal cavity, consistent with sinonasal polyps.

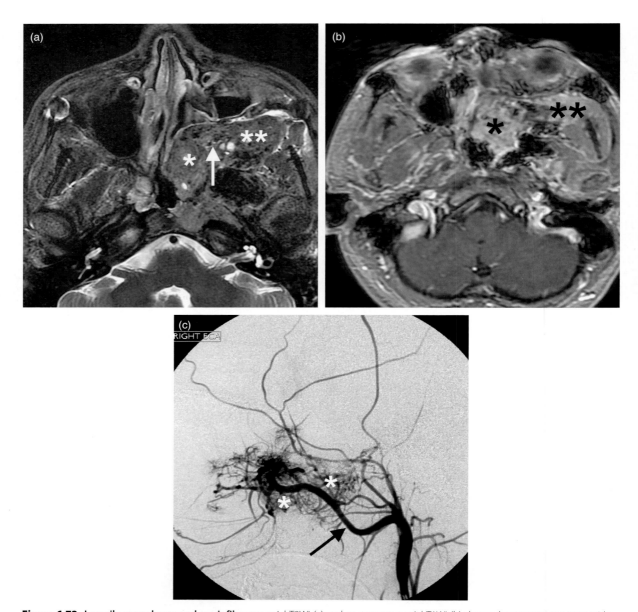

Figure 6.73 Juvenile nasopharyngeal angiofibroma: axial T2WI (a) and post-contrast axial T1WI (b) show a heterogeneous mass with multiple flow voids and enhancement extending from the posterior nasal cavity (single asterisk) laterally, through the sphenopalatine foramen (arrow in [a]) into the masticator space (double asterisks). Lateral external carotid digital subtraction angiogram (c) shows the hypervascularity (asterisks) of the tumor arising from the distal internal maxillary artery (black arrow). *Source:* Used with permission from Barrow Neurological Institute.

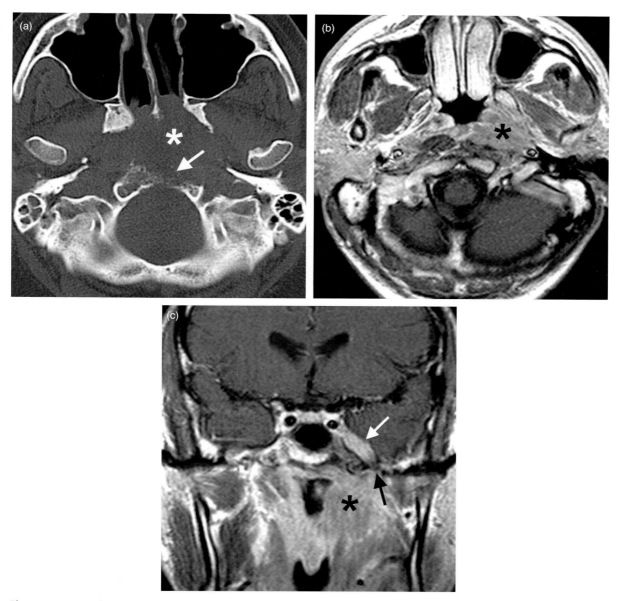

Figure 6.74 Nasopharyngeal carcinoma: axial CT bone window (a) shows a nasopharyngeal mass (asterisk) invading and destroying the skull base/clivus (arrow). Post-contrast axial T1WI (b) reveals the left sided nasopharyngeal mass (asterisk) involving the fossa of Rosenmuller. Contrast enhanced coronal T1WI (c) shows the mass (asterisk), which demonstrates perineural spread along the mandibular division (V3) of the trigeminal nerve (white arrow) via the foramen ovale (black arrow).

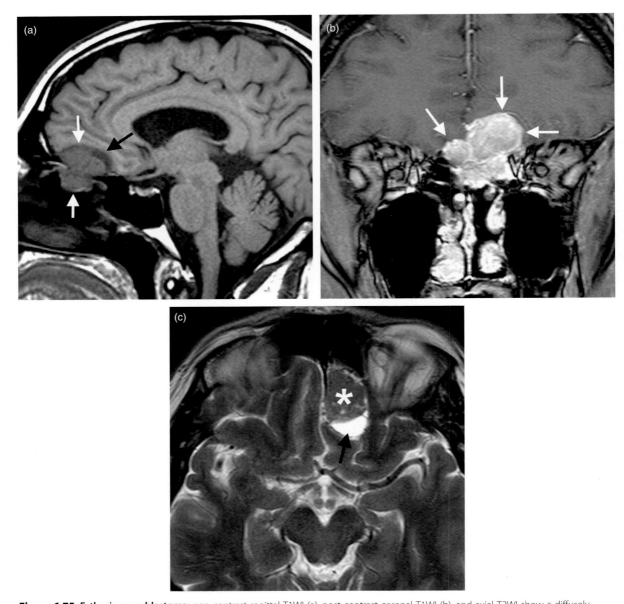

Figure 6.75 Esthesioneuroblastoma: non-contrast sagittal T1WI (a), post-contrast coronal T1WI (b), and axial T2WI show a diffusely enhancing mass in the upper nasal cavity/ethmoid complex (white arrows in [a,b]), destroying the cribriform plate and extending into the anterior cranial fossa. In (c) note the mass (asterisk) and the cyst adjacent to the brain parenchyma (black arrows in [a,c]).

Intracranial tumors
Primary intra-axial neoplasms
Neuroepithelial (glial) tumors
Astrocytic diffuse

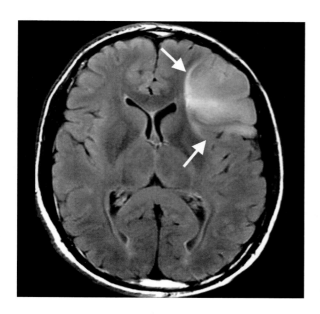

Figure 6.76 Astrocytoma: axial FLAIR image shows a relatively well-circumscribed and homogeneous mass-like region (arrows) of increased signal intensity, involving cortical gray and underlying white matter, with only mild mass effect. There was no contrast enhancement (not shown); a biopsy proven WHO grade II astrocytoma.

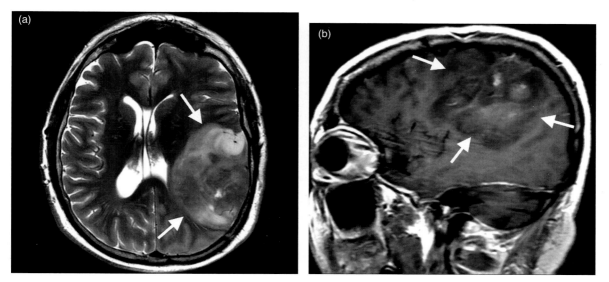

Figure 6.77 Anaplastic astrocytoma: axial T2WI (a) and post-contrast sagittal T1WI (b) show a heterogeneous mass (arrows) in the left parietal lobe, involving white matter and overlying gray matter, with patchy enhancement and mass effect; a biopsy proven WHO grade III (anaplastic) astrocytoma.

117

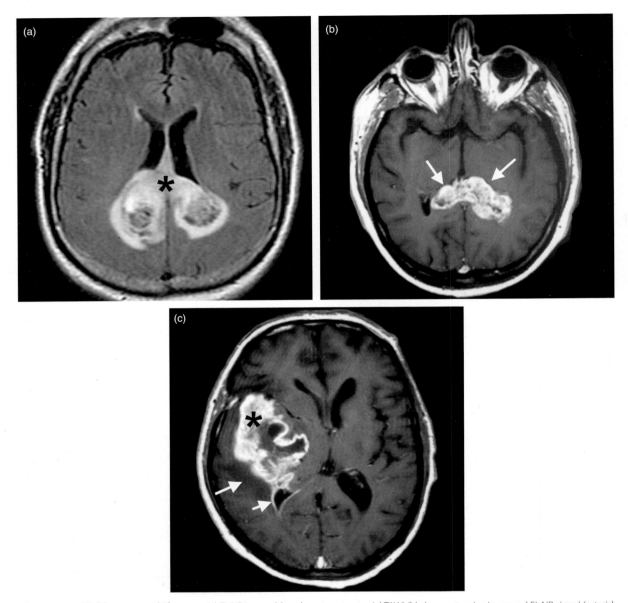

Figure 6.78 **Glioblastoma multiforme:** axial FLAIR image (a) and post-contrast axial T1WI (b) show extensive increased FLAIR signal (asterisk in [a]) and heterogeneous enhancement (arrows in [b]) extending across the splenium of the corpus callosum, representing a WHO grade IV astrocytoma/glioblastoma multiforme (butterfly glioma). Post-contrast axial T1WI in a second patient (c) shows an extensive glioblastoma multiforme (asterisk) with surrounding edema (long arrow) and subependymal spread (short arrow). *Source:* Figure 6.78a used with permission from Barrow Neurological Institute.

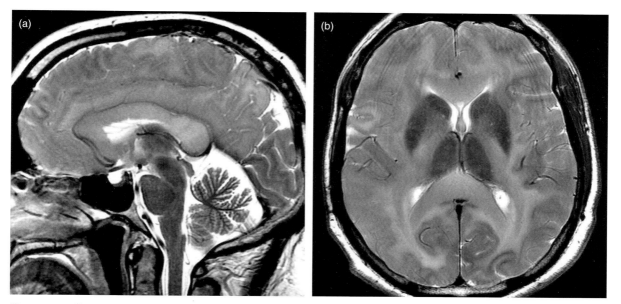

Figure 6.79 **Gliomatosis cerebri:** sagittal (a) and axial (b) T2WI show diffuse infiltration of the white matter of both cerebral hemispheres, including the corpus callosum, without contrast enhancement (not shown), representing gliomatosis cerebri (WHO grade III neoplasm). *Source:* Used with permission from Barrow Neurological Institute.

Astrocytic focal

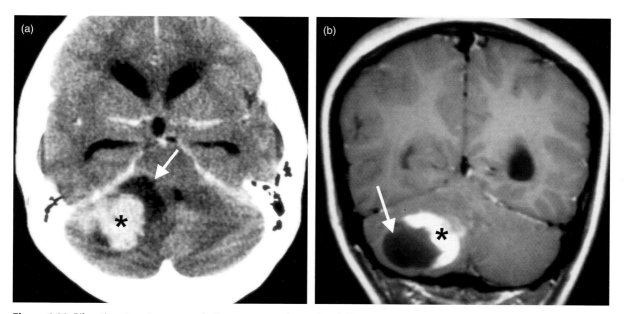

Figure 6.80 **Pilocytic astrocytoma – cerebellum:** contrast enhanced axial CT image (a) and coronal T1WI (b) reveal a cystic mass (arrow) with enhancing nodular component (asterisk) along the periphery, typical for this WHO grade I neoplasm.

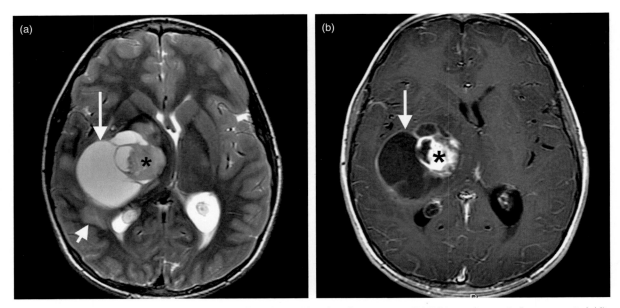

Figure 6.81 Pilocytic astrocytoma – supratentorial: axial T2WI (a) and axial post-contrast T1WI (b) reveals a cystic (long arrows in [a,b]) and solid enhancing mass (asterisk) within the right basal ganglia/internal capsule region. Mild associated vasogenic edema is noted by the short arrow in (a).

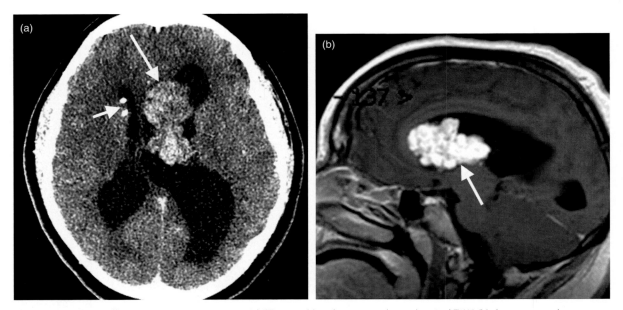

Figure 6.82 Giant cell astrocytoma: non-contrast axial CT image (a) and contrast enhanced sagittal T1WI (b) demonstrate a large, multilobulated enhancing intraventricular mass (long arrows) in this patient with tuberous sclerosis. Calcified subependymal tubers are indicated by the short arrow in (a).

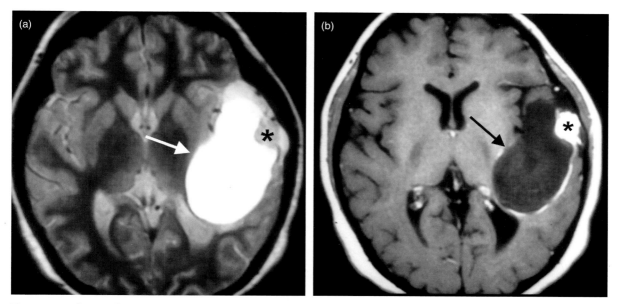

Figure 6.83 **Pleomorphic xanthoastrocytoma:** axial T2WI (a) and post-contrast axial T1WI (b) show a cystic temporal lobe mass (arrows) with an enhancing solid nodule (asterisk) along the pial surface, with adjacent remodeling of the inner table (best seen in [b]). *Source:* Used with permission from Barrow Neurological Institute.

Brainstem glioma

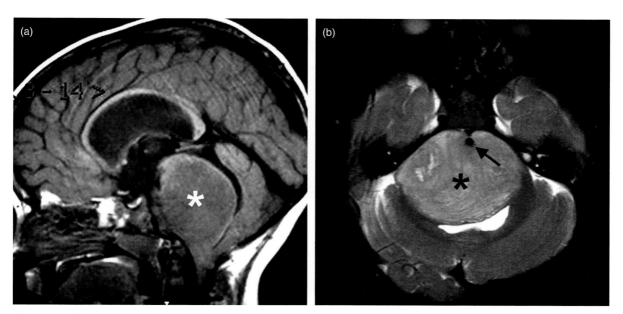

Figure 6.84 **Brainstem glioma:** non-contrast sagittal T1WI (a) and axial T2WI (b) demonstrate marked expansion of the brainstem (asterisk) with increased T2 signal (b). Exophytic growth ventrally surrounds and engulfs the basilar artery (arrow in [b]).

Non-astrocytic glial

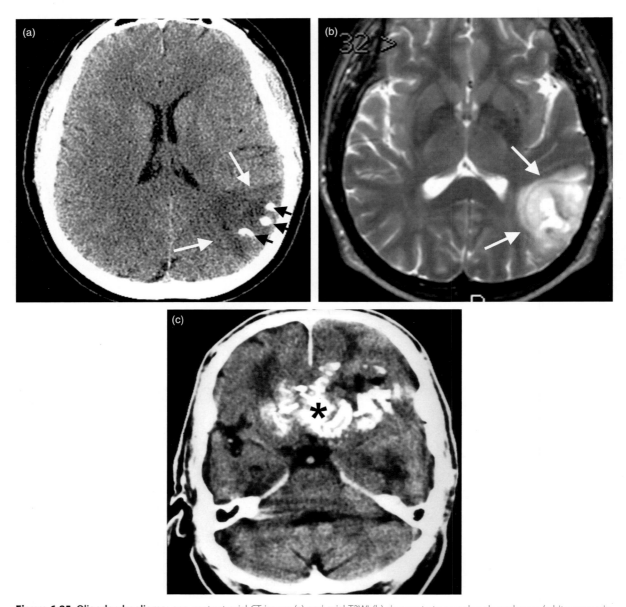

Figure 6.85 Oligodendroglioma: non-contrast axial CT image (a) and axial T2WI (b) demonstrate a wedge shaped mass (white arrows in [a,b]), involving the cortex and underlying white matter, with calcifications (black arrows in [a]). There was no significant contrast enhancement (not shown). Non-contrast axial CT image (c) shows a large extensively calcified mass in both frontal lobes in a second patient with oligodendroglioma.

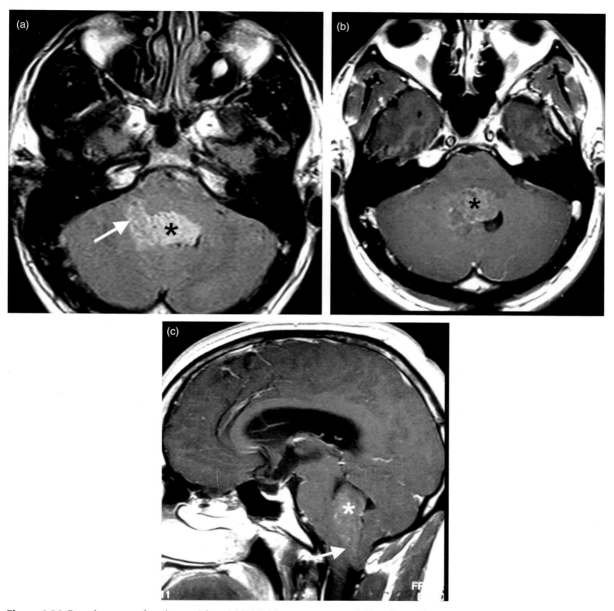

Figure 6.86 Ependymoma – fourth ventricle: axial FLAIR (a), post-contrast axial (b) and sagittal (c), T1WI images show a large mildly enhancing fourth ventricular mass (asterisks) extending through the foramen of Luschka (arrow in [a]) and the foramen of Magendie (arrow in [c]).

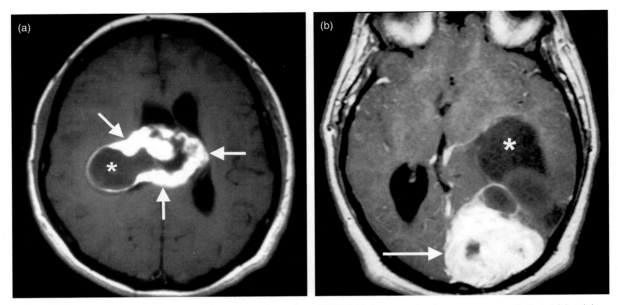

Figure 6.87 Ependymoma – supratentorial: contrast enhanced axial T1WI (a,b) demonstrating heterogeneous, cystic (asterisks), solid partially enhancing masses (arrows) with associated mass effect, in two different patients.

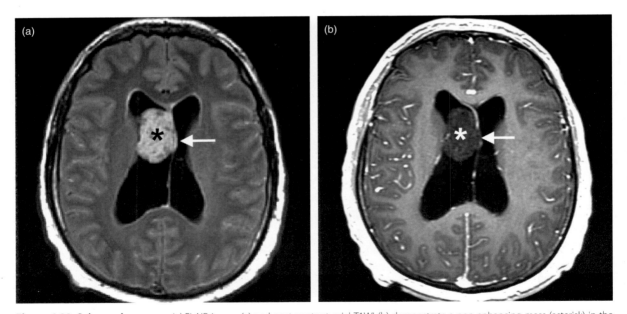

Figure 6.88 Subependymoma: axial FLAIR image (a) and post-contrast axial T1WI (b) demonstrate a non-enhancing mass (asterisk) in the anterior body of the right lateral ventricle, attached to the septum pellucidum (arrow).

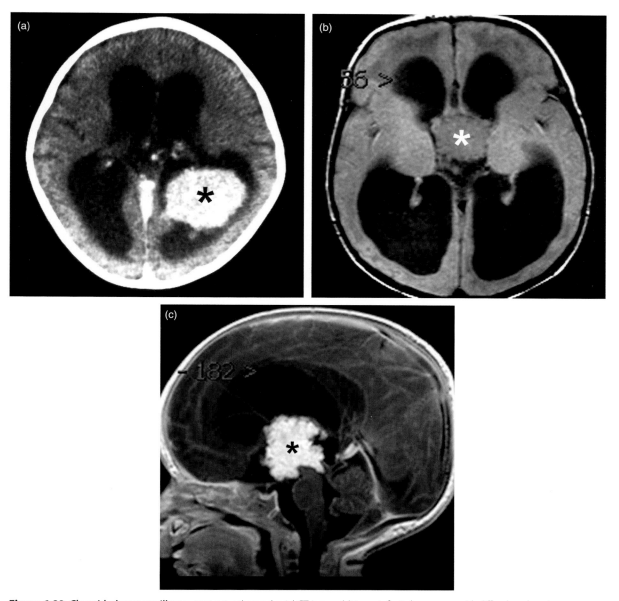

Figure 6.89 Choroid plexus papilloma: contrast enhanced axial CT image (a) in an infant shows an ovoid, diffusely enhancing mass (asterisk) within the atrium of the left lateral ventricle, and hydrocephalus from CSF overproduction. Non-contrast axial T1WI (b) and contrast enhanced sagittal T1WI (c) in a different patient show a multilobulated, densely enhancing third ventricular mass (asterisk), extending into the aqueduct of Sylvius, and obstructive hydrocephalus.

Neuronal and mixed neuronal-glial tumors

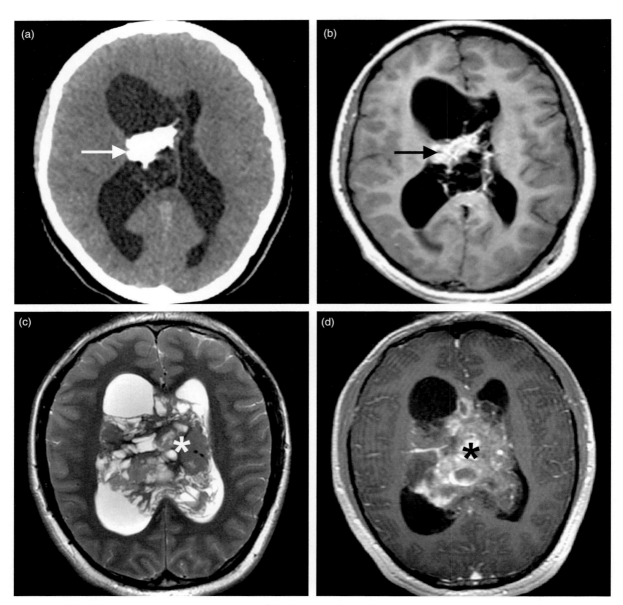

Figure 6.90 Central neurocytoma: non-contrast axial CT image (a) and contrast enhanced T1WI (b) show an irregularly shaped, partially calcified and partially enhancing mass (arrow) in the body of the right lateral ventricle, attached to the septum pellucidum. Axial T2WI (c) and contrast enhanced axial T1WI (d) show a large, heterogeneous mass with heterogeneous enhancement in both lateral ventricles (asterisks) in a different patient. *Source:* used with permission from Barrow Neurological Institute.

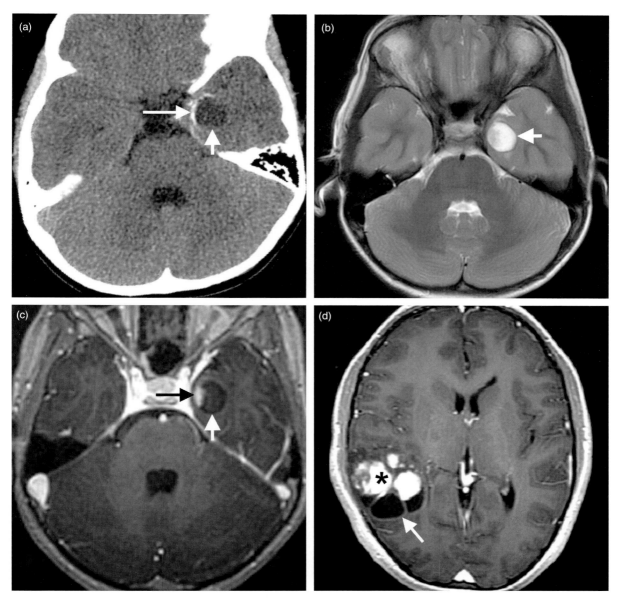

Figure 6.91 **Ganglioglioma:** non-contrast axial CT image (a), axial T2WI (b), and post-contrast axial T1WI (c) demonstrate a partially calcified (long arrow in [a]), cystic (short white arrows in [a,b,c]), and partially enhancing (black arrow in [c]) mass in the medial left temporal lobe. Post-contrast axial T1WI (d) in another patient shows a partially cystic (arrow) and solid enhancing (asterisk) parietal ganglioglioma. *Source:* Figure 6.91a,b,c used with permission from Barrow Neurological Institute.

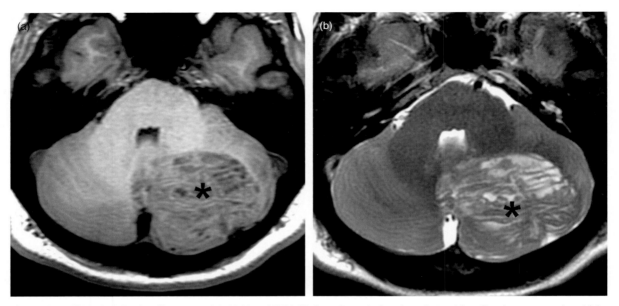

Figure 6.92 Lhermitte–Duclos disease: axial T1WI (a) and T2WI (b) show the typical corduroy/striated/lamellated appearance (asterisks) of this disorder, which is also referred to as dysplastic cerebellar gangliocytoma. *Source:* used with permission from Barrow Neurological Institute.

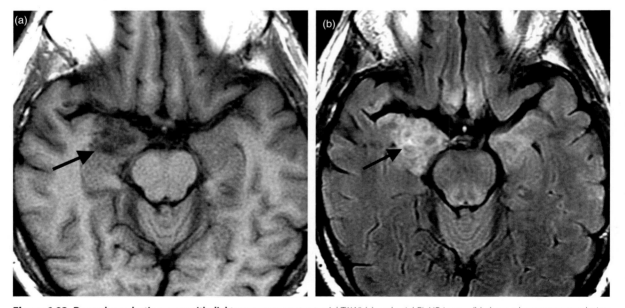

Figure 6.93 Dysembryoplastic neuroepithelial tumor: non-contrast axial T1WI (a) and axial FLAIR image (b) show a heterogeneous lesion in the anteromedial right temporal lobe (arrows), without contrast enhancement (not shown).

Embryonal tumors

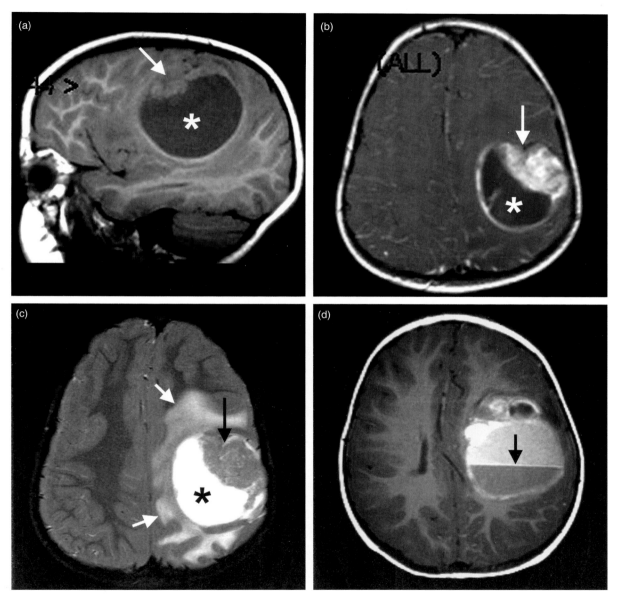

Figure 6.94 Primitive neuroectodermal tumors – supratentorial: non-contrast sagittal T1WI (a), contrast enhanced axial T1WI (b), and axial T2WI (c) show a large partially cystic/necrotic (asterisk) parietal mass with solid enhancing nodular components (long white arrows in [a,b] and black arrow in [c]), with surrounding vasogenic edema (short white arrows in [c]). Non-contrast T1WI (d) in another child with a primitive neuroectodermal tumor shows a large hemorrhagic mass with a blood level (arrow).

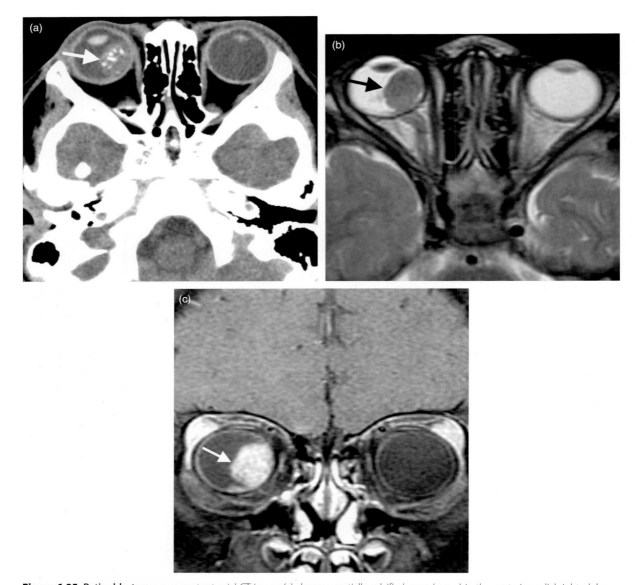

Figure 6.95 **Retinoblastoma:** non-contrast axial CT image (a) shows a partially calcified mass (arrow) in the posteriomedial right globe, which demonstrates hypointensity (arrow) on T2WI (b), and diffuse enhancement on contrast enhanced T1WI (arrow in [c]). *Source:* used with permission from Barrow Neurological Institute.

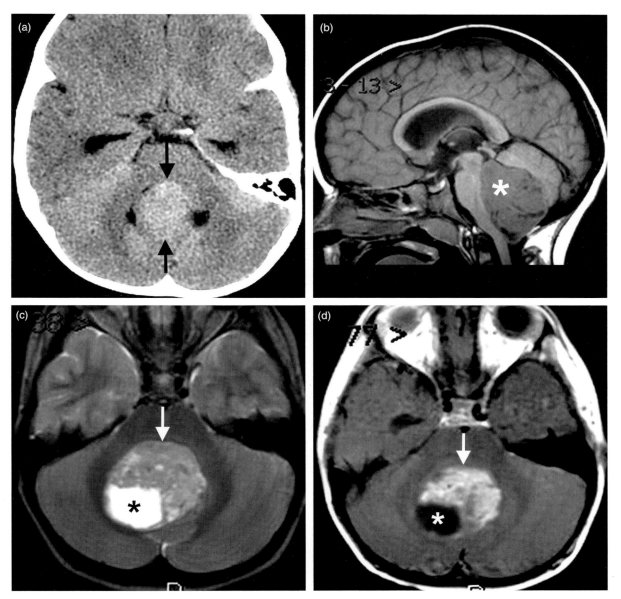

Figure 6.96 **Medulloblastoma:** non-contrast axial CT image (a) shows a relatively dense mass filling the fourth ventricle (arrows). Non-contrast sagittal T1WI (b), axial T2WI (c), and post-contrast axial T1WI (d) in another patient show a large mildly heterogeneous mass with a cystic component (asterisks in [c,d]) and solid, nodular enhancement (asterisk in [b] and arrows in [c,d]), filling and obliterating the fourth ventricle.

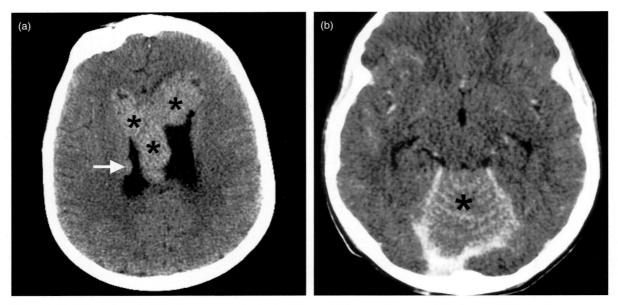

Figure 6.97 Metastatic medulloblastoma: non-contrast axial CT image (a) shows bulky masses infiltrating and thickening the subependymal regions of both lateral ventricles (asterisks), with an additional subependymal nodule (white arrow). Post-contrast axial CT image (b) in another patient shows pathologic enhancement along the pial surfaces of the cerebellum, and along the tentorium cerebelli (asterisk).

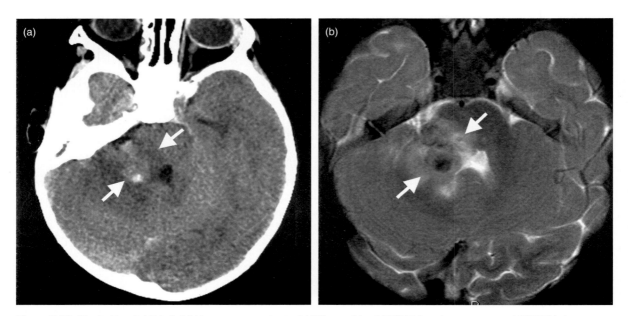

Figure 6.98 Atypical teratoid/rhabdoid tumor: non-contrast axial CT image (a), axial T2WI (b), and post-contrast axial T1WI (c) show a mass (arrows) in the right middle cerebellar peduncle, with a small area of calcification or hemorrhage (area of increased density in [a] and hypointensity in [b]), which diffusely enhances (arrow in [c]) with surrounding vasogenic edema.

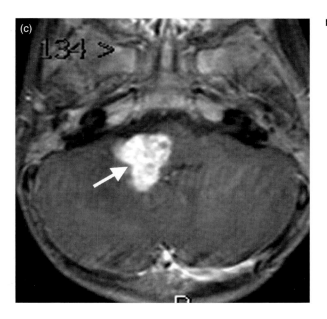

Figure 6.98 (*cont.*)

Other primary intra-axial neoplasms

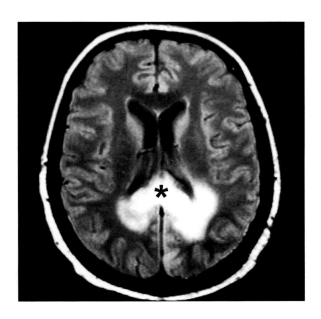

Figure 6.99 **Lymphoma:** axial FLAIR image shows lymphoma infiltrating both cerebral hemispheres via the splenium of the corpus callosum. This demonstrated diffuse enhancement and restricted diffusion (not shown).

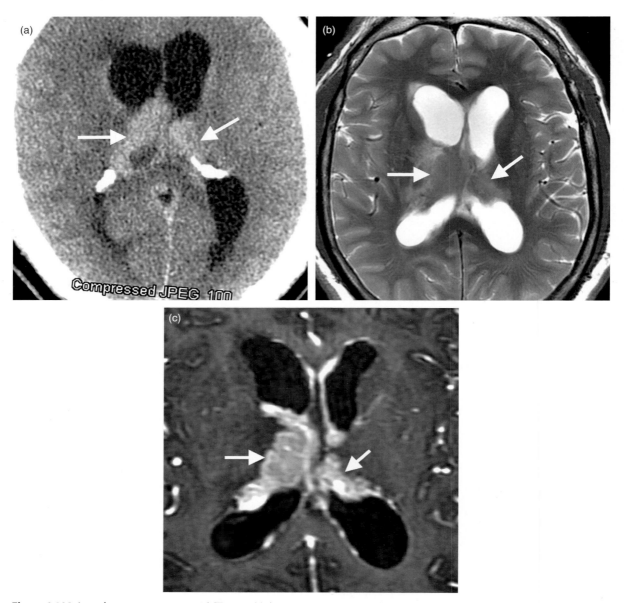

Figure 6.100 Lymphoma: non-contrast axial CT image (a) demonstrates intraventricular/periventricular masses of increased density (arrows). Axial T2WI (b) shows the masses to be hypointense, and on post-contrast axial T1WI (c) there is diffuse enhancement of the masses (arrows) with infiltration along the ependyma and septum pellucidum. *Source:* used with permission from Barrow Neurological Institute.

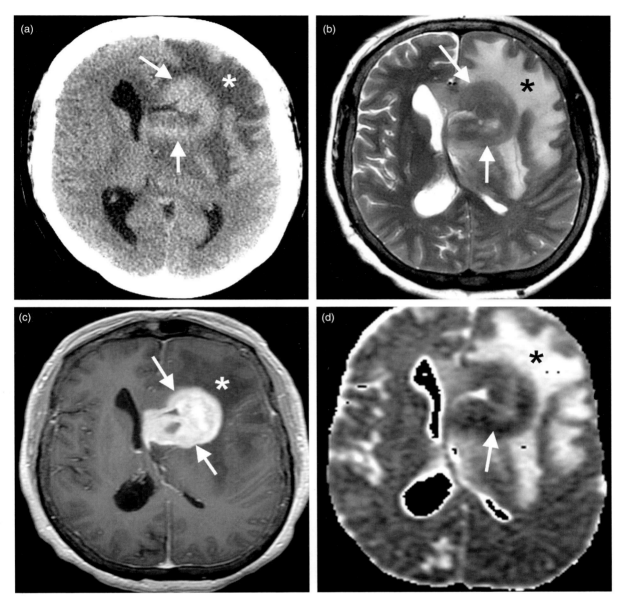

Figure 6.101 Lymphoma: axial non-contrast CT image (a) shows a mass surrounding/engulfing the left frontal horn and anterior body of the left lateral ventricle, which is high density (arrows), with surrounding edema (asterisk). Axial T2WI (b) shows the mass is hypointense, and on post-contrast axial T1WI (c) it shows extensive enhancement. ADC map (d) shows diffusion restriction. *Source:* used with permission from Barrow Neurological Institute.

Miscellaneous tumors/tumor-like lesions

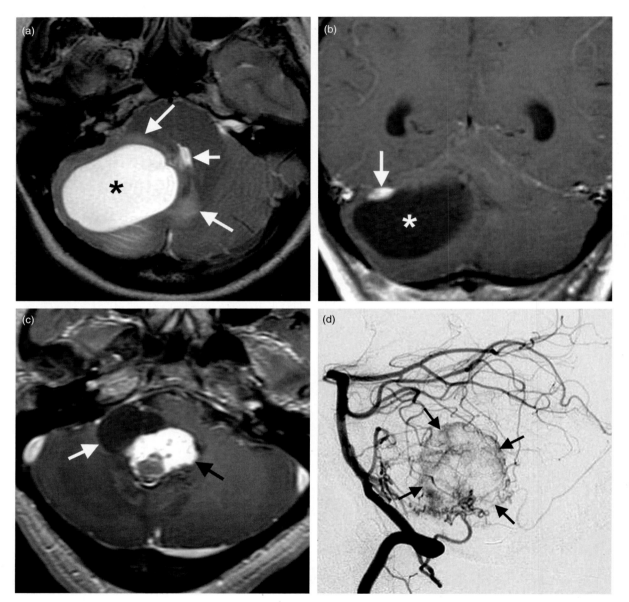

Figure 6.102 Hemangioblastomas: axial T2WI (a) and post-contrast coronal T1WI (b) show a predominantly cystic cerebellar mass (asterisk) with a small superficially located enhancing nodule (arrow in [b]) and surrounding edema (long arrows in [a]). There is mass effect on the fourth ventricle (short arrow in [a]). Post-contrast axial T1WI (c) in a second patient shows a complex cystic (white arrow)/ solid (black arrow) hemangioblastoma. Lateral vertebral artery angiograms (d,e) show the marked hypervascularity (arrows) of this lesion. Post-contrast axial T1WI (f) in a third patient shows a predominantly solid, enhancing hemangioblastoma of the dorsal medulla (arrow). *Source:* Figure 6.102c,d,e used with permission from Barrow Neurological Institute.

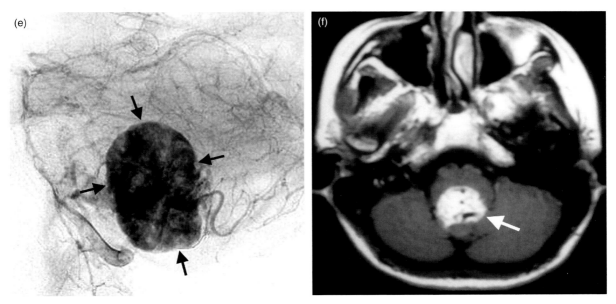

Figure 6.102 (*cont.*)

Pineal region tumors/masses

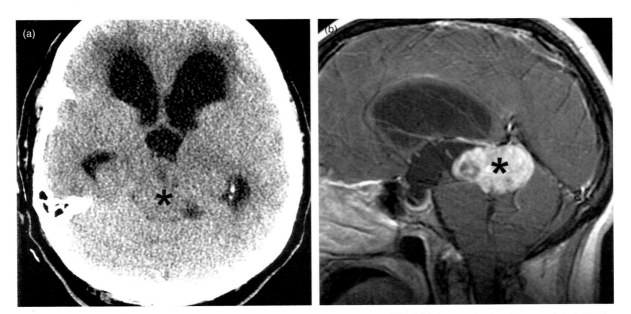

Figure 6.103 **Pineocytoma:** non-contrast axial CT image (a) and post-contrast sagittal T1WI (b) show a pineal region mass (asterisk) with diffuse but mildly heterogeneous enhancement. There is obliteration of the tectal plate and obstructive hydrocephalus.
Source: Used with permission from Barrow Neurological Institute.

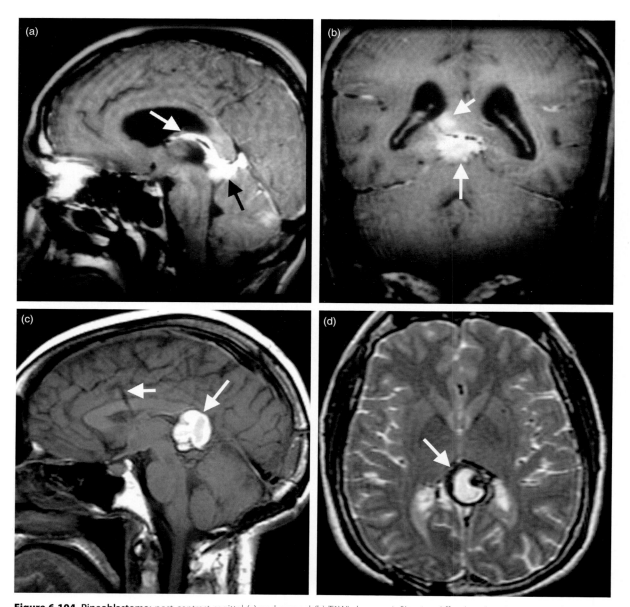

Figure 6.104 Pineoblastoma: post-contrast sagittal (a) and coronal (b) T1WI show an infiltrative diffusely enhancing mass in the pineal region, spreading into the cistern of the velum interpositum (white arrow in [a]), the tectal plate, quadrigeminal plate cistern (black arrow in [a] and long arrow in [b]), and the right side of the splenium of the corpus callosum (short arrow in [b]). Non-contrast sagittal T1WI (c) and axial T2WI (d) in another patient show a hemorrhagic mass (long arrow in [c] and arrow in [d]) in the pineal region. A ventricular shunt is seen (short arrow) in (c). *Source:* Figure 6.104c,d used with permission from Barrow Neurological Institute.

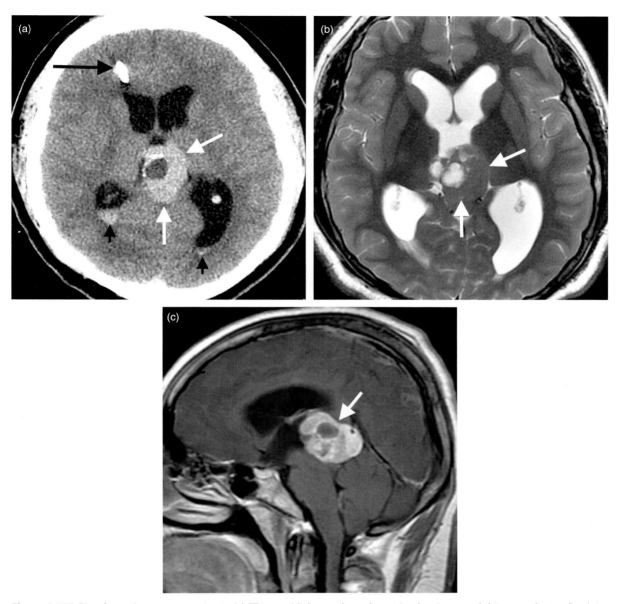

Figure 6.105 **Pineal germinoma:** non-contrast axial CT image (a) shows a hyperdense pineal region mass (white arrows) extending into the third ventricle, with cystic change that is engulfing the pineal calcification. Intraventricular blood (short black arrows) secondary to placement of a ventricular drainage catheter for obstructive hydrocephalus (long black arrow) is seen. Axial T2WI (b) and post-contrast sagittal T1WI (c) show the low signal of the mass on T2WI (arrows in [b]) and the diffuse enhancement with cystic change and compression of the tectal plate (arrow in [c]). *Source:* Used with permission from Barrow Neurological Institute.

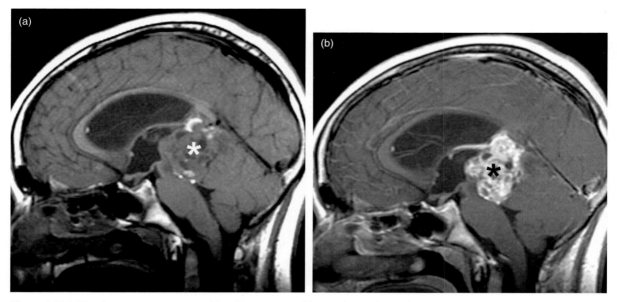

Figure 6.106 Pineal teratoma: pre-contrast (a) and post-contrast (b) sagittal T1WI show a large heterogeneous pineal region mass (asterisks), with areas of T1 shortening on the pre-contrast image consistent with areas of fat signal. Compression of the tectal plate and cerebral aqueduct with obstructive hydrocephalus is present. *Source:* Used with permission from Barrow Neurological Institute.

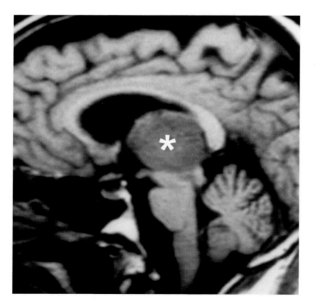

Figure 6.107 Thalamic glioma: this non-contrast T1WI shows a thalamic glioma (asterisk) that could be mistaken for a pineal region mass, although it is more anterior than would be expected for a mass of pineal origin. Other imaging planes would help distinguish these two entities.

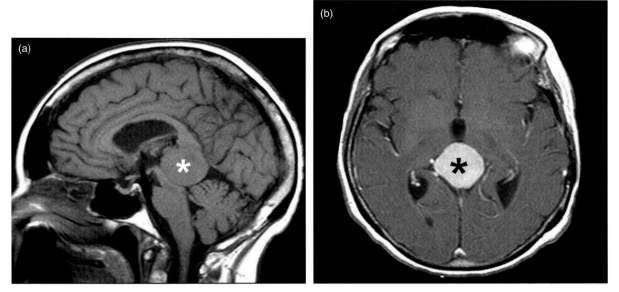

Figure 6.108 Pineal region meningioma: pre-contrast sagittal (a) and post-contrast axial (b) T1WI show a homogeneous mass with diffuse homogeneous enhancement (asterisk). T2WI (not shown) showed signal similar to gray matter.

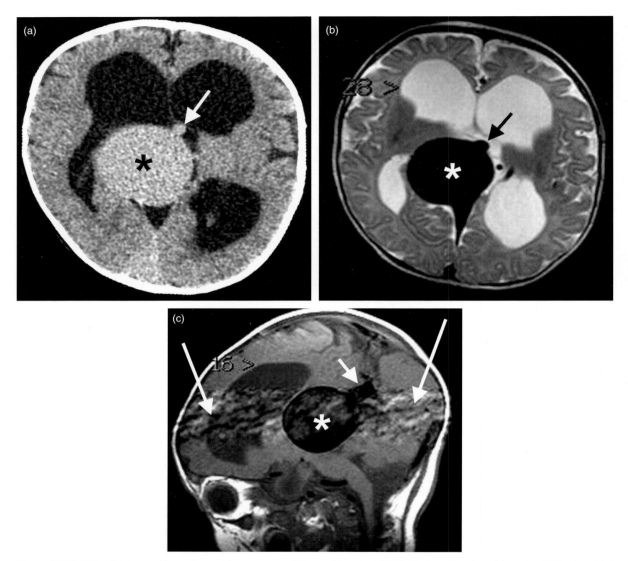

Figure 6.109 Vein of Galen malformation: axial non-contrast CT image (a) and axial T2WI (b) show dilatation of the vein of Galen (asterisks) with a mural type arterial feeder (arrows in [a,b]). In (b) note the stenosis of the straight sinus. Sagittal non-contrast T1WI (c) shows the dilated vein of Galen (asterisk) and a persistent falcine sinus (short arrow). A pulsatile motion artifact related to the high-flow vascular malformation is seen along the phase encoding direction (long arrows).

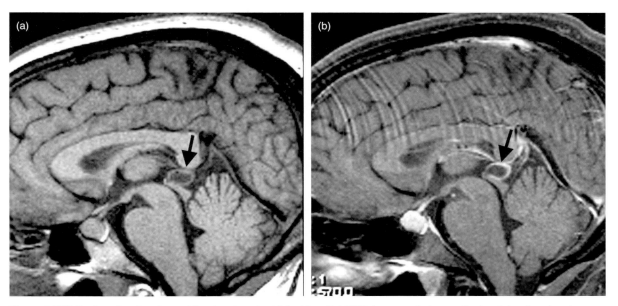

Figure 6.110 Benign pineal cyst: pre- (a) and post-contrast (b) mid-sagittal T1WI show a well-circumscribed peripherally enhancing benign pineal cyst (arrows).

Primary pituitary tumors

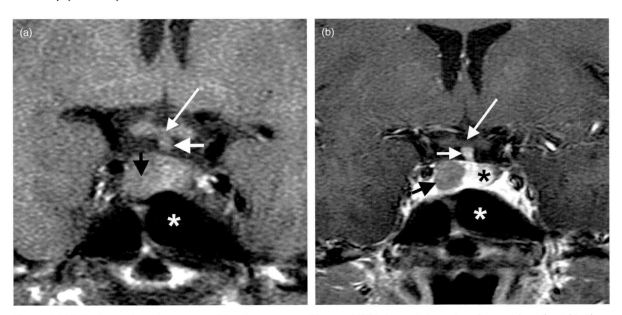

Figure 6.111 Pituitary microadenoma: pre- (a) and post-contrast (b) coronal T1WI demonstrate a microadenoma along the right side of the pituitary gland, which is hypointense (short black arrows). The infindibulum (short white arrow) is slightly displaced to the left. A normal enhancing pituitary gland is indicated by the black asterisk in (b). The optic chiasm is indicated by the long arrow and the sphenoid sinus by white asterisks in (a,b).

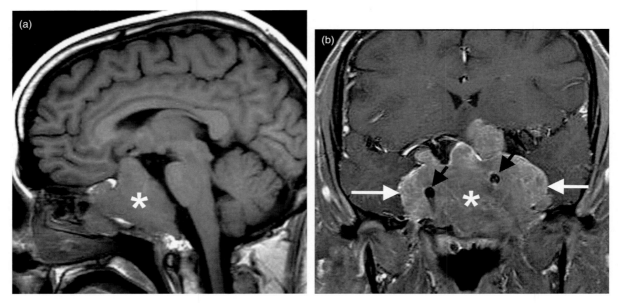

Figure 6.112 Invasive pituitary macroadenoma: non-contrast sagittal T1WI (a) shows a large mass (asterisk in [a,b]) destroying and replacing the sphenoid bone and clivus, and extending into the prepontine cistern, suprasellar cistern, and sphenoid sinus. Post-contrast coronal T1WI (b) shows invasion into the cavernous sinuses (long white arrows) with encasement of the carotid arteries (black arrows).

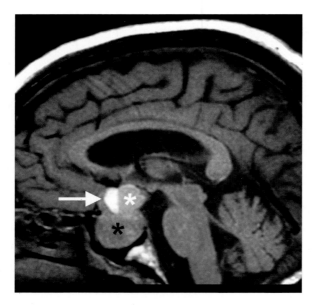

Figure 6.113 Hemorrhagic pituitary macroadenoma: non-contrast sagittal T1WI shows an intrasellar macroadenoma (black asterisk) extending into the suprasellar region (white asterisk), with a blood level (arrow).

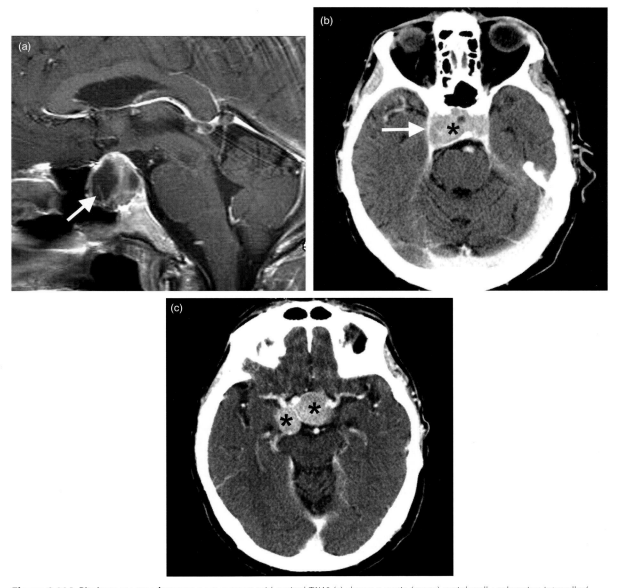

Figure 6.114 **Pituitary macroadenoma:** post-contrast mid-sagittal T1WI (a) shows a cystic (arrow) peripherally enhancing intrasellar/suprasellar macroadenoma. Post-contrast axial CT image (b,c) in another patient shows a macroadenoma (asterisks in [b,c]) invading the right cavernous sinus (arrow in [b]), with multilobulated suprasellar extension (c).

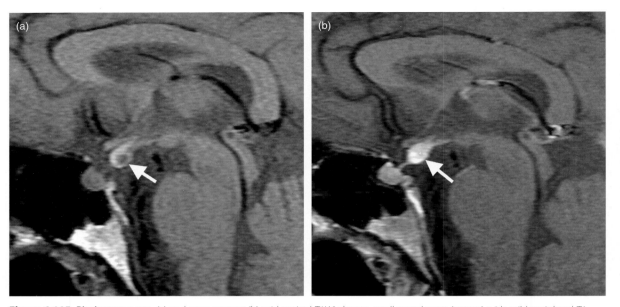

Figure 6.115 Pituicytoma: pre- (a) and post-contrast (b) mid-sagittal T1WI show a small round mass (arrows) with mild peripheral T1 hyperintensity on pre-contrast images (a), with diffuse homogeneous enhancement (b) along the pituitary stalk (infindibulum). *Source:* Used with permission from Barrow Neurological Institute.

Tumors/tumor-like lesions related to the craniopharyngeal duct

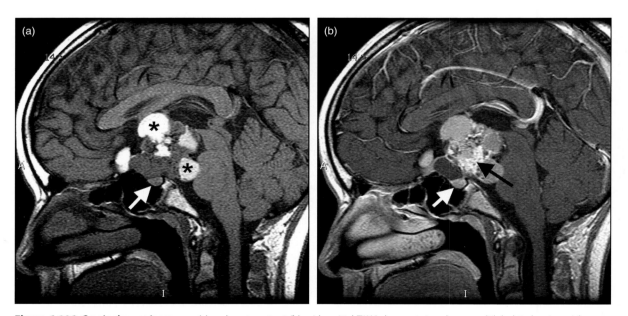

Figure 6.116 Craniopharyngioma: pre- (a) and post-contrast (b) mid-sagittal T1WI demonstrate a large, multilobulated, extra-axial mass with the epicenter in the suprasellar region. Hyperintense cysts on the pre-contrast image (asterisks in [a]) and areas of enhancement (black arrow in [b]) are visible. A normal pituitary gland is indicated by short white arrows in (a,b). Non-contrast sagittal T1WI (c) in a second patient shows a very large, lobulated craniopharyngioma with extensive hyperintense cysts (asterisk). *Source:* Figure 6.116c used with permission from Barrow Neurological Institute.

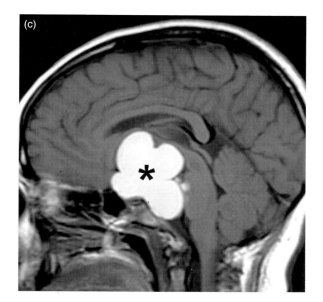

Figure 6.116 (*cont.*)

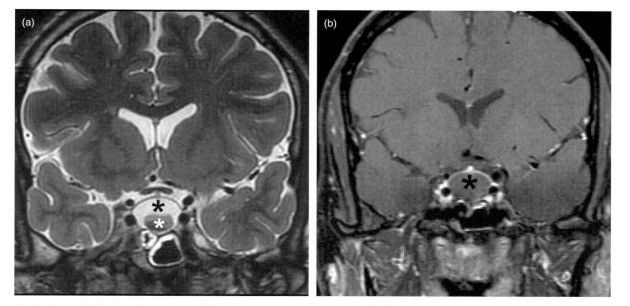

Figure 6.117 Rathke's cleft cyst: coronal T2WI (a) and post-contrast coronal T1WI (b) show an intrasellar/suprasellar cyst (black asterisk) with a hypointense intracystic nodule (white asterisk in [a]) and only thin peripheral enhancement post-contrast (b). *Source:* Used with permission from Barrow Neurological Institute.

Other suprasellar masses/mass-like lesions: SATCHMOE

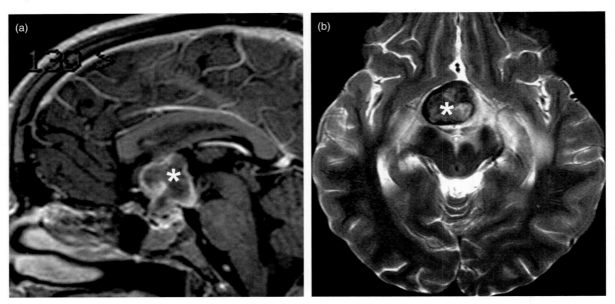

Figure 6.118 Suprasellar germinoma: post-contrast sagittal T1WI (a) and axial T2WI (b) show a heterogeneous suprasellar mass (asterisk) extending into the third ventricle, with mixed signal on T2WI (b) and peripheral enhancement on the post-contrast image (a).

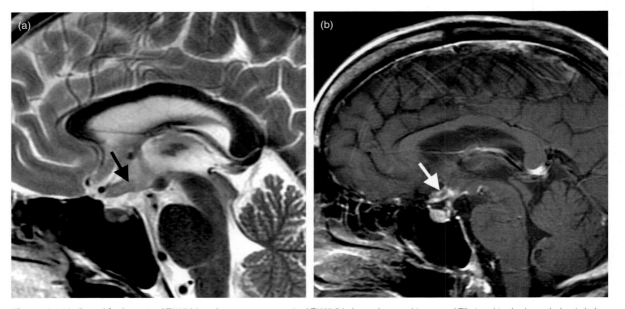

Figure 6.119 Sarcoidosis: sagittal T2WI (a) and post-contrast sagittal T1WI (b) show abnormal increased T2 signal in the hypothalamic/tuber cinereum/optic chiasm region (arrow in [a]) with contrast enhancement (arrow in [b]). *Source:* Used with permission from Barrow Neurological Institute.

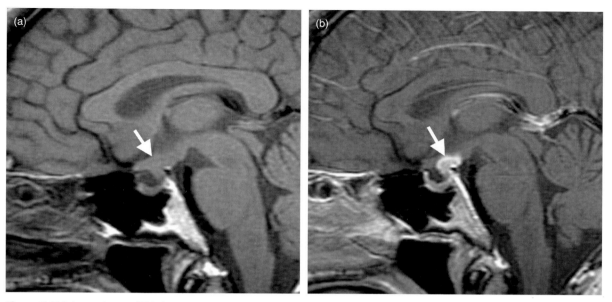

Figure 6.120 **Langerhans cell histiocytosis:** pre- (a) and post-contrast (b) mid-sagittal T1WI show thickening and pathologic enhancement along the hypothalamic/tuber cinereum region (arrow) and pituitary stalk. *Source:* Used with permission from Barrow Neurological Institute.

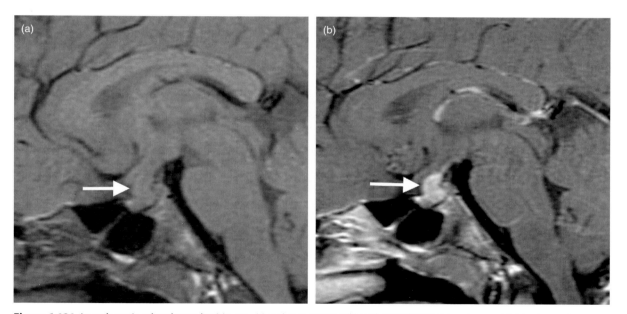

Figure 6.121 **Lymphocytic adenohypophysitis:** pre- (a) and post-contrast (b) mid-sagittal T1WI show abnormal thickening and enhancement (arrows) of the pituitary stalk (infindibulum). *Source:* Used with permission from Barrow Neurological Institute.

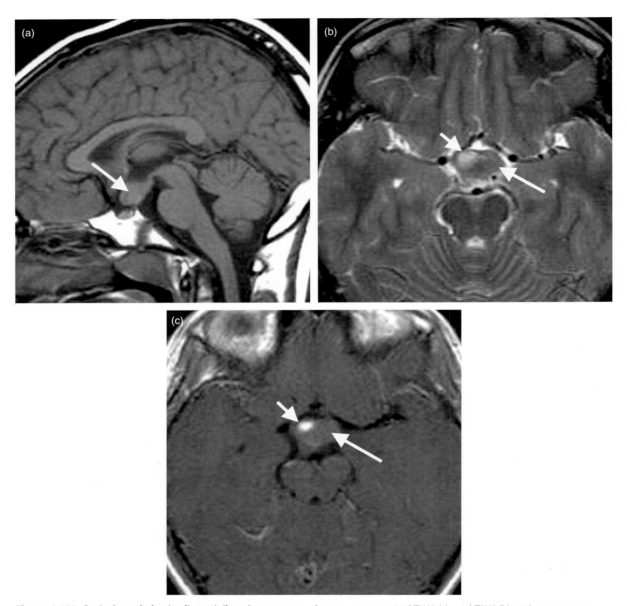

Figure 6.122 Opticohypothalamic glioma (pilocytic astrocytoma): non-contrast sagittal T1WI (a), axial T2WI (b), and post-contrast axial T1WI (c) show mass-like enlargement of the optic chiasm/hypothalamus (long arrow) projecting into the inferior third ventricle (arrow in [a]). There is a focal region of increased T2 signal with enhancement along the right anterior margin (short arrow in [b,c]).

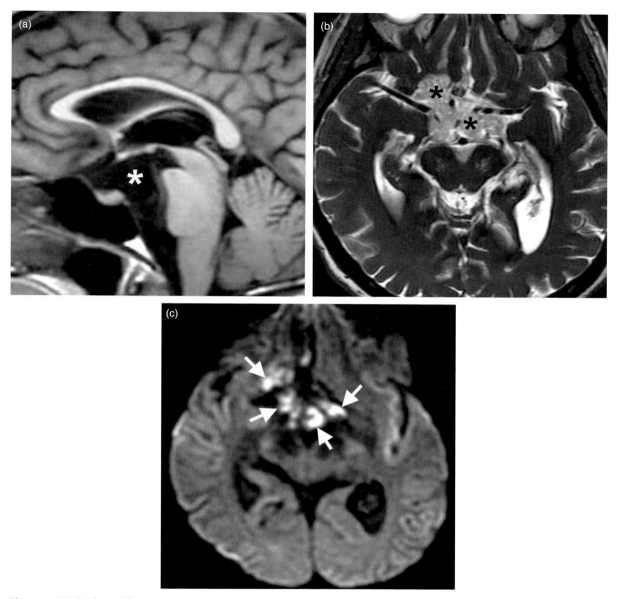

Figure 6.123 **Epidermoid cyst:** non-contrast sagittal T1WI (a), axial T2WI (b), and diffusion trace image (c) demonstrate a CSF-similar extra-axial lesion (asterisk in [a]), with mass effect in the suprasellar, interpeduncular, and prepontine cisterns, and with complex internal architecture (asterisks in [b]) and diffusion restriction (arrows in [c]).

Intraventricular tumors

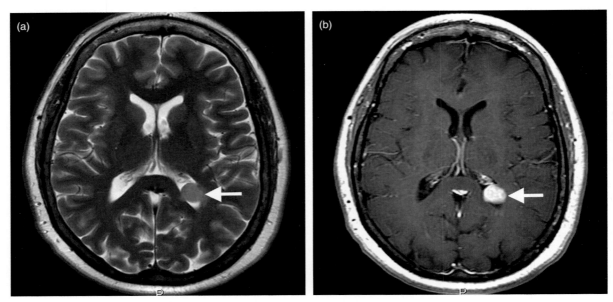

Figure 6.124 Intraventricular meningioma: axial T2WI (a) and post-contrast axial T1WI (b) show a well-circumscribed rounded mass, with signal similar to gray matter (arrow in [a]) and diffuse homogeneous enhancement (arrow in [b]), in the atrium of the left lateral ventricle.

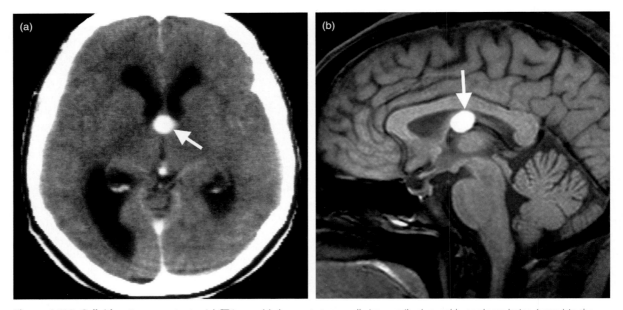

Figure 6.125 Colloid cyst: non-contrast axial CT image (a) demonstrates a well-circumscribed round hyperdense lesion (arrow) in the anterior third ventricle at the level of the foramen of Monroe, with dilatation of both lateral ventricles. Non-contrast fat suppressed sagittal T1WI (b) demonstrates a well-circumscribed round hyperintense mass (arrow) in the anteriosuperior third ventricular region.

Primary extra-axial neoplasms

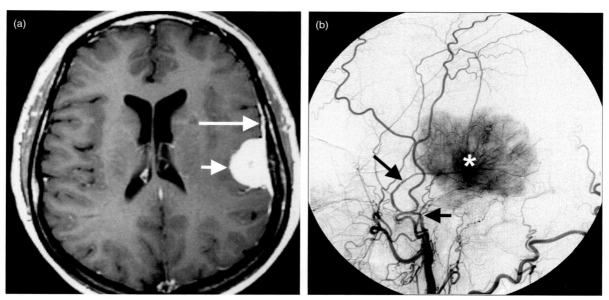

Figure 6.126 Meningioma WHO grade I (convexity): post-contrast axial T1WI (a) and lateral external carotid angiogram (b) show an extra-axial mass with diffuse homogeneous contrast enhancement (short arrow in [a]), with thickening and enhancement of the adjacent dura (dural tail) indicated by the long arrow in (a). The lateral angiographic image (b) shows a prominent tumor stain (asterisk) supplied by the middle meningeal artery (black arrows).

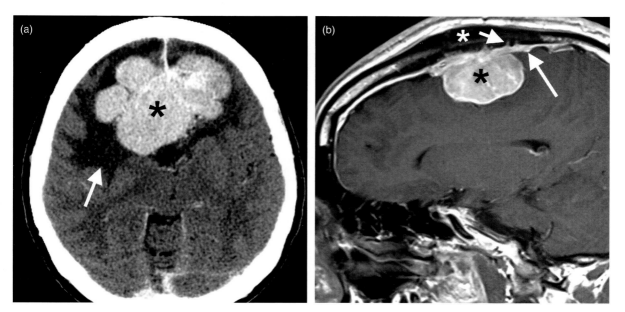

Figure 6.127 Meningiomas: post-contrast axial CT image in patient #1 (a) shows a large diffusely enhancing multilobulated bilateral mass, straddling the falx cerebri (asterisk), with prominent vasogenic edema (arrow). Patient #2, post-contrast sagittal T1WI (b) shows a diffusely enhancing high convexity meningioma (black asterisk) and dural tail (long arrow) with invasion of the inner table (short arrow) and marked hyperostosis of the skull (white asterisk).

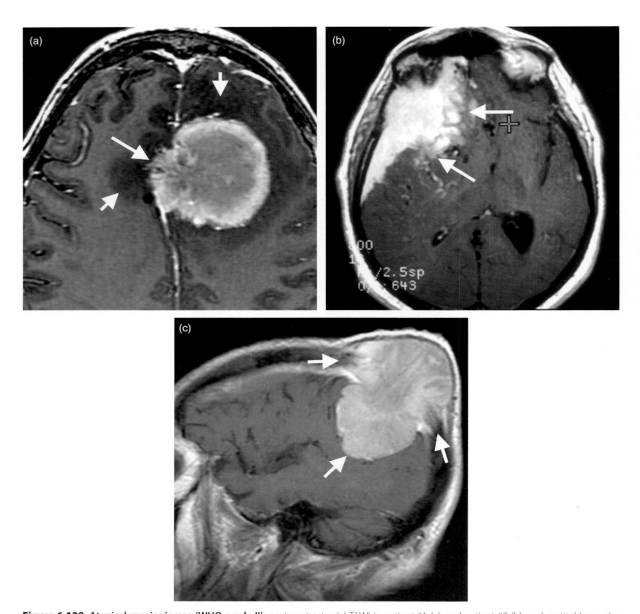

Figure 6.128 Atypical meningiomas (WHO grade II): post-contrast axial T1WI in patient #1 (a), and patient #2 (b), and sagittal image in patient #3 (c) demonstrate enhancing meningiomas with irregular, infiltrative appearing margins (long arrows in [a,b]) and vasogenic edema (short arrows in [a]). In (c) the meningioma is destroying the bone and extending through the parietal skull into the overlying scalp. *Source:* Figure 6.128c used with permission from Barrow Neurological Institute.

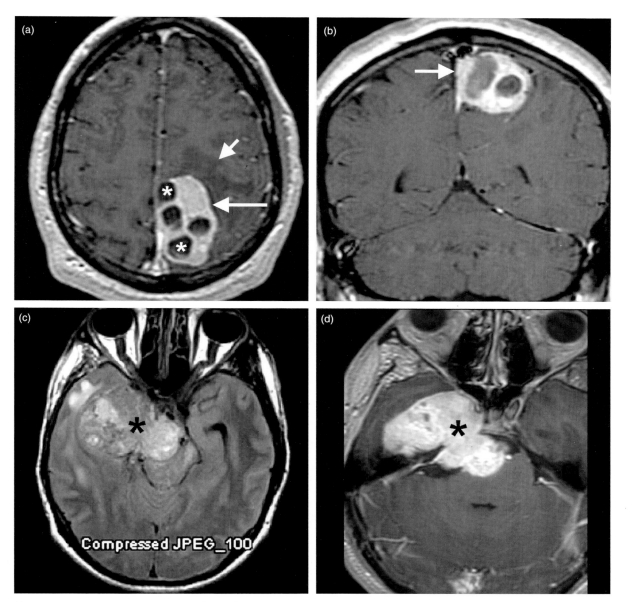

Figure 6.129 Hemangiopericytoma: axial (a) and coronal (b) post-contrast T1WI in patient #1 show a dural based extra-axial enhancing mass (long arrow in [a] and arrow in [b]), with cystic/necrotic changes (asterisks in [a]) and vasogenic edema (short arrow in [a]). In patient #2, axial FLAIR image (c) and axial post-contrast T1WI (d) show an extra-axial mass with heterogeneous signal (asterisk in [c]) and enhancement in the middle and posterior cranial fossa (asterisk in [d]). *Source:* Used with permission from Barrow Neurological Institute.

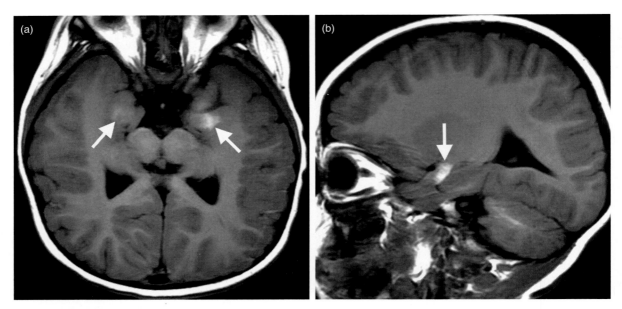

Figure 6.130 Melanocytic deposits: axial (a) and sagittal (b) non-contrast T1WI show hyperintense foci in the amygdaloid nuclei (arrows). Similar appearing deposits were present along the leptomeningeal surfaces of the cerebellum (not shown) in this patient with neurocutaneous melanosis.

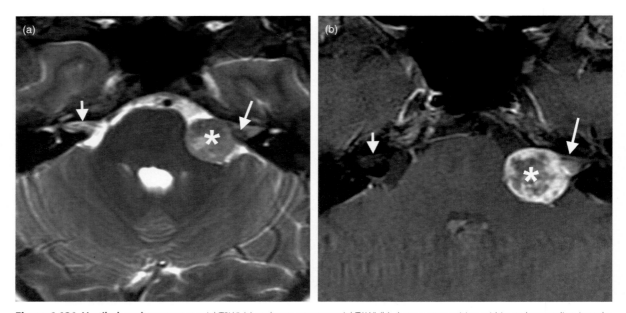

Figure 6.131 Vestibular schwannoma: axial T2WI (a) and post-contrast axial T1WI (b) show a mass arising within and expanding into the left internal auditory canal (long white arrows on the left), extending through the porus acousticus into the CP angle cistern, and with associated mass effect. The CP angle cistern component is heterogeneous (asterisk). The short white arrow on the right indicates the normal size and contents within the right internal auditory canal.

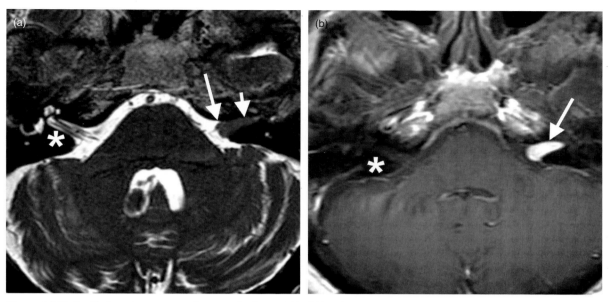

Figure 6.132 **Vestibular schwannoma – intracanalicular:** axial T2WI (a) and post-contrast axial T1WI (b) show a predominantly intracanalicular lesion (short arrow in [a] and arrow in [b]), extending to the porus acousticus (long arrow in [a]). The asterisk is just posterior to the normal appearing right internal auditory canal.

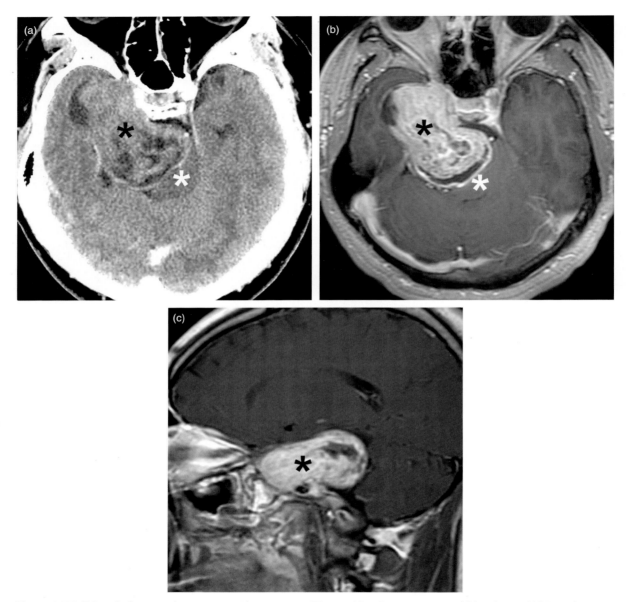

Figure 6.133 Trigeminal nerve schwannoma: axial non-contrast CT image (a) and post-contrast axial (b) and sagittal (c) T1WI show a heterogeneous tubular enhancing mass (black asterisk) extending along the expected course of the trigeminal nerve, with marked compression of the pons (white asterisk in [a,b]). *Source:* Used with permission from Barrow Neurological Institute.

Secondary intracranial neoplasms

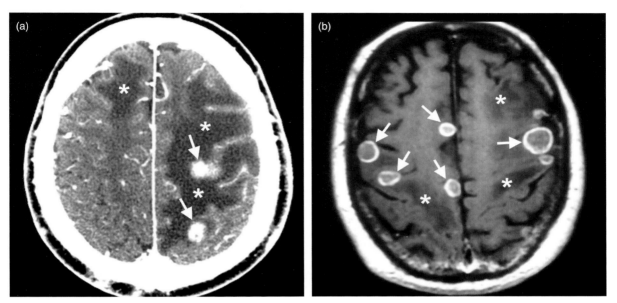

Figure 6.134 Intra-axial metastatic disease to the brain: post-contrast axial CT image of patient #1 (a) and post-contrast axial T1WI of patient #2 (b) show multiple enhancing cerebral lesions (arrows) with associated vasogenic edema (asterisks).

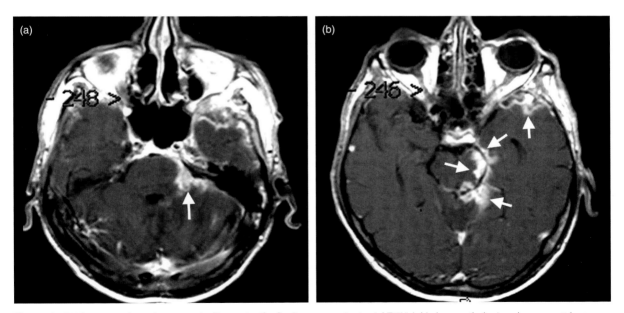

Figure 6.135 Leptomeningeal metastatic disease to the brain: post-contrast axial T1WI (a,b) show pathologic enhancement (arrows in [b]) along the pial surfaces of the left side of the brainstem and the medial and anterior pial surfaces of the left temporal lobe. The metastatic deposits are seen to extend into the underlying brain parenchyma. A focally prominent deposit in the left CP angle cistern is noted (arrow in [a]).

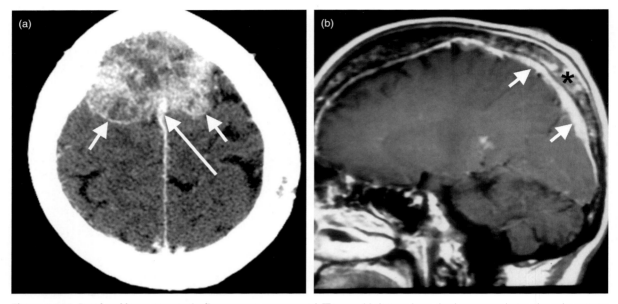

Figure 6.136 **Dural and bony metastatic disease:** post-contrast axial CT image (a) shows a large dural metastatic lesion along the anterior falx (long arrow) and frontal convexity (short arrows). Post-contrast sagittal T1WI (b) in a second patient shows dural (arrows) and bony (asterisk) metastatic lesions.

Non-neoplastic mass-like lesions

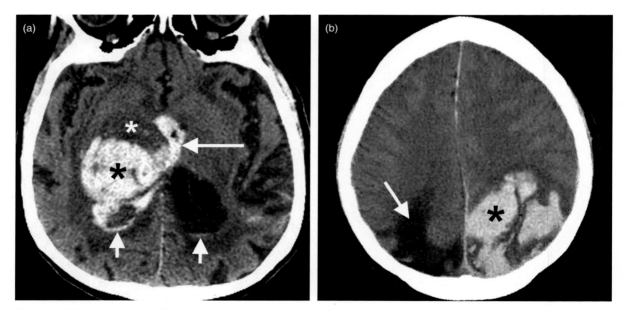

Figure 6.137 **Intraparenchymal hemorrhage:** non-contrast axial CT image (a) shows a large right thalamic hypertensive hemorrhage (black asterisk) with intraventricular extension (short and long arrows) and prominent surrounding edema (white asterisk). Non-contrast axial CT image (b) in a second patient shows a large cortical and subcortical hemorrhage on the left (black asterisk) and an old, resolved hemorrhage on the right (arrow) secondary to amyloid angiopathy. *Source:* Figure 6.137b used with permission from Barrow Neurological Institute.

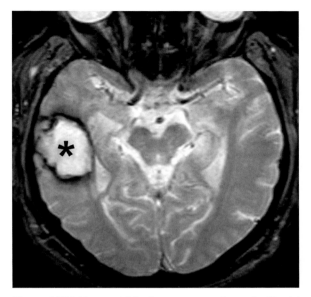

Figure 6.138 Temporal lobe hematoma: gradient echo T2 axial image shows a resolving subacute to chronic right temporal lobe hematoma (asterisk) with a peripheral rim of hemosiderin and central high signal from extra-cellular methemoglobin.

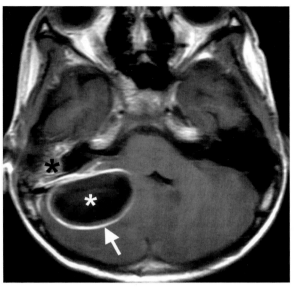

Figure 6.139 Cerebellar abscess: post-contrast axial T1WI shows a peripherally enhancing (arrow) cystic (white asterisk) mass in the right cerebellum, with associated mass effect. Note the pathologic enhancement in the right mastoid region (black asterisk) reflecting adjacent mastoiditis. The cerebellar mass demonstrated diffusion restriction (not shown).

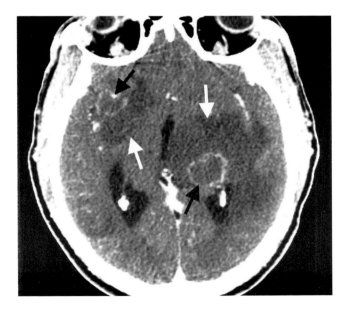

Figure 6.140 Toxoplasmosis: post-contrast axial CT image shows ring enhancing lesions (black arrows) in the left thalamus and right subinsular regions, with vasogenic edema (white arrows).

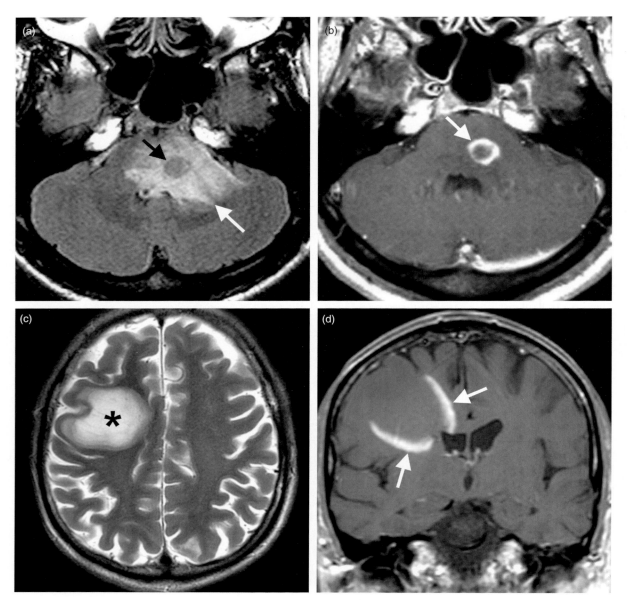

Figure 6.141 Tumefactive multiple sclerosis: axial FLAIR image (a) and post-contrast axial T1WI (b) in patient #1 shows a ring enhancing lesion in the left pons (black arrow in [a] and white arrow in [b]), with extensive surrounding edema (white arrow in [a]) and mass effect. Axial T2WI (c) and post-contrast coronal T1WI (d) in patient #2 shows a mass-like region of increased T2 signal (asterisk in [c]) and peripheral enhancement (arrows in [d]) with mass effect. *Source:* Figure 6.141c,d used with permission from Barrow Neurological Institute.

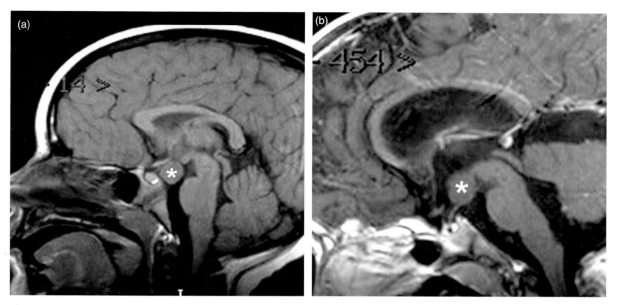

Figure 6.142 Hypothalamic hamartoma: non-contrast sagittal T1WI (a) in patient #1 and post-contrast sagittal T1WI (b) in patient #2 show a well-circumscribed pedunculated mass (asterisk in [a]) projecting inferiorly from the tuber cinereum, without contrast enhancement (not shown) and a non-enhancing hamartoma of the tuber cinereum (asterisk in [b]) projecting superiorly into the third ventricle.

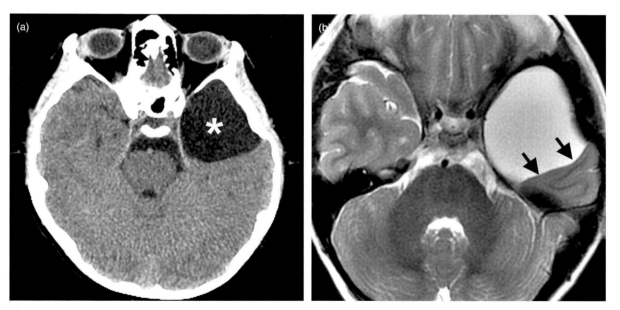

Figure 6.143 Arachnoid cyst – middle cranial fossa: non-contrast axial CT (a) and axial T2WI (b) show a well marginated extra-axial CSF-identical fluid collection (asterisk in [a]) in the anterior middle cranial fossa. Mass effect upon the left temporal lobe is noted, with gray matter at the interface (black arrows in [b]) indicating an extra-axial lesion.

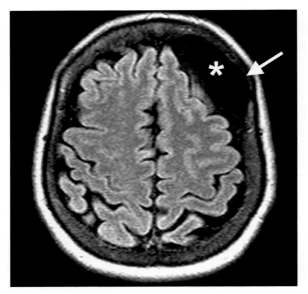

Figure 6.144 Arachnoid cyst – lateral convexity: axial FLAIR image shows a left frontal convexity arachnoid cyst (asterisk) with mass effect upon the frontal lobe and bony remodeling of the adjacent calvarium (arrow).

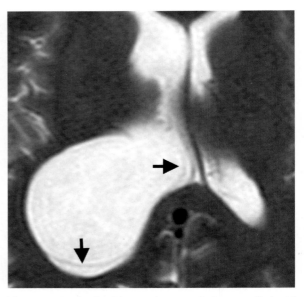

Figure 6.146 Arachnoid cyst – intraventricular: magnified axial T2WI shows a CSF-identical fluid collection within and expanding the atrium of the right lateral ventricle. Note the thin, subtle wall of the cyst (arrows).

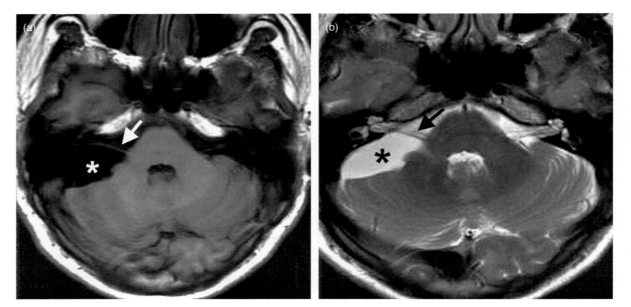

Figure 6.145 Arachnoid cyst – CP angle cistern: non-contrast axial T1WI (a) and axial T2WI (b) show a CSF-identical extra-axial fluid collection in the right CP angle cistern (asterisk) with stretching/mass effect upon the right seventh and eighth nerve complex (arrow).

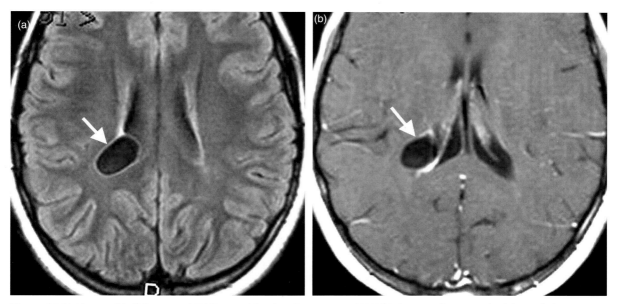

Figure 6.147 Neuroepithelial cyst: axial FLAIR image (a) and axial post-contrast T1WI (b) show a well-circumscribed thin-walled cyst (arrow) without significant contrast enhancement immediately adjacent to the superior trigone of the right lateral ventricle.

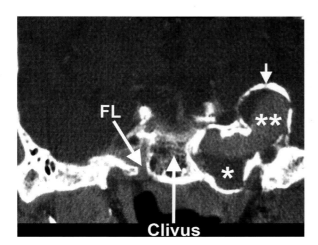

Figure 6.148 Fusiform atherosclerotic aneurysm: post-contrast coronal CT image shows a partially thrombosed (single asterisk), giant fusiform, atherosclerotic aneurysm with peripheral calcifications (small arrow), involving the horizontal petrous internal carotid artery and projecting superiorly into the left middle cranial fossa. The enhancing patent lumen is shown by double asterisks. FL indicates foramen lacerum.

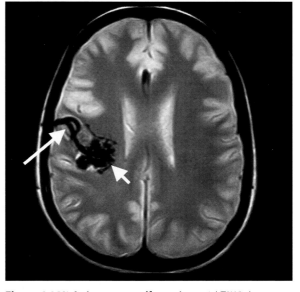

Figure 6.149 Atriovenous malformation: axial T2WI shows the typical appearance of a high-flow pial arteriovenous malformation with arterial feeders/draining veins (long arrow) and the nidus (short arrow).

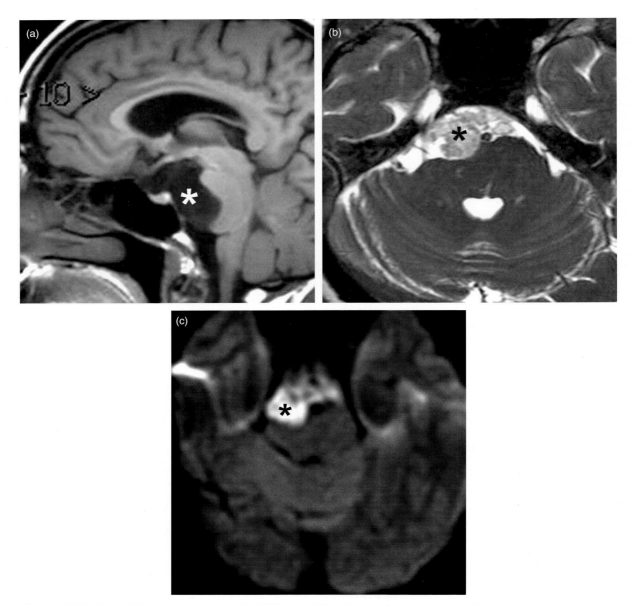

Figure 6.150 Epidermoid cyst: non-contrast sagittal T1WI (a), axial T2WI (b), and diffusion trace image (c) demonstrate a low signal intensity lesion (a) with internal architecture (b) and diffusion restriction (c) within the prepontine cistern (asterisks), with mass effect upon the pons.

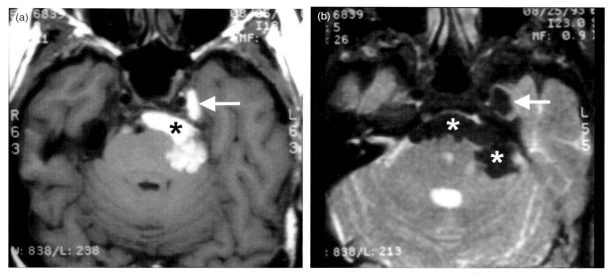

Figure 6.151 Bright epidermoid: non-contrast axial T1WI (a) and axial T2WI (b) show an extra-axial lesion (asterisks) within the prepontine cistern, extending into the left CP angle cistern and left Meckel's cave (arrow). It exhibits high T1 and low T2 signal and represents an atypical epidermoid.

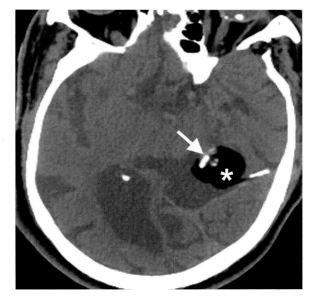

Figure 6.152 Dermoid cyst: non-contrast axial CT image shows a mixed density mass-like lesion with predominant fatty density (asterisk) but with smaller areas of calcification and soft tissue density (arrow).

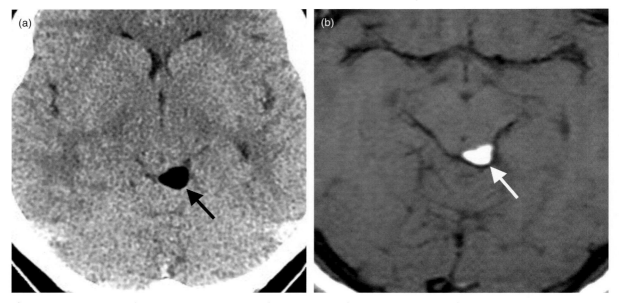

Figure 6.153 Lipoma: axial non-contrast CT image (a) and non-contrast axial T1WI (b) show a simple fatty density/signal intensity mass (arrow) in the left side of the quadrigeminal plate cistern.

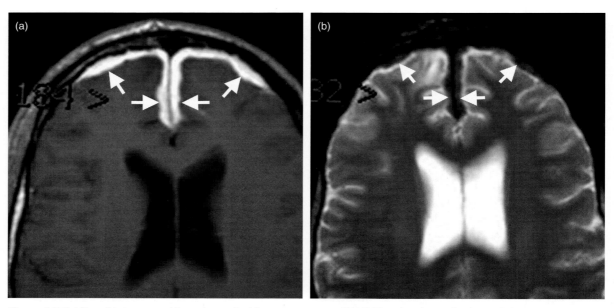

Figure 6.154 Idiopathic hypertrophic pachymeningitis: post-contrast axial T1WI (a) and axial T2WI (b) show mildly irregular dural thickening and pathologic contrast enhancement (arrows).

Intracranial infectious/inflammatory lesions

Pediatric infectious diseases

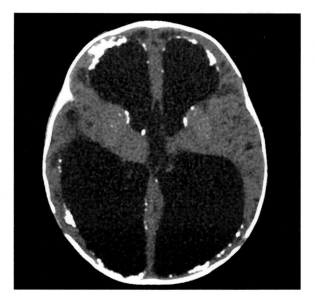

Figure 6.155 Neonatal cytomegalovirus: non-contrast axial CT image demonstrates ventriculomegaly with multifocal, segmental areas of pathologic calcification in the ependymal/subependymal regions surrounding the lateral ventricles. There is also parenchymal volume loss.

Pyogenic

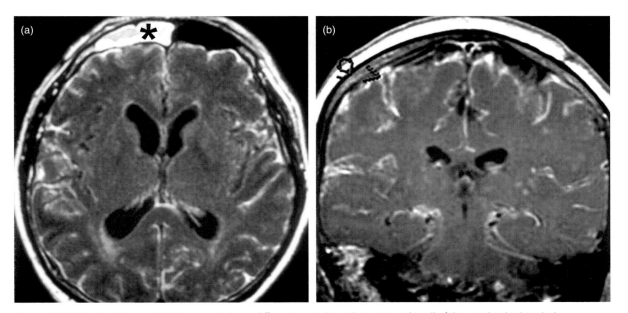

Figure 6.156 Meningitis: axial FLAIR image (a) shows diffuse increased signal intensity within all of the visualized sulci, which demonstrates contrast enhancement on the coronal post-contrast T1WI (b). The pattern of enhancement represents an infectious leptomeningitis. Note the associated frontal sinusitis (asterisk in [a]).

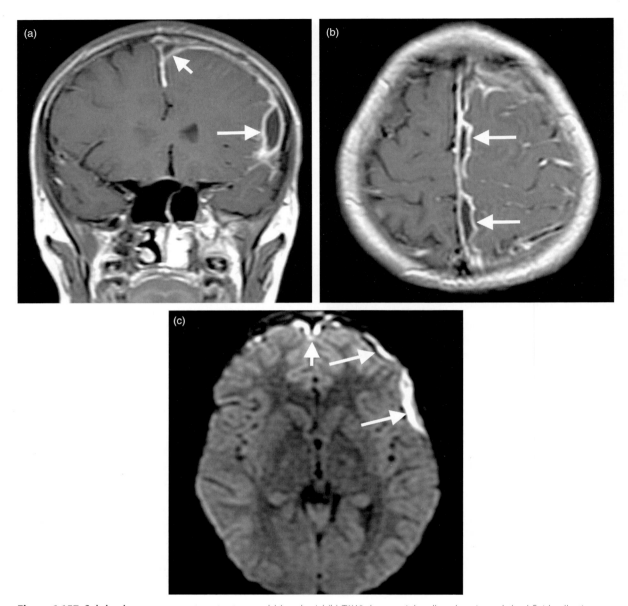

Figure 6.157 Subdural empyema: post-contrast coronal (a) and axial (b) T1WI show peripherally enhancing subdural fluid collections (arrows) along the lateral convexity and interhemispheric regions, which show diffusion restriction (arrows in [c]). Also note the leptomeningeal enhancement within the left hemispheric sulci in (b). *Source:* Used with permission from Barrow Neurological Institute.

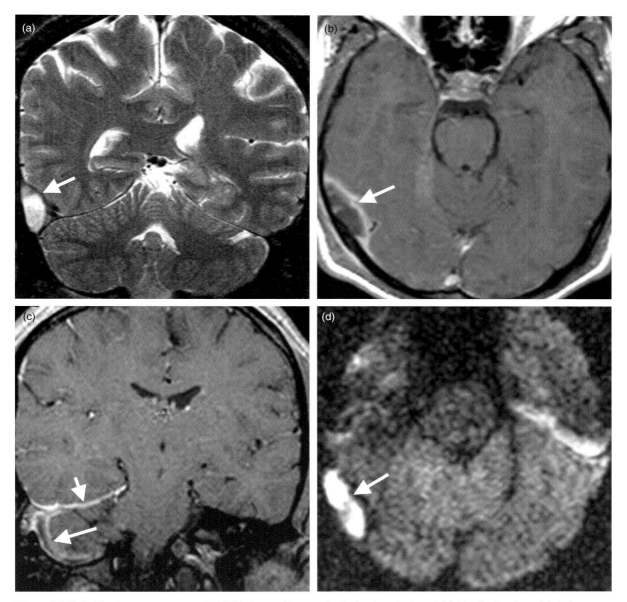

Figure 6.158 Epidural empyema: coronal T2WI (a) shows a biconvex, lenticular shaped extra-axial fluid collection (arrow) just above the lateral aspect of the tentorium cerebelli. Post-contrast axial T1WI (b) shows peripheral enhancement (arrow). Post-contrast coronal T1WI (c) shows pathologic enhancement and mild thickening of the tentorium cerebelli (short arrow) and peripheral enhancement surrounding the thrombosed sigmoid sinus (long arrow). Diffusion trace image (d) shows prominent diffusion restriction (arrow). This epidural empyema was a complication of right mastoiditis.

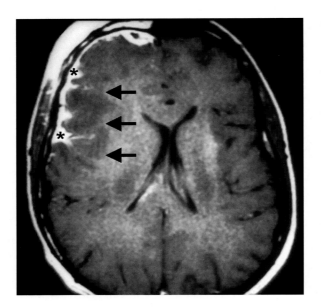

Figure 6.159 Meningitis and cerebritis: post-contrast axial T1WI shows pathologic thickening and enhancement of the dura and leptomeninges (asterisks) associated with non-enhancing decreased signal intensity in the underlying frontal lobe parenchyma (black arrows), which showed diffuse increased T2 signal (not shown).

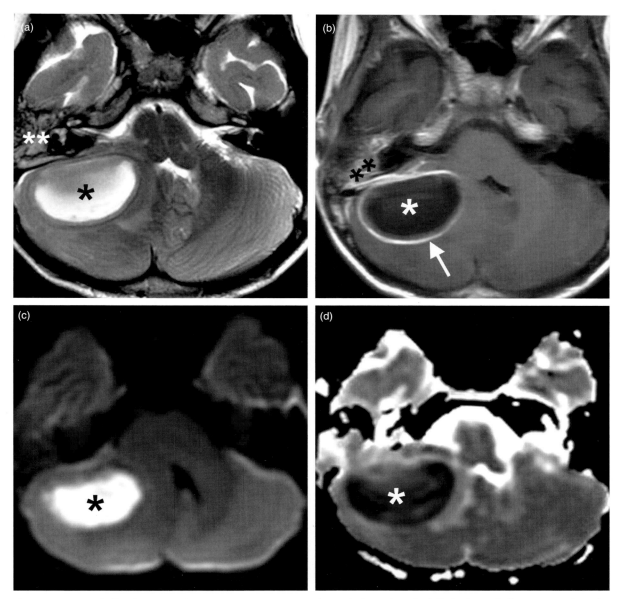

Figure 6.160 Cerebellar abscess: axial T2WI (a) and post-contrast axial T1WI (b) show a large fluid-filled right cerebellar mass (asterisk in [a,b]) with surrounding edema and mass effect with associated right mastoiditis (double asterisks in [a,b]). Thin, uniform peripheral enhancement is seen in (b) (arrow). Diffusion trace image (c) and ADC map (d) show prominent diffusion restriction. The abscess was a complication of mastoiditis.

Viral infection
Acute infective encephalitis

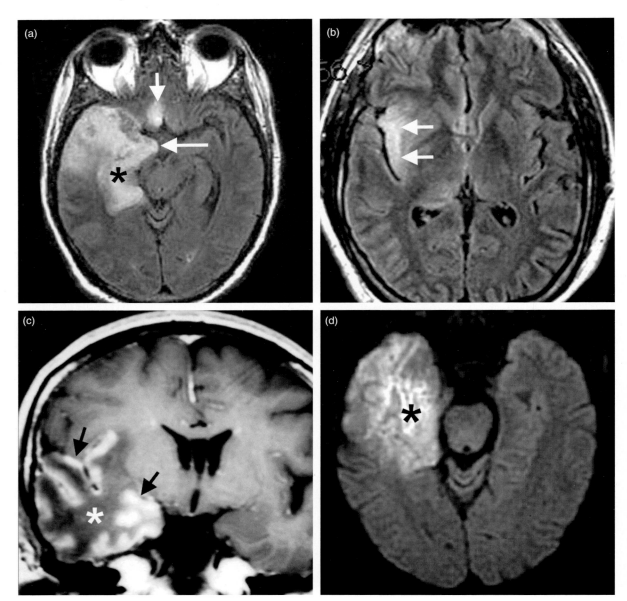

Figure 6.161 Herpes simplex encephalitis: axial FLAIR images (a,b) show increased signal and expansion of the right temporal lobe with uncal herniation (long arrow in [a]) and involvement of the right hippocampus (asterisk in [a]), insular/subinsular region (arrows in [b]), and posterior gyrus rectus (small arrow in [a]). Post-contrast coronal T1WI (c) shows gyriform enhancement (arrows), underlying parenchymal signal abnormality (asterisk), and swelling. Diffusion trace image (d) shows diffusion restriction (asterisk). Follow-up axial T2WI (e) one year later shows marked encephalomalacia with cystic change (single asterisk), marked hippocampal atrophy with enlargement of the temporal horn (double asterisk), and hemosiderin staining along the uncus (arrow).

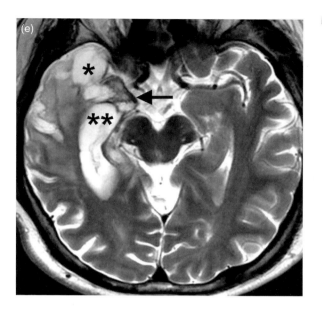

Figure 6.161 (*cont.*)

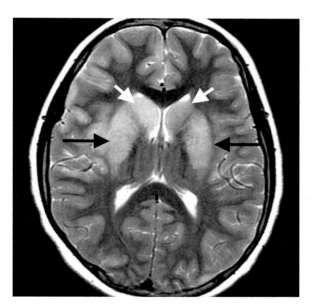

Figure 6.162 **Epstein-Barr encephalitis:** axial T2WI shows bilateral symmetric increased signal and swelling involving the lentiform nuclei (black arrows) and the caudate head (white arrows). *Source:* Used with permission from Barrow Neurological Institute.

Subacute encephalitis

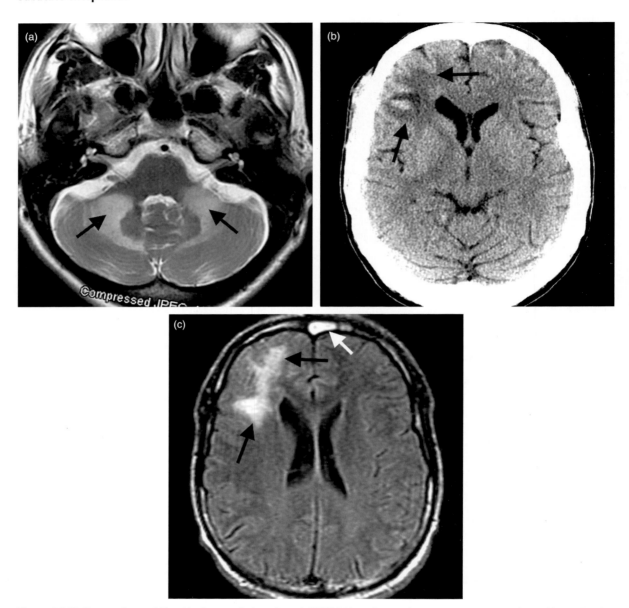

Figure 6.163 Progressive multifocal leukoencephalopathy: axial T2WI (a) in patient #1 shows symmetric increased signal (arrows) within the posterior middle cerebellar peduncles and adjacent anterior cerebellum without mass effect. There was no enhancement (not shown). Non-contrast axial CT (b) and axial FLAIR image (c) in patient #2 show decreased density and increased signal (black arrows) without mass effect in the right frontal white matter, extending to the subcortical U-fibers. There is no enhancement (not shown). Frontal sinusitis is indicated by the white arrow in (c). *Source:* Figure 6.163b,c used with permission from Barrow Neurological Institute.

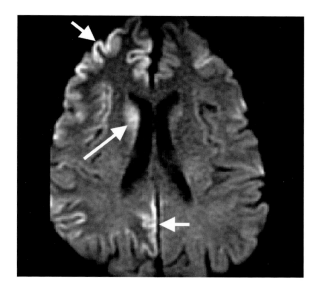

Figure 6.164 **Creutzfeldt-Jakob disease:** axial diffusion trace image shows increased signal intensity along the cortical surfaces (short arrows) in the right frontal and mesial right parietal lobes and in the right caudate nucleus (long arrow). *Source:* Used with permission from Barrow Neurological Institute.

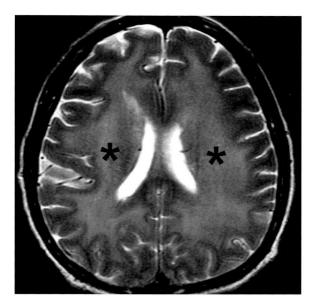

Figure 6.165 **HIV encephalitis:** axial T2WI shows diffuse increased T2 signal (asterisks) within the white matter of both cerebral hemispheres and generalized cortical atrophy in this 45-year-old HIV-positive patient.

Non-infectious encephalitis

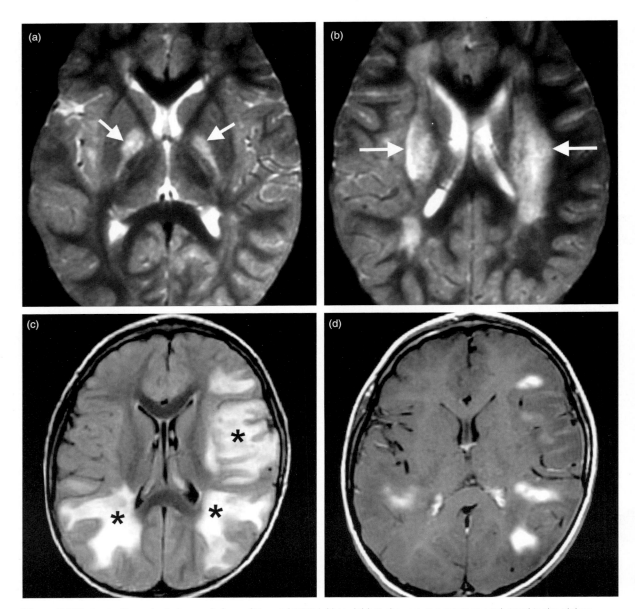

Figure 6.166 Acute disseminated encephalomyelitis: axial T2WI (a,b) in child #1 shows symmetric increased signal in the globus palladi (arrows in [a]) and increased signal intensity in the white matter (arrows in [b]). Axial FLAIR image (c), post-contrast axial T1WI (d), and sagittal T2WI (e) of the cervicothoracic spine in child #2 show asymmetric areas of increased T2 signal in the white matter (asterisks in [c]), with multifocal areas of enhancement (d) and increased T2 signal within the cervical and thoracic spinal cord (arrows in [e]). *Source:* Used with permission from Barrow Neurological Institute.

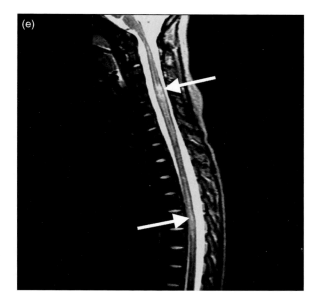

Figure 6.166 (*cont.*)

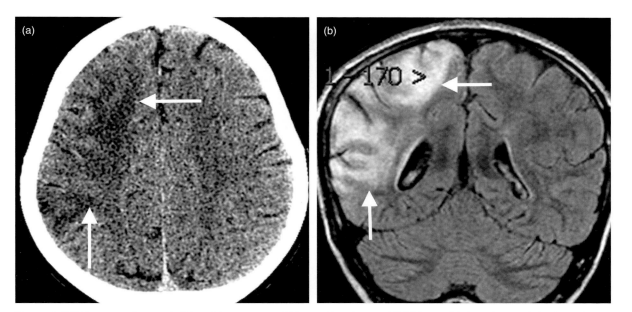

Figure 6.167 Rasmussen's encephalitis: axial non-contrast CT image (a) and coronal FLAIR image (b) show decreased density and increased signal intensity (arrows) in the right cerebral hemisphere. There was progressive involvement of the entire right hemisphere, progressing to atrophy in this patient, with intractable seizures. Eventually, a right hemispherectomy was performed.

Granulomatous infections/inflammatory lesions

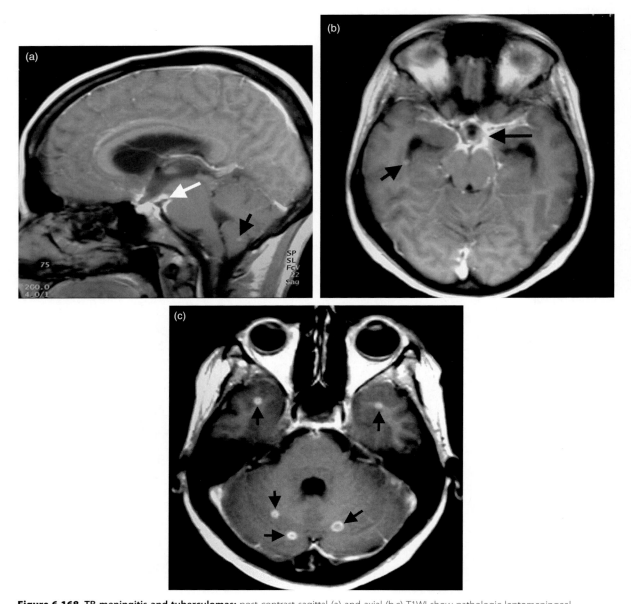

Figure 6.168 **TB meningitis and tuberculomas:** post-contrast sagittal (a) and axial (b,c) T1WI show pathologic leptomeningeal enhancement in the basal cisterns (white arrow in [a], long black arrow in [b]) with numerous enhancing parenchymal nodules (tuberculomas – short black arrows).

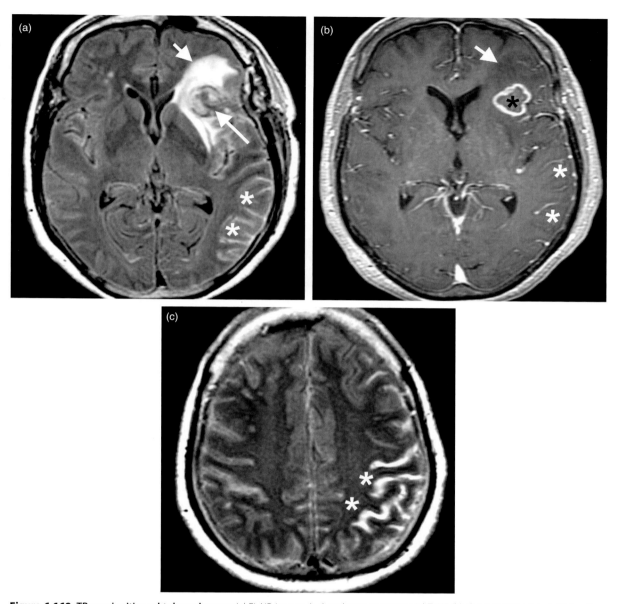

Figure 6.169 **TB meningitis and tuberculoma:** axial FLAIR images (a,c) and post-contrast axial T1WI (b) show increased signal intensity and leptomeningeal enhancement in the convexity sulci (most prominent on the left) (asterisks). Long white arrow (a) and black asterisk (b) show a ring enhancing tuberculoma with associated vasogenic edema (short white arrow in [a,b]). *Source:* Used with permission from Barrow Neurological Institute.

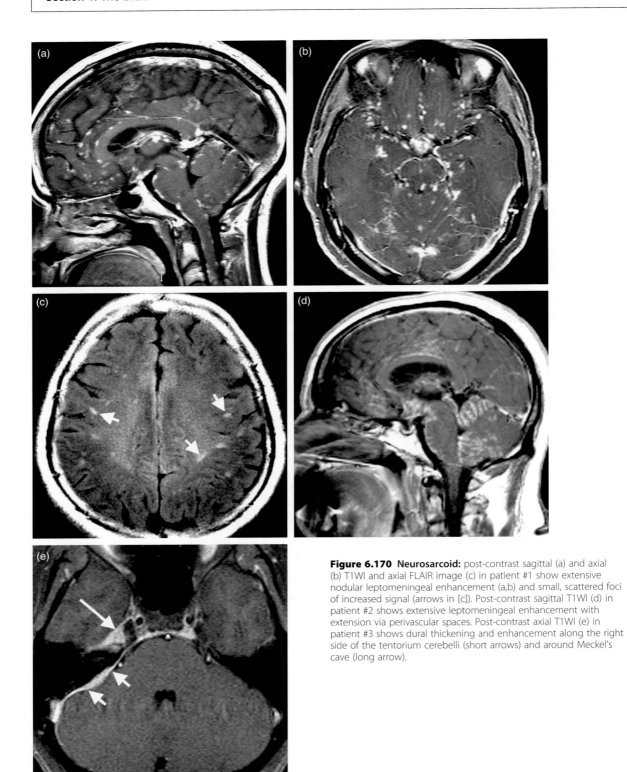

Figure 6.170 Neurosarcoid: post-contrast sagittal (a) and axial (b) T1WI and axial FLAIR image (c) in patient #1 show extensive nodular leptomeningeal enhancement (a,b) and small, scattered foci of increased signal (arrows in [c]). Post-contrast sagittal T1WI (d) in patient #2 shows extensive leptomeningeal enhancement with extension via perivascular spaces. Post-contrast axial T1WI (e) in patient #3 shows dural thickening and enhancement along the right side of the tentorium cerebelli (short arrows) and around Meckel's cave (long arrow).

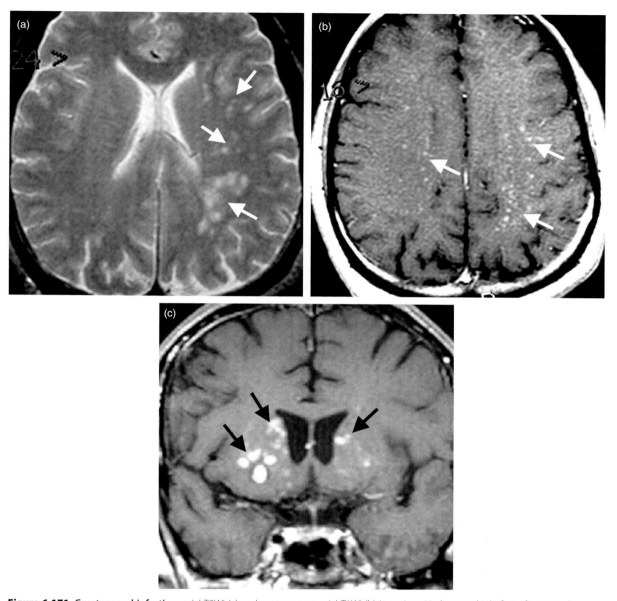

Figure 6.171 **Cryptococcal infection:** axial T2WI (a) and post-contrast axial T1WI (b) in patient #1 show multiple foci of increased signal within the white matter of the left cerebral hemisphere (a), with diffuse nodular enhancement (b) representing cryptococcomas extending through perivascular spaces. Post-contrast coronal T1WI (c) in patient #2 shows multiple enhancing cryptococcomas in the basal ganglia regions (arrows). *Source:* Used with permission from Barrow Neurological Institute.

Parasitic infections

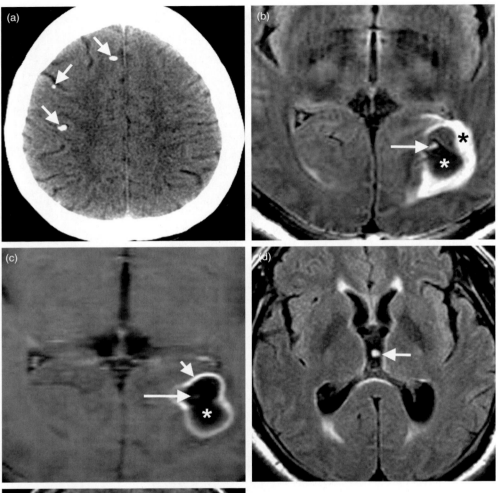

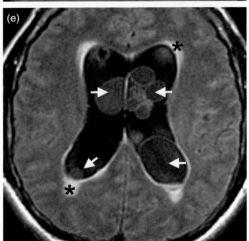

Figure 6.172 Cysticercosis: non-contrast axial CT image (a), magnified axial FLAIR image (b), and magnified post-contrast axial T1WI (c) of patient #1 show multiple cortical calcifications (arrows in [a]) representing old, healed lesions. An active lesion (white asterisk in [b,c]) with peripheral enhancement (short arrow in [c]), surrounding edema (black asterisk in [b]), and the scolex (long arrow in [b,c]) are present in the occipital lobe. Axial FLAIR image (d) in patient #2 shows a scolex within the third ventricle (arrow). Axial FLAIR image (e) in patient #3 shows the racemose form within the lateral ventricle without identifiable scolices (arrows). Hydrocephalus with transependymal CSF resorption is noted (black asterisks). *Source:* Figure 6.172d,e used with permission from Barrow Neurological Institute.

Infections in immunocompromised patients

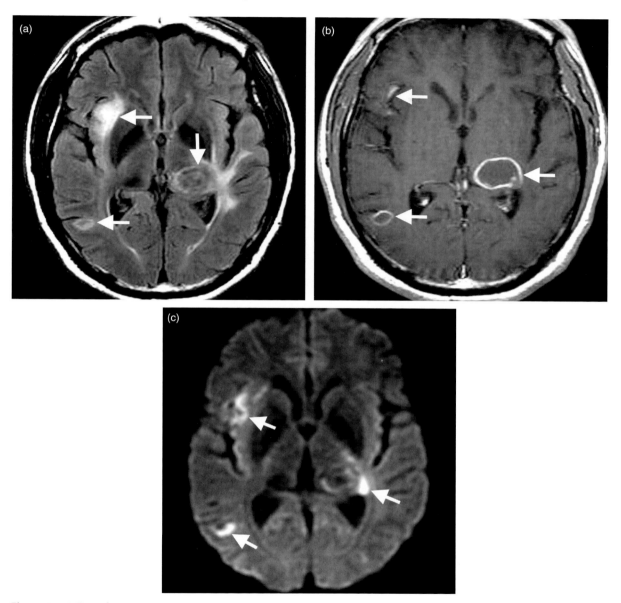

Figure 6.173 **Toxoplasmosis:** axial FLAIR image (a), post-contrast axial T1WI (b), and diffusion trace image (c) show multiple focal lesions (arrows) with ring enhancement, surrounding edema, and diffusion restriction in this patient with AIDS.

Intraventricular infection

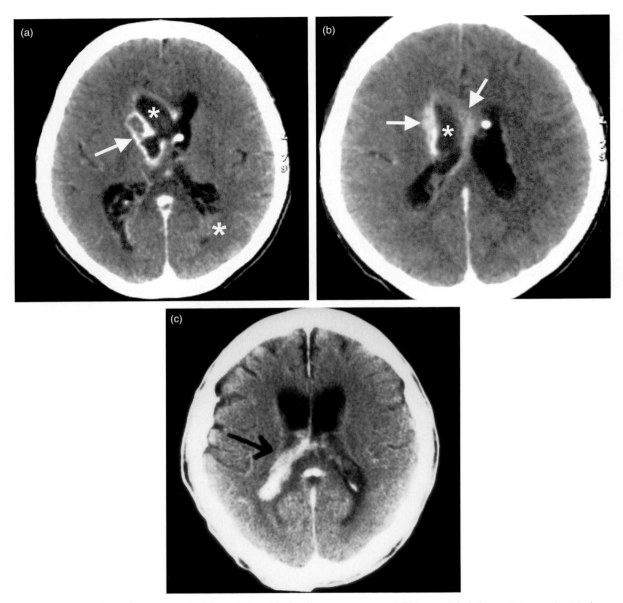

Figure 6.174 Cerebral abscess, ventriculitis, and choroid plexitis: post-contrast axial CT images (a,b,c) demonstrate a periventricular abscess (arrow in [a]) with a thicker lateral wall, which has ruptured through the thinner medial wall into the ventricle, showing ventricular exudate (asterisks in [a,b]), ventriculitis (short arrows in [b]), and choroid plexitis (black arrow in [c]).

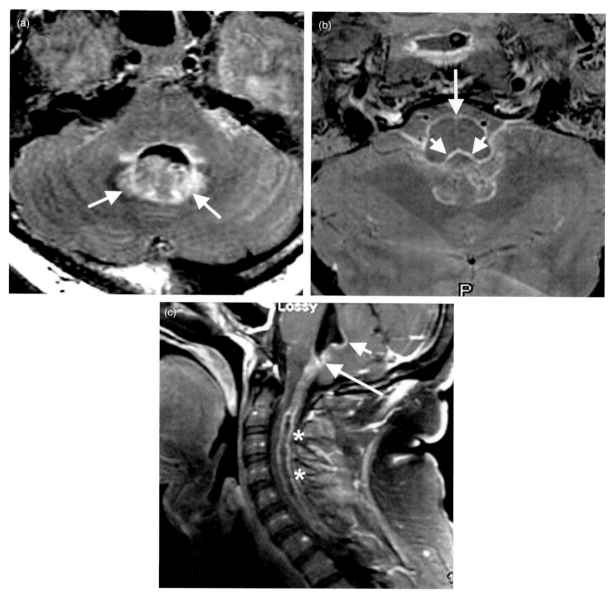

Figure 6.175 Leptomeningitis and ventriculitis: axial FLAIR image (a), fat suppressed post-contrast axial (b) and sagittal (c) T1WI reveal ventriculitis with enhancement (short arrows in [b,c]), increased FLAIR signal surrounding the fourth ventricle (arrows in [a]), and leptomeningeal enhancement (long arrow in [b]). The long arrow in (c) indicates pathologic enhancement extending through the obex, resulting in abscess formation and ependymitis within the central canal of the cervical cord (asterisks in [c]).

Demyelinating disorders

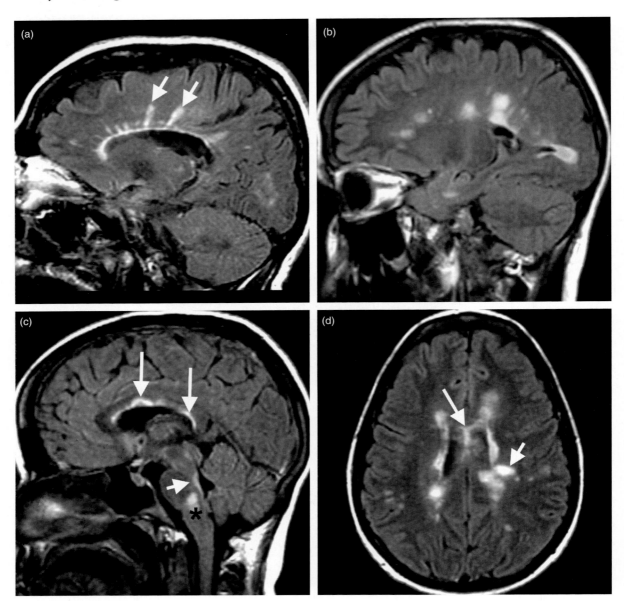

Figure 6.176 Multiple sclerosis: sagittal (a,b,c) and axial (d) FLAIR images show typical findings in MS. Linear foci of increased signal (Dawson's fingers) are noted emanating from the corpus callosum into the deep white matter (arrows in [a]). In (b) the periventricular lesions are fluffier in appearance. In (c) lesions are seen along the inferior aspect of the corpus callosum (long arrows), with a lesion along the floor of the fourth ventricle (short arrow), and a pontine lesion is visible (asterisk). In (d) lesions within the corpus callosum (long arrow) and periventricular zones (short arrow) are seen.

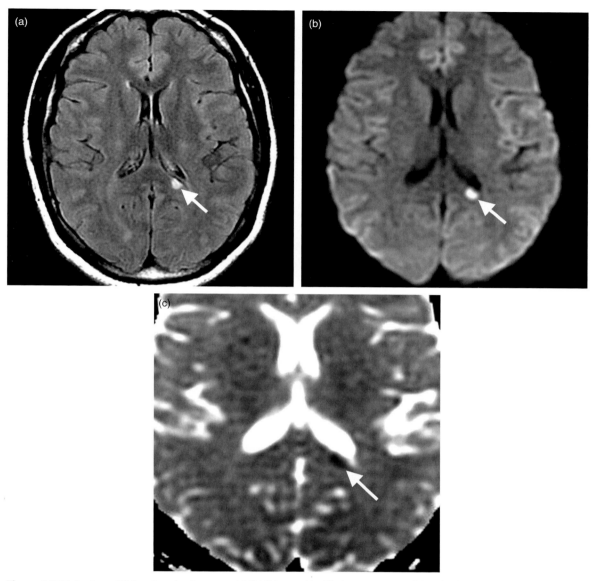

Figure 6.177 Acute multiple sclerosis plaques: axial FLAIR image (a), diffusion trace image (b), and ACD map (c) show a focal MS lesion (arrows) in the lateral aspect of the splenium of the corpus callosum with diffusion restriction, indicative of an acute MS lesion.

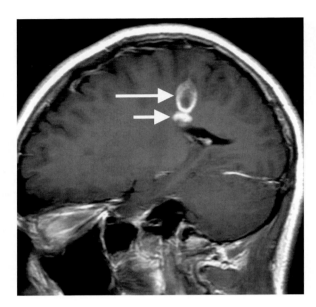

Figure 6.178 Acute multiple sclerosis plaques: post-contrast sagittal T1WI shows ring and nodular enhancing lesions in the periatrial white matter, representing areas of acute inflammation/demyelination in MS.

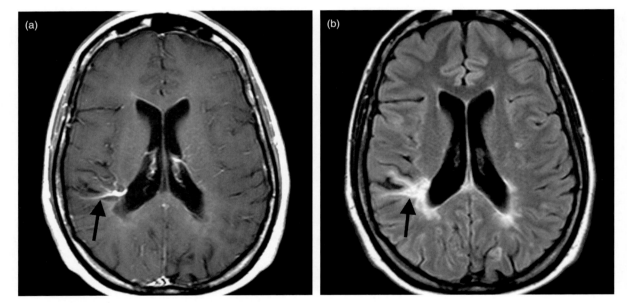

Figure 6.179 Multiple sclerosis and developmental venous anomaly: post-contrast axial T1WI (a) and axial FLAIR image (b) in a patient with MS and a developmental venous anomaly (arrow in [a]) show the presence of demyelination surrounding the developmental venous anomaly (arrow in [b]), illustrating the underlying pathology of perivenular demyelination.

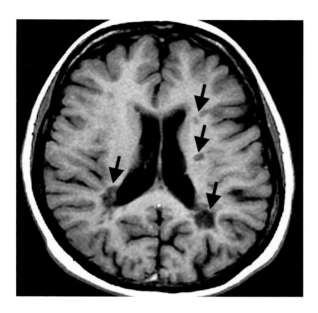

Figure 6.180 **Black holes in multiple sclerosis:** non-contrast axial T1WI shows multiple focal regions of prominent T1 hypointensity (black holes), indicative of chronic MS.

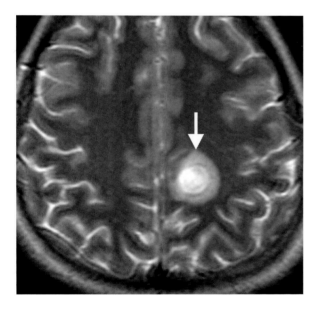

Figure 6.181 **Balo's concentric sclerosis:** magnified axial T2WI shows a focal demyelinating lesion with an onion-layered appearance (arrow) in Balo's concentric sclerosis.

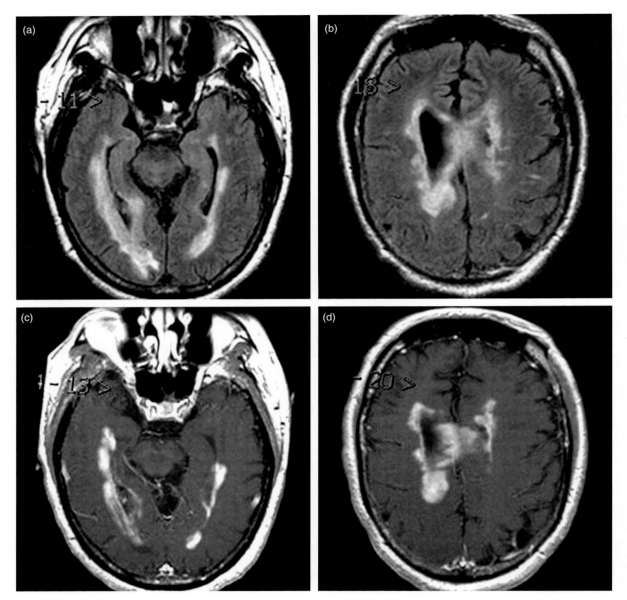

Figure 6.182 Marburg variant multiple sclerosis: axial FLAIR images (a,b) and post-contrast axial T1WI (c,d) show extensive, confluent abnormal signal intensity in the periventricular white matter, including the corpus callosum, with extensive enhancement. This was a monophasic presentation leading rapidly to death.

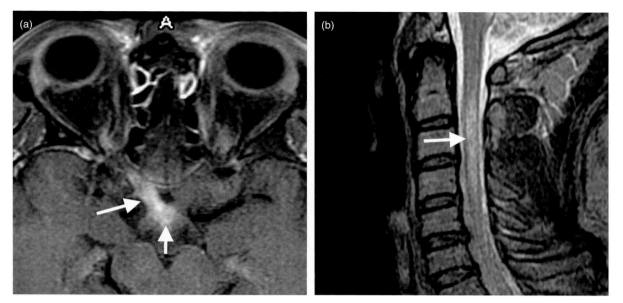

Figure 6.183 Devic's disease (neuromyelitis optica): axial post-contrast fat suppressed T1WI (a) and gradient echo T2 sagittal image (b) of the cervical spine show pathologic enhancement of the intracranial right optic nerve (long arrow in [a]) and the optic chiasm (short arrow in [a]) with concurrent myelitis of the cervical cord (arrow in [b]). *Source:* Used with permission from Barrow Neurological Institute.

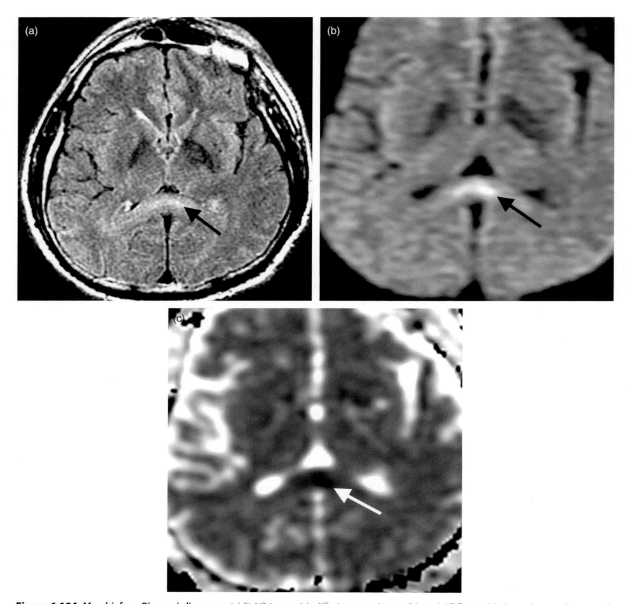

Figure 6.184 Marchiafava-Bignami disease: axial FLAIR image (a), diffusion trace image (b), and ADC map (c) show abnormal increased FLAIR signal with diffusion restriction in the splenium of the corpus callosum (arrows). *Source:* Used with permission from Barrow Neurological Institute.

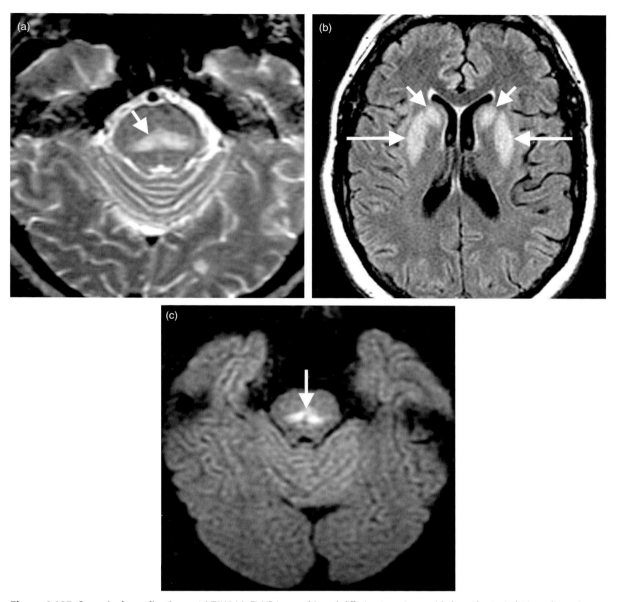

Figure 6.185 **Osmotic demyelination:** axial T2WI (a), FLAIR image (b), and diffusion trace image (c) show the typical triangular region of increased signal (arrow in [a]) in the pons, with extra-pontine myelinolysis in the basal ganglia region (arrows in [b]) and diffusion restriction in the pons (arrow in [c]). *Source:* Used with permission from Barrow Neurological Institute.

Traumatic lesions

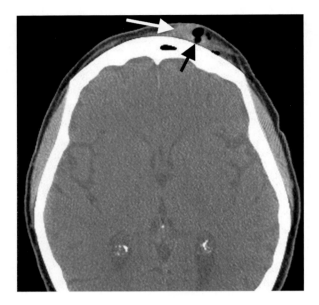

Figure 6.186 Traumatic scalp laceration: non-contrast axial CT image shows a left frontal scalp hematoma (white arrow) with soft tissue air (black arrow) typical of a scalp laceration.

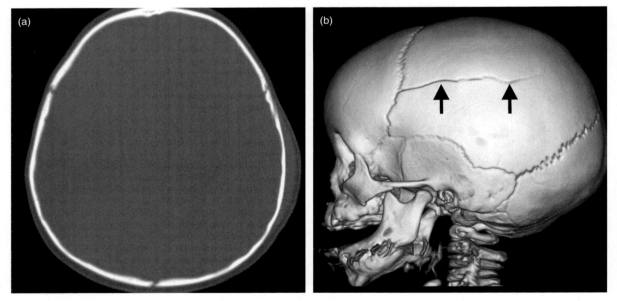

Figure 6.187 Linear skull fracture: axial CT bone window in a child (a) fails to reveal any definite fracture. 3D volume rendered CT reconstruction (b) clearly reveals a linear parietal skull fracture (arrows). Linear skull fractures in the plane of imaging may not be detected and 3D volume rendered images may be a helpful tool.

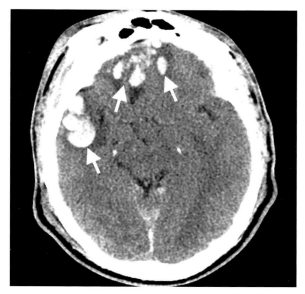

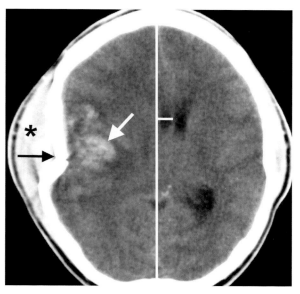

Figure 6.188 Cerebral contusions: non-contrast axial CT image shows numerous hemorrhagic contusions (arrows) with surrounding edema in the inferior frontal lobes and right temporal lobe.

Figure 6.189 Depressed skull fracture: non-contrast axial CT image shows a depressed right parietal skull fracture (black arrow), with an overlying scalp hematoma (asterisk) and underlying hemorrhagic contusions with edema (white arrow). There is mass effect with subfalcine herniation/midline shift indicated by the line placements.

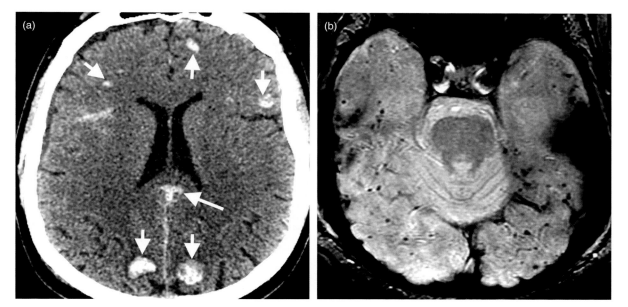

Figure 6.190 Diffuse axonal injury/shear injuries: non-contrast axial CT image (a) shows multiple hemorrhagic foci at the gray–white matter junction (small arrows) and in the splenium of the corpus callosum (long white arrow). Gradient echo T2 axial image (b) in a different patient shows innumerable punctate areas of hypointensity (magnetic susceptibility), representing diffuse axonal injury in a post-traumatic patient where the routine imaging was unremarkable.

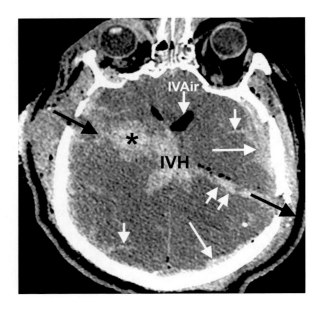

Figure 6.191 Gunshot injury to the head: non-contrast axial CT image shows the trajectory of the bullet (black arrows), the hemorrhage along the bullet tract, intraventricular hemorrhage (IVH), intraparenchymal hemorrhage (asterisk), subarachnoid blood (small white arrows), subdural hematoma (long white arrows), intraventricular air (IVAir), and diffuse cytotoxic edema reflected by loss of gray–white matter differentiation.

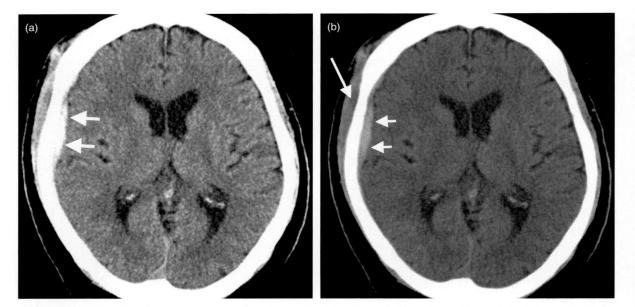

Figure 6.192 Epidural/subdural hematoma: non-contrast axial CT image with routine brain window (a) and subdural window (b) shows a small hyperdense extracerebral hemorrhage (small white arrows) and overlying scalp hematoma (long arrow in [b]), better seen on the subdural window (b).

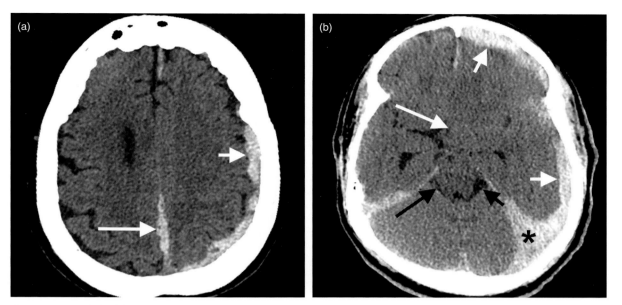

Figure 6.193 Subdural hematomas: non-contrast axial CT images (a,b). In (a) there are small acute convexity (short arrow) and interhemispheric (long arrow) subdural hematomas. In (b) there are acute lateral convexity subdural hematomas (short white arrows), which extend to the left tentorium cerebelli (asterisk), with marked uncal herniation (long white arrow) and downward transtentorial herniation with widening of the left (short black arrow) and narrowing of the right (long black arrow) perimesencephalic cisterns.

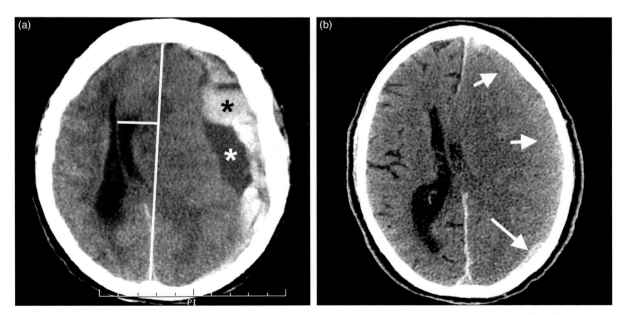

Figure 6.194 Subdural hematomas of varying ages: non-contrast axial CT image (a) shows a large acute (black asterisk) on chronic (white asterisk) left subdural hematoma, with marked mass effect and subfalcine herniation/midline shift (lines). Non-contrast axial CT image (b) shows a subacute/isodense left subdural hematoma (arrows) with midline shift. Non-contrast axial CT image (c) shows balancing, bilateral subacute/isodense subdural hematomas (arrows) without midline shift. Non-contrast axial CT image (d) shows bilateral subacute to chronic frontal subdural hematomas (arrows). Non-contrast axial CT image (e) shows balancing, bilateral chronic subdural hematomas or hygromas (arrows). Non-contrast sagittal T1WI (f) shows a thin holohemispheric subacute subdural hematoma (arrows).

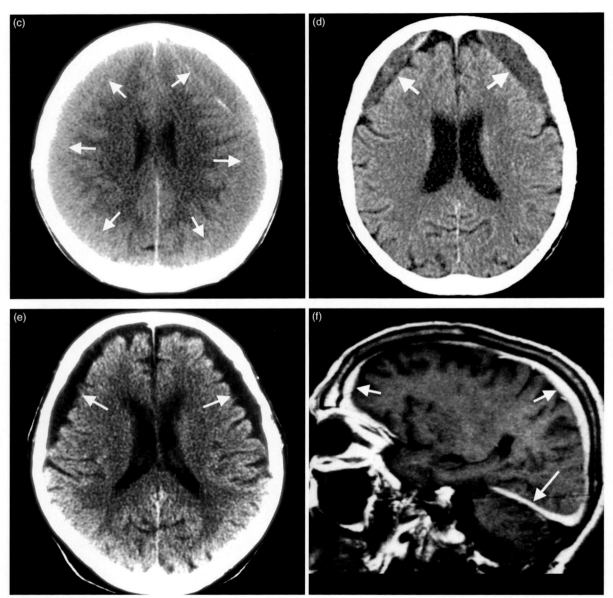

Figure 6.194 (*cont.*)

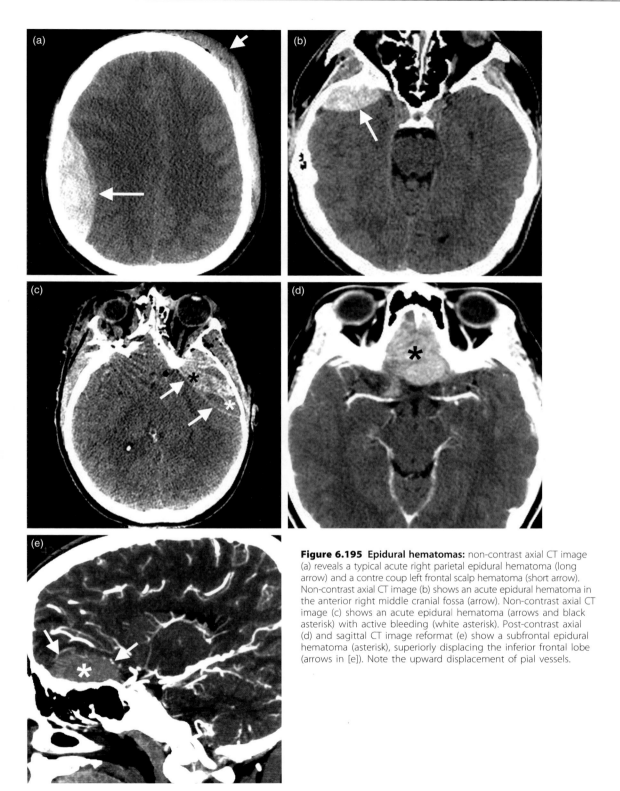

Figure 6.195 Epidural hematomas: non-contrast axial CT image (a) reveals a typical acute right parietal epidural hematoma (long arrow) and a contre coup left frontal scalp hematoma (short arrow). Non-contrast axial CT image (b) shows an acute epidural hematoma in the anterior right middle cranial fossa (arrow). Non-contrast axial CT image (c) shows an acute epidural hematoma (arrows and black asterisk) with active bleeding (white asterisk). Post-contrast axial (d) and sagittal CT image reformat (e) show a subfrontal epidural hematoma (asterisk), superiorly displacing the inferior frontal lobe (arrows in [e]). Note the upward displacement of pial vessels.

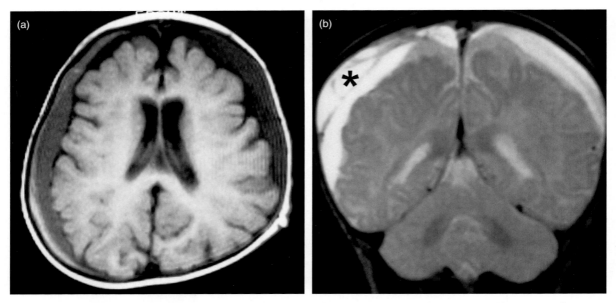

Figure 6.196 Non-accidental trauma (child abuse): axial T1WI (a) and coronal T2WI (b) show bilateral subdural hematomas of varying ages with membrane formation (asterisk in [b]) in an infant.

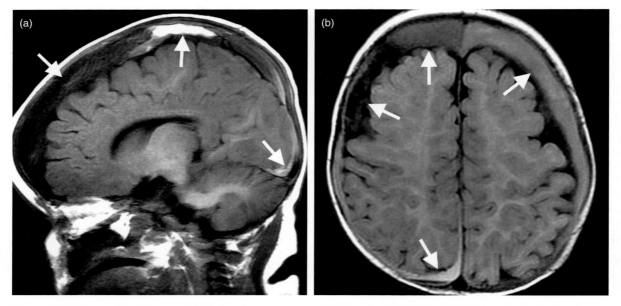

Figure 6.197 Non-accidental trauma (child abuse): non-contrast sagittal (a) and axial (b) T1WI, axial T2WI (c) and diffusion trace image (d) show multiple bilateral subdural hematomas of varying ages (white arrows in [a,b,c]), with membrane formation (long black arrow in [c]) and cytotoxic edema in the parietal lobes bilaterally (arrows in d). Short black arrow in (c) shows medial displacement of a superficial cortical vein.

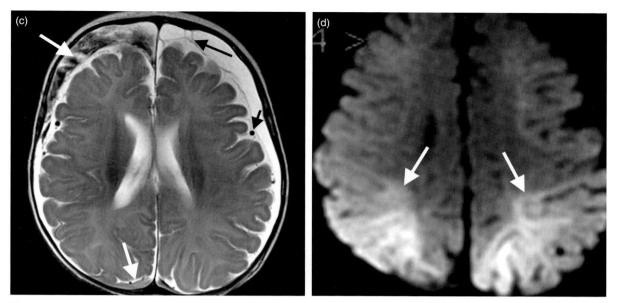

Figure 6.197 (cont.)

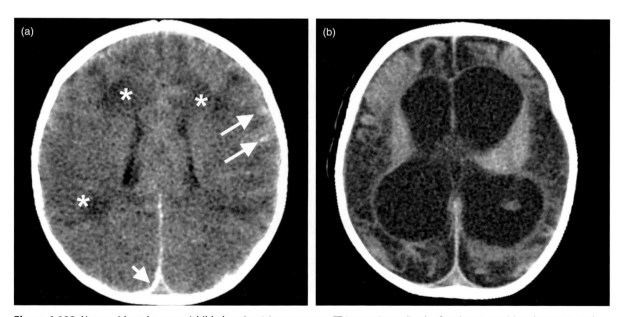

Figure 6.198 Non-accidental trauma (child abuse): axial non-contrast CT images immediately after the trauma (a) and approximately three months later (b) show a small area of acute subdural blood (short arrow in [a]), subarachnoid blood (long arrows in [a]), and areas of cytotoxic edema (asterisks in [a]); (b) demonstrates marked encephalomalacia and compensatory enlargement of the lateral ventricles as a sequelae of the trauma.

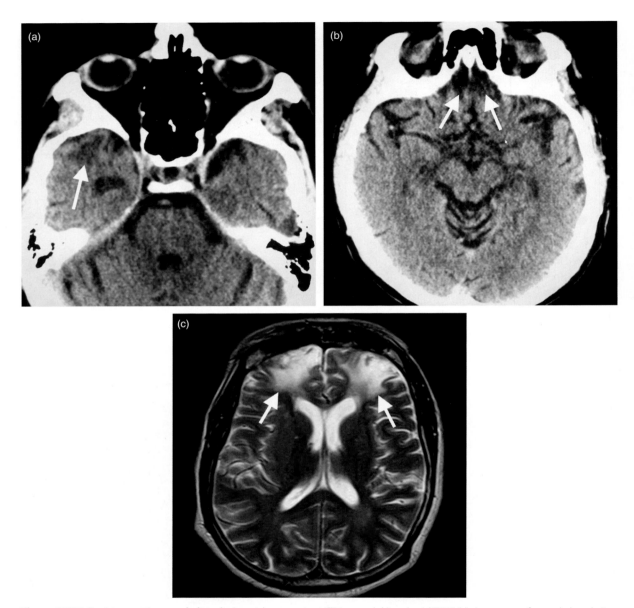

Figure 6.199 Post-traumatic encephalomalacia: axial non-contrast CT images (a,b) and axial T2WI (c) show areas of encephalomalacia (arrows) in the anterior right temporal lobe (a), the inferior frontal lobes (b), and both frontal lobes (c), secondary to remote trauma.

Vascular lesions

Hemorrhage

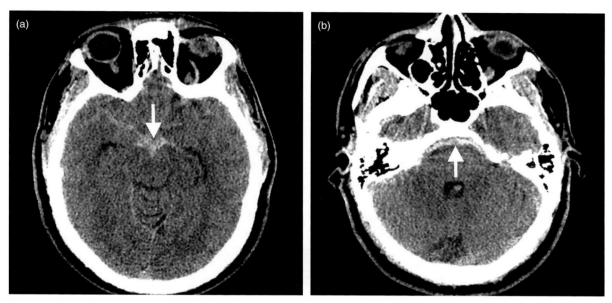

Figure 6.200 **Benign non-aneurysmal subarachnoid hemorrhage:** non-contrast axial CT images (a,b) reveal focal subarachnoid hemorrhage in the interpeduncular and prepontine cisterns (arrows). No aneurysm was found on angiography.

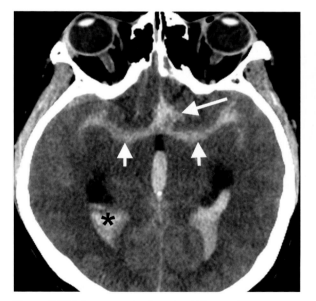

Figure 6.201 **Aneurysmal subarachnoid hemorrhage:** non-contrast axial CT image shows extensive subarachnoid hemorrhage in the horizontal Sylvian cisterns (short arrows), intraventricular blood (asterisk), and a focal collection of hemorrhage in the cistern of the lamina terminalis (long arrow) secondary to a ruptured anterior communicating artery aneurysm.

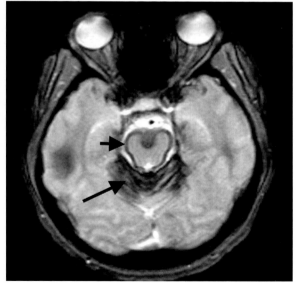

Figure 6.202 **Superficial siderosis:** axial gradient echo T2 image shows hemosiderin deposition along the pial surfaces of the cerebellar folia (long arrow) and midbrain (short arrow).

205

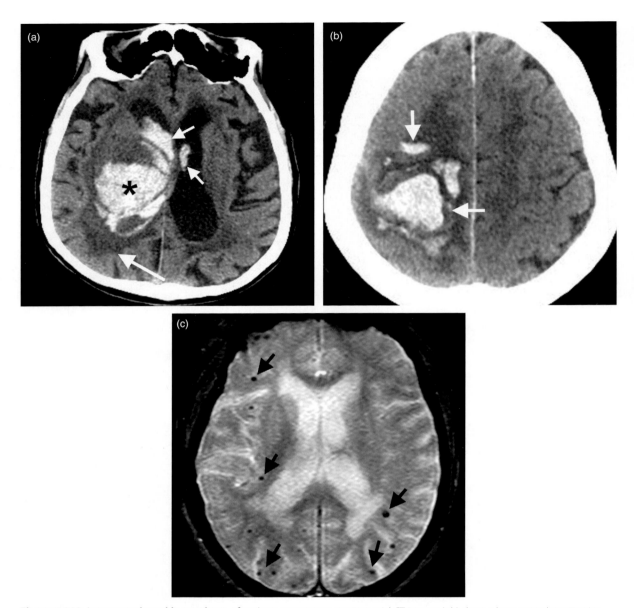

Figure 6.203 **Intraparenchymal hemorrhage of various causes:** non-contrast axial CT images (a,b) show a large acute hypertensive hemorrhage (asterisk in [a]) with surrounding edema (long arrow in [a]) and intraventricular extension (short arrows in [a]). Hemorrhage secondary to amyloid angiopathy (arrows in [b]), which extends from the subcortical region into the deep white matter, is seen. Gradient echo T2 axial image (c) shows numerous microbleeds (arrows) secondary to uncontrolled hypertension.

Aneurysms

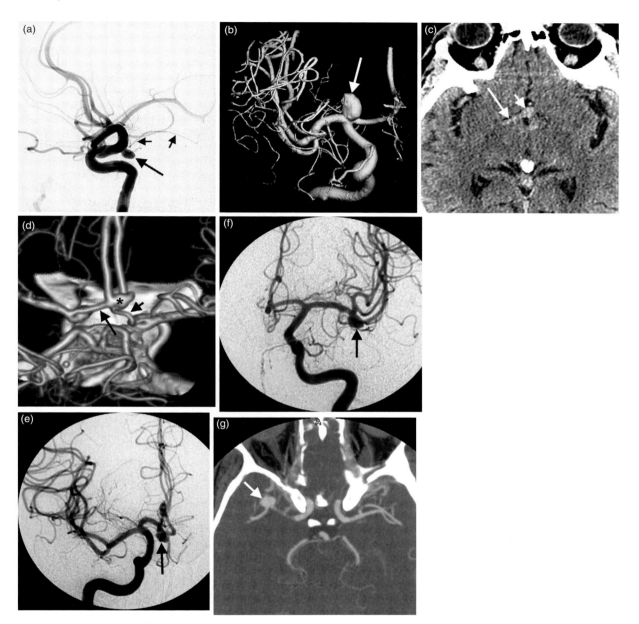

Figure 6.204 Anterior circulation aneurysms: lateral internal carotid angiogram (a) shows an aneurysm arising from the posterior wall of the supraclinoid internal carotid artery at the level of the posterior communicating artery (long arrow). Note the normal appearance of the anterior choroidal artery (short arrows). 3D catheter angiogram (b) shows an internal carotid artery terminus aneurysm (arrow). Axial non-contrast CT image (c) shows a suspected anterior communicating artery aneurysm (short arrow) extending from a prominent right A1 segment (long arrow). CT angiogram (d) in the same patient confirms an anterior communicating artery aneurysm (asterisk), a hypoplastic left A1 segment (short arrow), and a large right A1 segment (long arrow). Anteroposterior right internal carotid angiogram (e) shows an anterior communicating artery aneurysm (arrow). Anteroposterior left internal carotid angiogram (f) shows a left middle cerebral artery bifurcation aneurysm (arrow). Source image from a CTA (g) shows a right middle cerebral artery bifurcation region aneurysm (arrow). *Source:* Figure 6.204g used with permission from Barrow Neurological Institute.

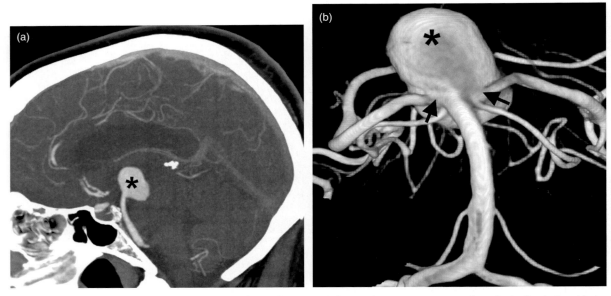

Figure 6.205 Giant basilar tip aneurysm: sagittal reformat from CTA (a) shows a large aneurysm arising from the basilar tip (asterisks in [a,b]), which is confirmed on the 3D rotational catheter angiogram (b). In (b) note the incorporation of the P1 segments into the base of the giant aneurysm (arrows). *Source:* Used with permission from Barrow Neurological Institute.

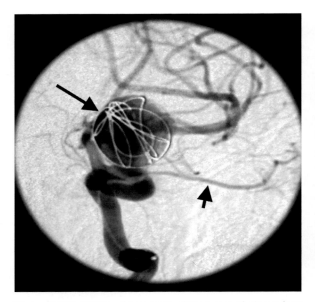

Figure 6.206 Coiling of aneurysm: oblique, magnified view from an internal carotid artery angiogram shows placement of the first GDC coil into this giant para-ophthalmic artery aneurysm (long arrow). Note the ophthalmic artery (short arrow).

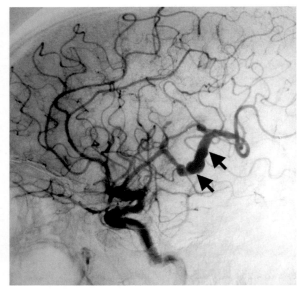

Figure 6.207 Serpentine aneurysm: lateral view internal carotid artery angiogram shows a serpentine aneurysm (arrows) of the angular branch of the middle cerebral artery. *Source:* Used with permission from Barrow Neurological Institute.

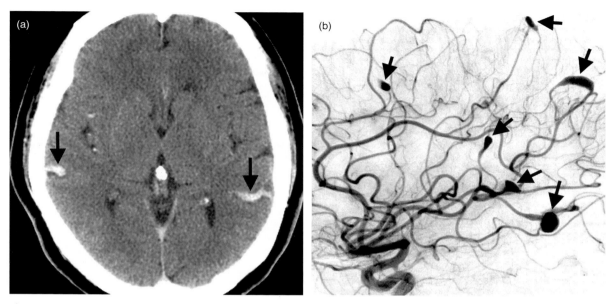

Figure 6.208 **Neoplastic aneurysms – atrial myxoma:** contrast enhanced axial CT image (a) shows a sausage-shaped dilatation of the peripheral branches of the middle cerebral arteries (arrows). Lateral internal carotid angiogram (b) shows numerous aneurysms of the distal vascular branches (arrows). *Source:* Used with permission from Barrow Neurological Institute.

Vascular malformations

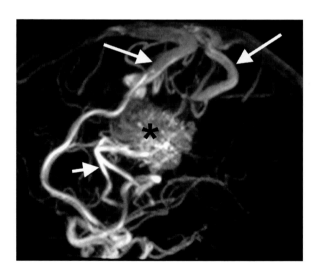

Figure 6.209 **Arteriovenous malformation:** lateral view from an intracranial MRA shows the three components of a high-flow pial arteriovenous malformation: the middle cerebral arterial feeders (short arrow), the nidus (asterisk), and the draining veins (long arrows).

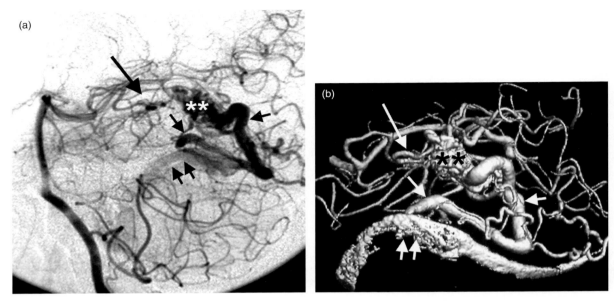

Figure 6.210 **Arteriovenous malformation:** lateral view from a vertebral angiogram (a) and lateral view from a 3D rotational catheter angiogram (b) show a temporal lobe arteriovenous malformation with supply from the posterior temporal branches of the posterior cerebral artery (long arrows), the nidus (double asterisk), and the main draining vein (short arrows). Double short arrows indicate the distal transverse sinus.

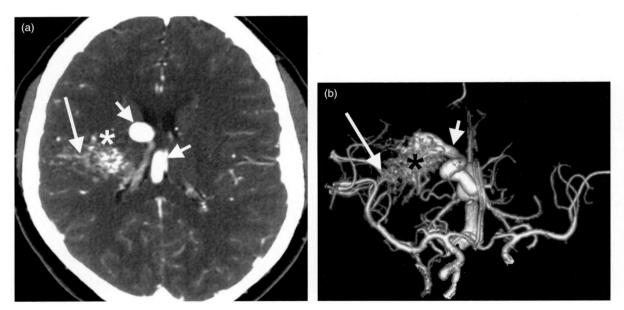

Figure 6.211 **CTA of arteriovenous malformation:** axial source images (a) and 3D volume rendered reconstruction from a CTA shows middle cerebral arterial feeders (long arrow), the nidus (asterisk), and the deep draining veins extending into the internal cerebral vein (short arrows).

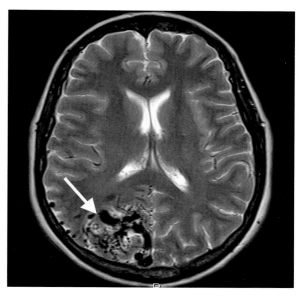

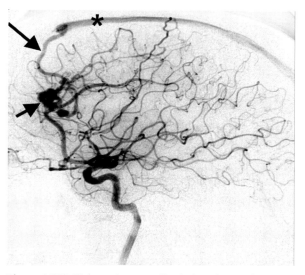

Figure 6.212 MRI of arteriovenous malformation: axial T2WI shows pathologically enlarged vessels (arrow) in the parietal/occipital region, representing an arteriovenous malformation.

Figure 6.213 Pial arteriovenous fistula: lateral internal carotid angiogram shows a fistulous connection (short arrow) (note there is no true nidus) between a branch of the anterior cerebral artery and a draining vein (long arrow), extending to the superior sagittal sinus (asterisk).

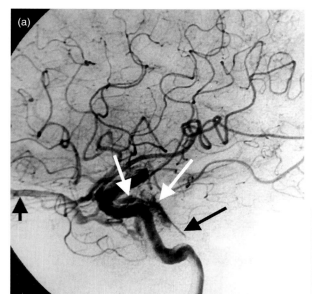

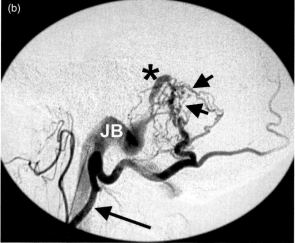

Figure 6.214 Dural arteriovenous fistulas: lateral internal carotid angiogram (a) shows a slow flow carotid–cavernous sinus dural arteriovenous fistula supplied by numerous small internal carotid artery branches, with drainage into the cavernous sinus (white arrows), the inferior petrosal sinus (long black arrow), and superior ophthalmic vein (short black arrow). Lateral view (b) from a selective occipital artery (long arrow) injection in another patient shows a dural fistula between multiple transmastoid branches (short arrows) of the occipital artery and a small pouch (asterisk) within an occluded transverse sinus. Venous outflow is into the sigmoid sinus and jugular bulb (JB).

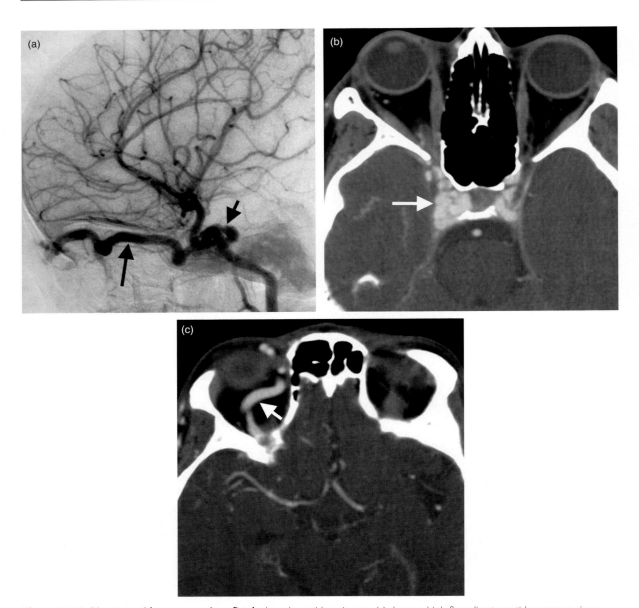

Figure 6.215 Direct carotid cavernous sinus fistula: lateral carotid angiogram (a) shows a high-flow direct carotid cavernous sinus fistula secondary to trauma. Arterial venous shunting into the cavernous sinus (short arrow) and dilated superior ophthalmic vein (long arrow) are noted. Contrast enhanced axial CT images (b,c) in the same patient show asymmetric enhancement of the right cavernous sinus (arrow in [b]) and dilatation of the superior ophthalmic vein (arrow in [c]).

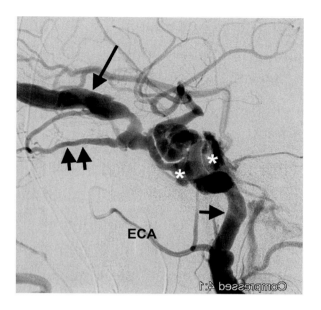

Figure 6.216 Direct carotid cavernous sinus fistula: magnified lateral carotid angiogram shows a high-flow direct carotid cavernous sinus fistula. The internal carotid artery is indicated by a single short arrow, and cavernous sinus opacification by asterisks. Superior (long arrow) and inferior (double short arrows) ophthalmic veins are seen to drain from the cavernous sinus. *Source:* Used with permission from Barrow Neurological Institute.

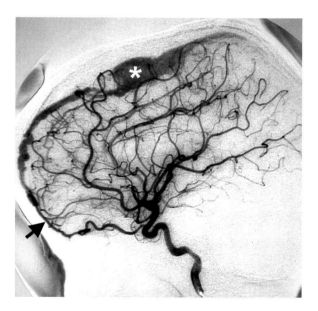

Figure 6.217 Pediatric dural arteriovenous fistula: lateral internal carotid artery angiogram shows a high-flow dural arteriovenous fistula supplied by the anterior falcine branch (arrow) of the ophthalmic artery, which drains into a dilated superior sagittal sinus (asterisk). *Source:* Used with permission from Barrow Neurological Institute.

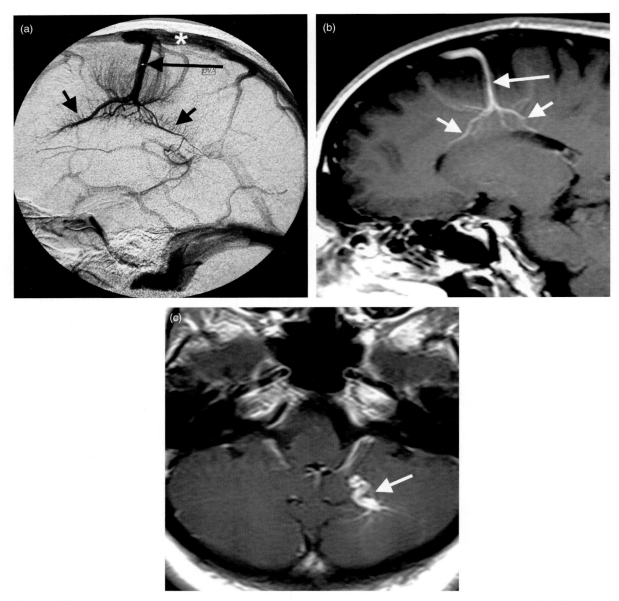

Figure 6.218 Developmental venous anomalies: lateral venous phase carotid artery injection (a) and post-contrast sagittal T1WI (b) show a large typical developmental venous anomaly with multiple small venous radicles (short arrows) draining through a large single venous stem (long arrow) into the superior sagittal sinus (asterisk in [a]). Post-contrast axial T1WI (c) shows similar features of a developmental venous anomaly in the left cerebellum (arrow).

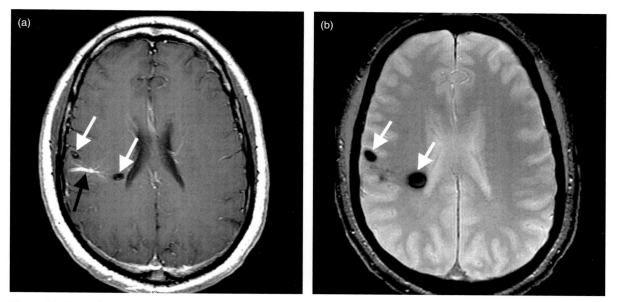

Figure 6.219 Developmental venous anomaly and cavernous malformations: post-contrast axial T1WI (a) and axial gradient echo T2 image (b) show a developmental venous anomaly (black arrow in [a]) associated with cavernous malformations (white arrows in [a,b]), which are more conspicuous in (b) owing to magnetic susceptibility effects on gradient echo T2 images.

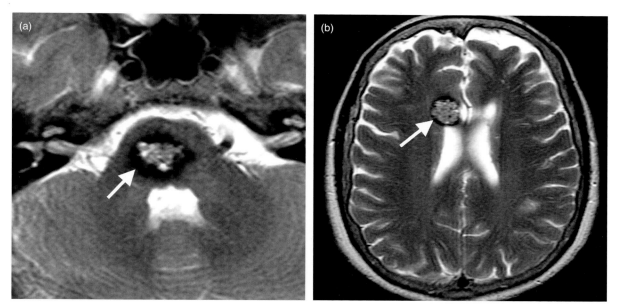

Figure 6.220 Cavernous malformations: axial T2WI through the posterior fossa (a) and supratentorial compartment (b) show the typical appearance of a cavernous malformation (arrow) with heterogeneous, popcorn-like appearance and a complete peripheral rim of hemosiderin. No edema is seen unless there is recent bleeding/expansion.

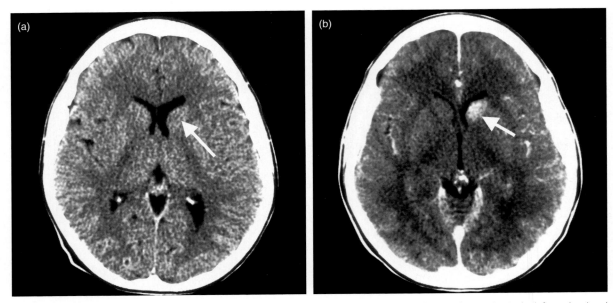

Figure 6.221 Capillary telangiectasia: axial pre- (a) and post-contrast (b) CT images show no obvious abnormality in the left caudate head on pre-contrast (a), but diffuse enhancement conforming to the shape of the caudate head on post-contrast (b) images (arrows).

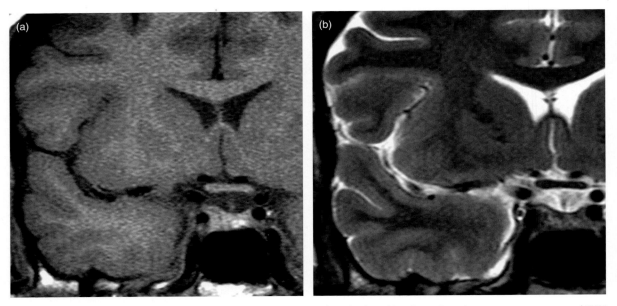

Figure 6.222 Capillary telangiectasia: no signal abnormality is seen in the inferolateral basal ganglia region on non-contrast coronal T1WI (a) or T2WI (b), but brush-like enhancement (arrow) is visible on post-contrast coronal T1WI (c).

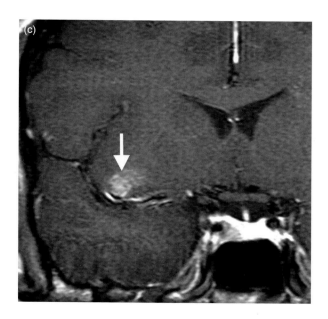

(c)

Figure 6.222 (*cont.*)

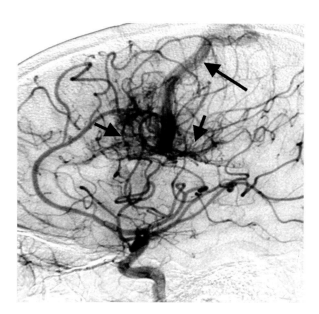

Figure 6.223 Transitional vascular malformation: lateral carotid angiogram in the arterial phase shows filling of a large, typical appearing developmental venous anomaly (arrows) indicating that there is arteriovenous shunting.

Cerebral infarction (stroke)

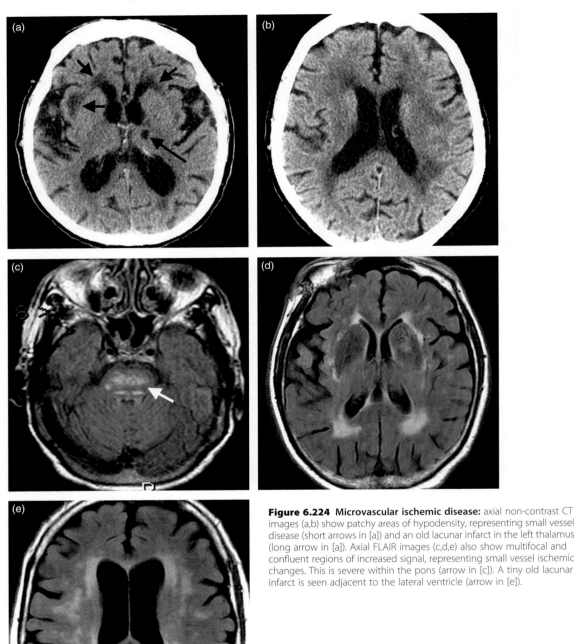

Figure 6.224 Microvascular ischemic disease: axial non-contrast CT images (a,b) show patchy areas of hypodensity, representing small vessel disease (short arrows in [a]) and an old lacunar infarct in the left thalamus (long arrow in [a]). Axial FLAIR images (c,d,e) also show multifocal and confluent regions of increased signal, representing small vessel ischemic changes. This is severe within the pons (arrow in [c]). A tiny old lacunar infarct is seen adjacent to the lateral ventricle (arrow in [e]).

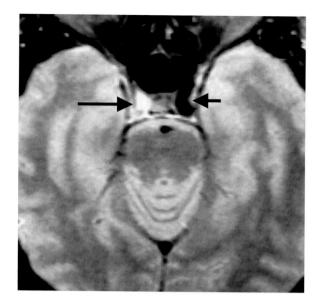

Figure 6.225 Carotid occlusion MRI: axial T2WI shows absent flow void of the cavernous segment of the internal carotid artery on the right (long arrow) compared with normal flow void on the left (short arrow).

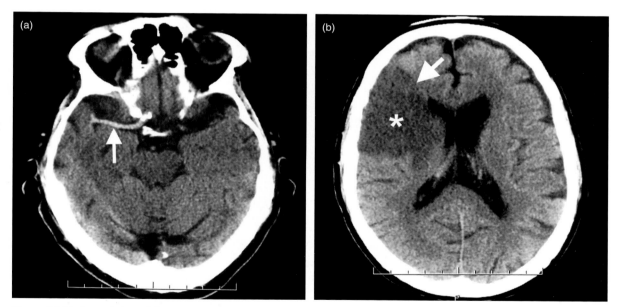

Figure 6.226 Acute right middle cerebral artery infarct: non-contrast axial CT images (a,b) show the hyperdense middle cerebral artery sign (arrow in [a]), indicative of intraluminal thrombus, and the subsequent right middle cerebral artery territory infarct (asterisk in [b]) on follow-up. The white arrow in (b) is the watershed zone between the anterior and middle cerebral arteries.

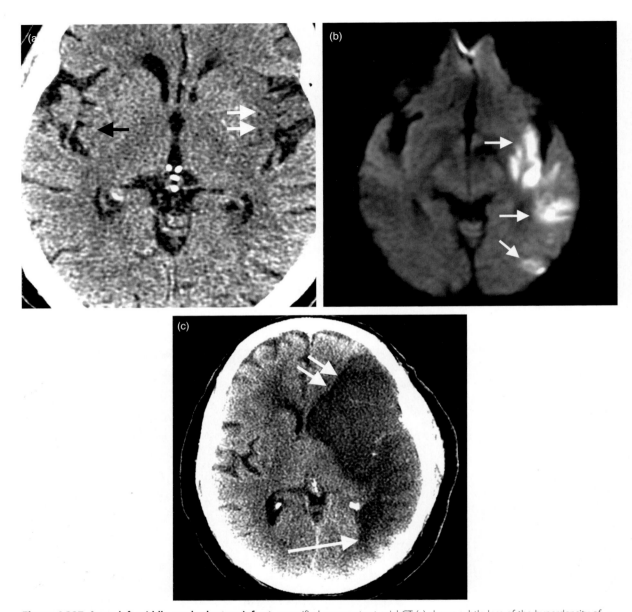

Figure 6.227 Acute left middle cerebral artery infarct: magnified non-contrast axial CT (a) shows subtle loss of the hyperdensity of the left insular cortex/subinsular region (double white arrows) compared with the normal right side (black arrow). Diffusion trace image (b) shows a larger region of diffusion restriction (arrows) with the follow-up CT image (c) showing the full extent of the middle cerebral artery infarct. The double arrows in (c) indicate the anterior/middle cerebral artery watershed region and the large arrow indicates the middle/posterior cerebral artery watershed zone.

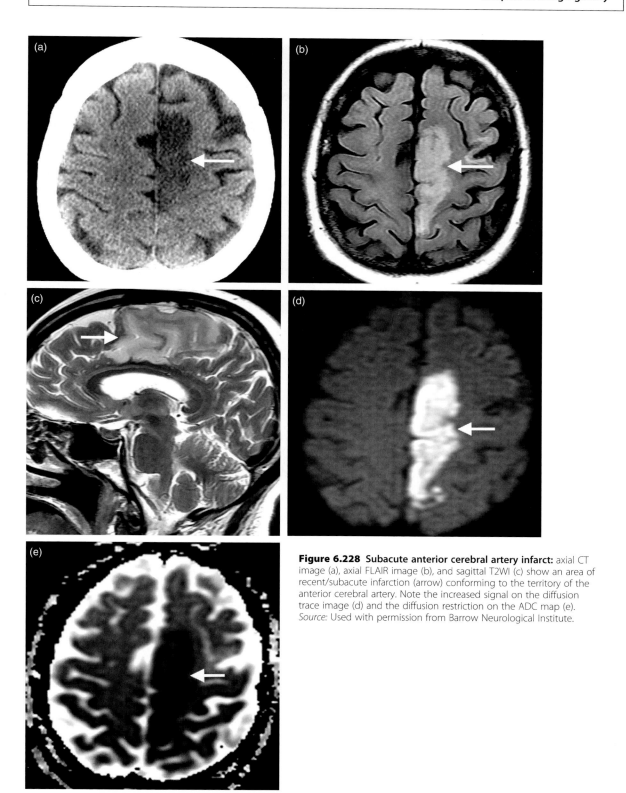

Figure 6.228 Subacute anterior cerebral artery infarct: axial CT image (a), axial FLAIR image (b), and sagittal T2WI (c) show an area of recent/subacute infarction (arrow) conforming to the territory of the anterior cerebral artery. Note the increased signal on the diffusion trace image (d) and the diffusion restriction on the ADC map (e). *Source:* Used with permission from Barrow Neurological Institute.

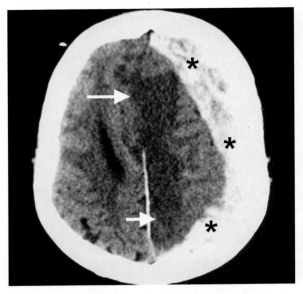

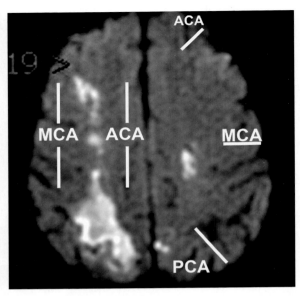

Figure 6.229 Traumatic anterior cerebral artery infarct: non-contrast axial CT image shows a large acute left subdural hematoma (asterisks) with underlying mass effect and midline shift. Hypodensity, representing a subacute anterior cerebral artery infarct (arrows), is present following compression/occlusion of the anterior cerebral artery upon the falx, secondary to the mass effect.

Figure 6.230 Watershed infarcts: axial diffusion trace image shows multiple areas of acute infarction in watershed distributions. The various watershed regions have been delineated.

Figure 6.231 Subacute posterior cerebral artery infarct: axial FLAIR image shows a subacute infarct conforming to the posterior cerebral artery vascular territory (long arrow). Note the inclusion of the dorsolateral right thalamus (small arrow) from involvement of thalamoperforator branches of the posterior cerebral artery.

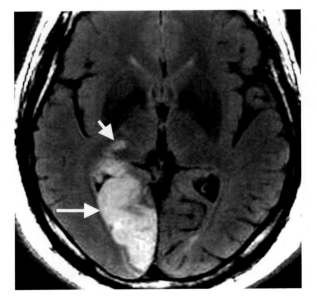

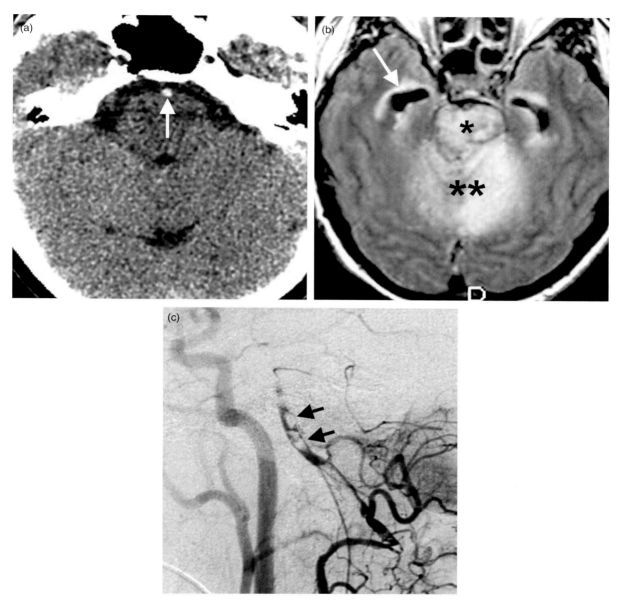

Figure 6.232 Basilar artery thrombosis: axial non-contrast CT image (a) shows hyperdensity of the basilar artery (arrow) representing thrombosis. Axial FLAIR image (b) shows evolving infarction of the brainstem (single asterisk) and cerebellum (double asterisks) with obstructive hydrocephalus and transependymal CSF resorption (arrow). Lateral view from an angiogram (c) shows extensive thrombus within the basilar artery (arrows).

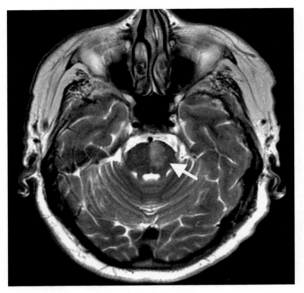

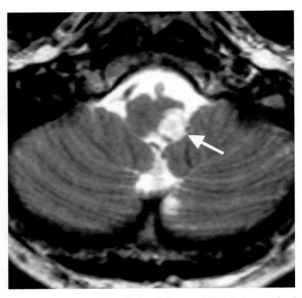

Figure 6.233 Pontine infarct: axial T2WI shows a left paramedian pontine infarct (arrow) representing a perforating artery territory infarct.

Figure 6.235 Lateral medullary infarct: axial T2WI shows a focal infarct involving the lateral medulla (arrow) in a patient with a Wallenberg syndrome. This results from a posterior inferior cerebellar artery or distal vertebral artery occlusion.

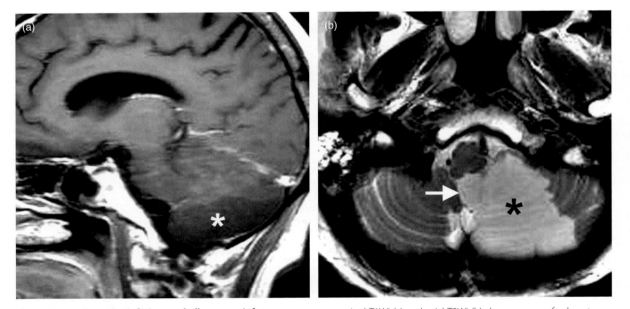

Figure 6.234 Posterior inferior cerebellar artery infarct: post-contrast sagittal T1WI (a) and axial T2WI (b) show an area of subacute infarction conforming to the territory of the posterior inferior cerebellar artery (asterisk). The arrow in (b) indicates involvement of the cerebellar tonsil.

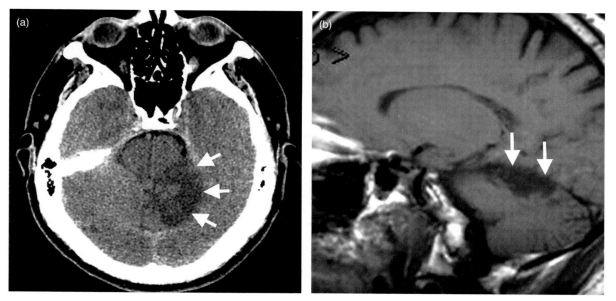

Figure 6.236 Superior cerebellar artery infarct: non-contrast axial CT image (a) and sagittal T1WI (b) show an area of infarction (arrows) along the superior surface of the cerebellum.

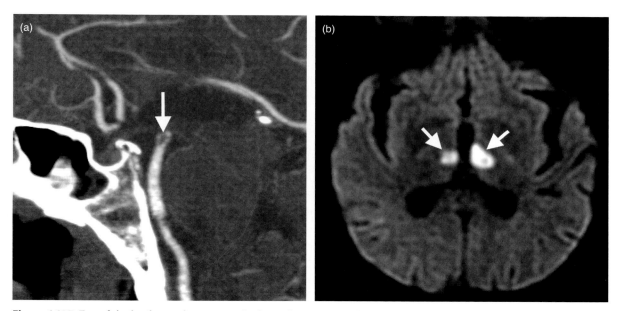

Figure 6.237 Top of the basilar syndrome: sagittal reformat from a CTA (a) shows a focal thrombus (arrow) within the top of the basilar artery. Diffusion trace image (b) shows bilateral medial thalamic infarcts (arrows) reflecting infarction of the artery of Percheron (solitary artery from a proximal posterior cerebral artery supplying both medial thalami). *Source:* Used with permission from Barrow Neurological Institute.

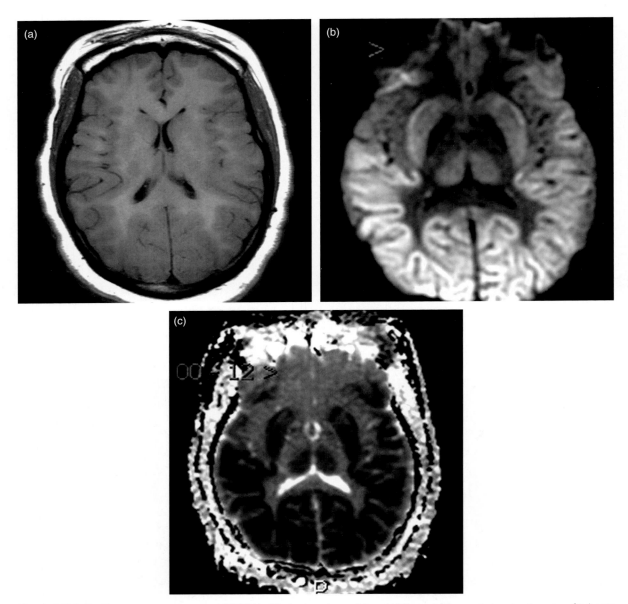

Figure 6.238 Cardiac arrest: non-contrast axial T1WI (a), diffusion trace image (b), and ADC map (c) demonstrate extensive areas of ischemic infarction involving cortical gray matter and deep gray matter nuclei. Note the subtle swelling of these regions in (a).

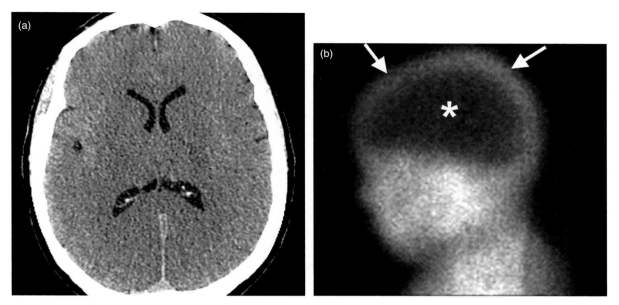

Figure 6.239 Diffuse anoxic injury: non-contrast axial CT image (a) shows diffuse loss of gray–white matter differentiation. The nuclear medicine study for brain death (b) shows complete absence of intracranial flow (asterisk). Note the flow related to the scalp (arrows in [b]). *Source:* Used with permission from Barrow Neurological Institute.

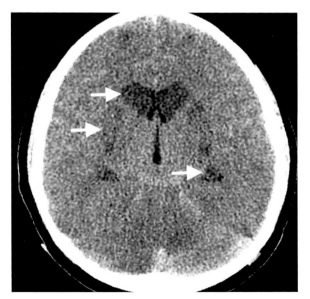

Figure 6.240 Diffuse anoxia: axial non-contrast CT image shows diffuse loss of gray–white matter differentiation from diffuse cytotoxic edema, with accentuated areas of discrete infarction in the deep gray matter nuclei (arrows). *Source:* Used with permission from Barrow Neurological Institute.

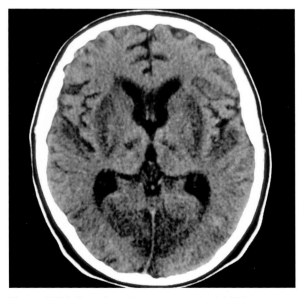

Figure 6.241 Near drowning: non-contrast axial CT image shows symmetric regions of infarction in the basal ganglia, ventrolateral thalami, and occipital lobes, representing areas of higher metabolic demand and greater susceptibility to severe, abrupt anoxic injury.

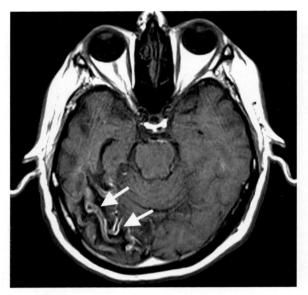

Figure 6.242 Cortical laminar necrosis: non-contrast axial T1WI shows serpiginous increased signal intensity along the cortical surfaces (arrows) in a region of previous infarction in the right posterior cerebral artery distribution.

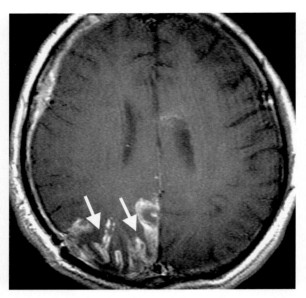

Figure 6.243 Enhancing subacute infarct: post-contrast axial T1WI shows a gyriform region of contrast enhancement (arrows) in the right parietal lobe in this patient with a subacute infarct.
Source: Used with permission from Barrow Neurological Institute.

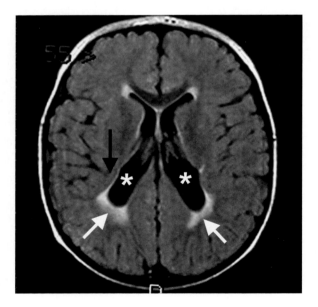

Figure 6.244 Periventricular leukomalacia: axial FLAIR image shows increased signal in the periatrial regions (white arrows) extending to the ependymal surfaces, enlargement of the posterior bodies/atria of the lateral ventricles (asterisks), and marked loss of white matter (black arrow) in this child with cerebral palsy.

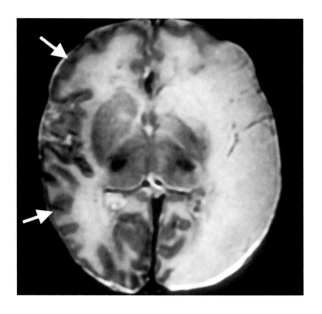

Figure 6.245 **Neonatal infarction:** axial T2WI shows a very large region of infarction in the left cerebral hemisphere with loss of a normally expected hypointense ribbon of gray matter and deep gray matter nuclei. Arrows indicate a normal cortical ribbon along the right hemisphere.

Non-atherosclerotic vasculopathies/vasculitis/CADASIL

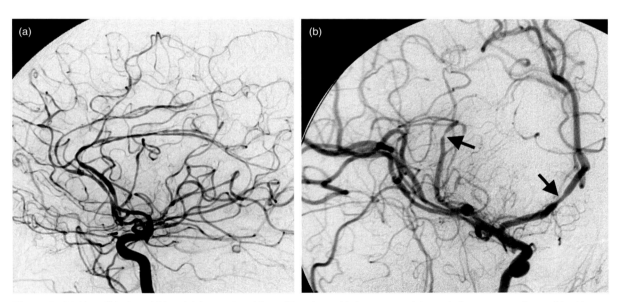

Figure 6.246 **Vasculitis:** lateral (a) and right anterior oblique (b) angiographic images reveal the typical appearance of vasculitis with multifocal areas of vascular narrowing. Changes are most severe in (a). Note the beaded appearance (arrows) in (b) owing to alternating regions of narrowing with non-stenotic segments. *Source:* Used with permission from Barrow Neurological Institute.

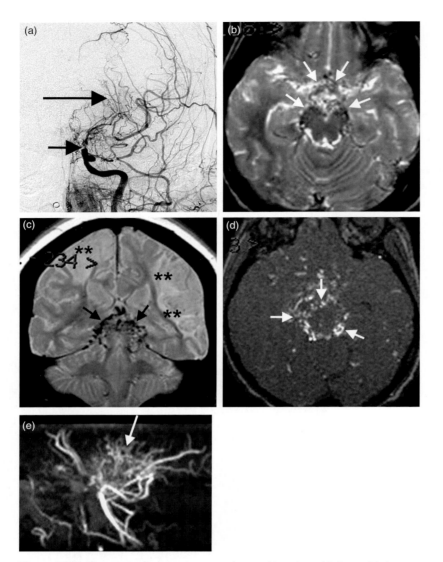

Figure 6.247 Moyamoya disease: anteroposterior carotid angiographic image (a) shows severe stenosis of the supraclinoid internal carotid artery (short arrow), and steno-occlusive change of the anterior and middle cerebral arteries with prominence of basal perforators (long arrow). Axial T2WI (b), coronal FLAIR image (c), and axial source image from MRA (d) show an increased number and prominence of the basal perforating arteries (arrows) and areas of infarction in both cerebral hemispheres (double asterisks in [c]). Maximum intensity projection image from MRA (e) shows the enlargement and increased number of perforating arteries giving the puff-of-smoke appearance (arrow). *Source:* Figure 6.247a Used with permission from Barrow Neurological Institute.

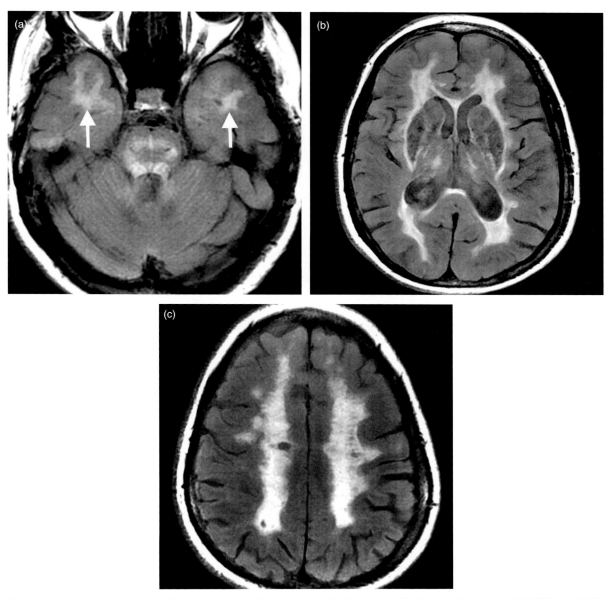

Figure 6.248 **Cerebral autosomal dominant arteriopathy with subcortical infarcts and leukoencephalopathy (CADASIL):** axial FLAIR images (a,b,c) reveal extensive symmetric increased signal in the white matter, including the external capsules, and in the anterior temporal lobe white matter (arrows in [a]).

Cortical venous/dural sinus thrombosis

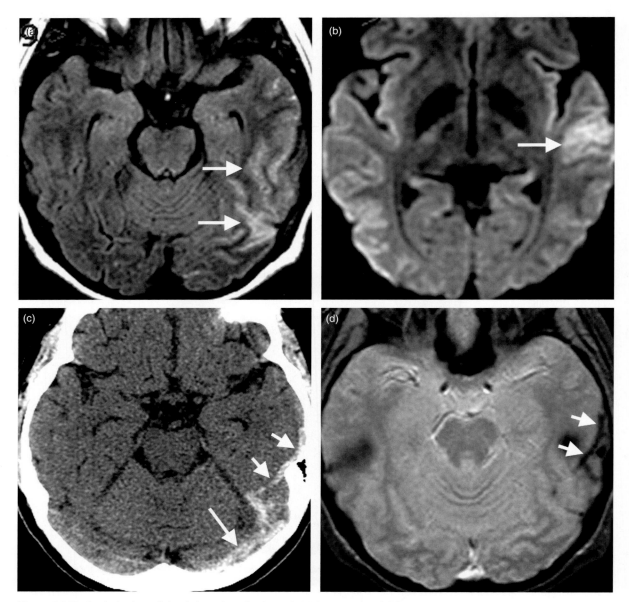

Figure 6.249 Cortical vein and dural sinus thrombosis: axial FLAIR image (a) and diffusion trace image (b) show increased signal (a) and diffusion restriction (b) in the left temporal lobe (arrows). Non-contrast axial CT images (c,e) and gradient echo T2 (d,f) show thrombosis of the left vein of Labbe (short arrows in [c,d,e,f]) and the left transverse sinus (long arrow in [c]). Maximum intensity projection image from MRV (g) shows occlusion of the left transverse sinus (short arrow); the long arrow indicates a patent right transverse sinus.

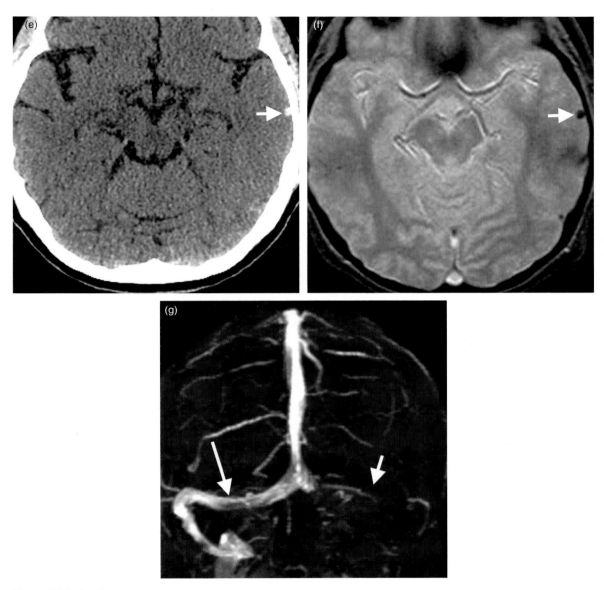

Figure 6.249 (cont.)

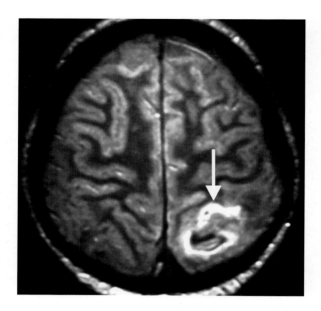

Figure 6.250 **Venous infarct:** axial T2WI shows a partially hemorrhagic, parasagittal region of abnormal signal intensity representing a venous infarct (arrow) secondary to cortical vein thrombosis (not shown).

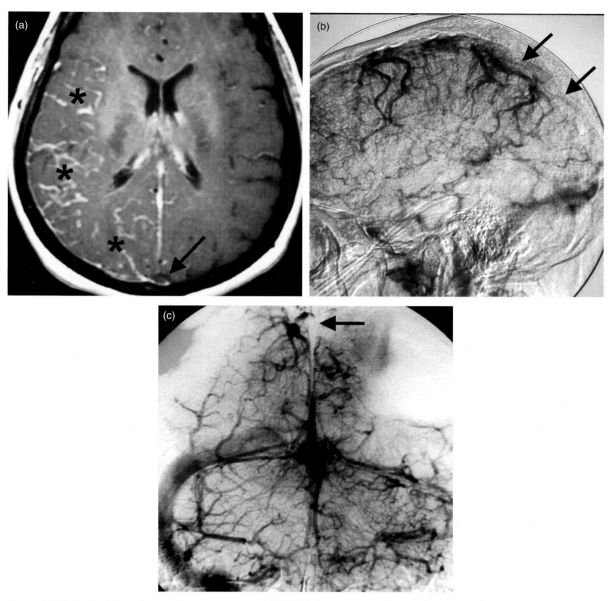

Figure 6.251 Sagittal sinus thrombosis: post-contrast axial T1WI (a) shows non-visualization of contrast in the superior sagittal sinus (arrow) associated with numerous venous collaterals in the right hemisphere (asterisks). Lateral (b) and anteroposterior (c) venous phase images from a carotid angiogram show the absence of the superior sagittal sinus (arrows) and an increased number of cortical and deep medullary veins.

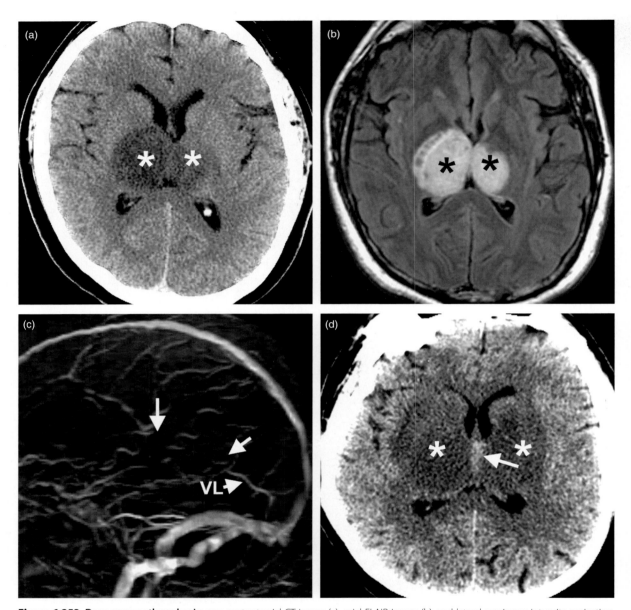

Figure 6.252 Deep venous thrombosis: non-contrast axial CT image (a), axial FLAIR image (b), and lateral maximum intensity projection image from MRV (c) in patient #1 show bilateral thalamic edema (asterisks in [a,b]) and absence of the internal cerebral veins, vein of Galen, and straight sinus (arrows in [c]). VL in (c) is the vein of Labbe. Axial non-contrast CT (d) in patient #2 shows bithalamic edema (asterisks), but also increased density in the midline (arrow), representing thrombosis of the internal cerebral veins. *Source:* Figure 6.252a,b,c used with permission from Barrow Neurological Institute.

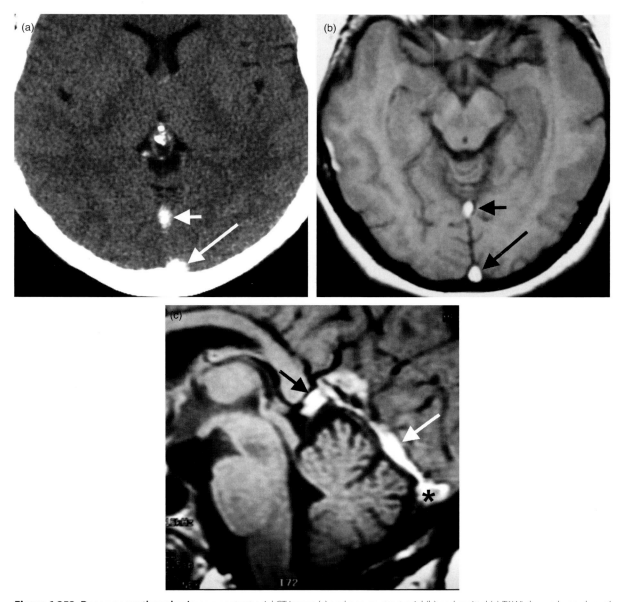

Figure 6.253 Deep venous thrombosis: non-contrast axial CT image (a) and non-contrast axial (b) and sagittal (c) T1WI show a hyperdense/ hyperintense clot in the straight sinus (short arrows in [a,b]) and superior sagittal sinus (long arrows in [a,b]). In (c) a hyperintense clot is seen in the vein of Galen (black arrow), the straight sinus (white arrow), and the torcular herophili (asterisk).

Vasospasm

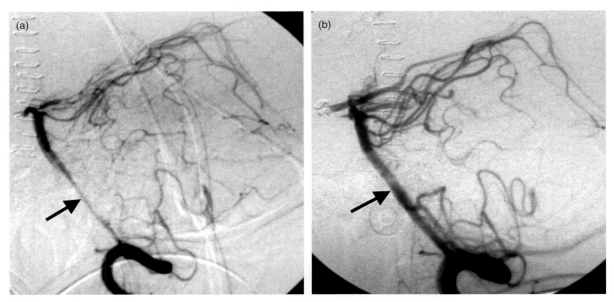

Figure 6.254 Vasospasm: lateral vertebral angiograms following aneurysm clipping show severe vasospasm (arrow) of the basilar artery (a) with a successful result following balloon angioplasty (b).

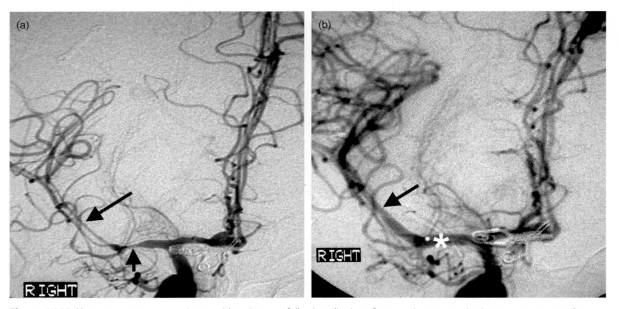

Figure 6.255 Vasospasm: anteroposterior carotid angiograms following clipping of an anterior communicating artery aneurysm show severe vasospasm of MI (short arrow in [a]) and M2 (long arrow in [a]). This was successfully treated with balloon angioplasty of MI (asterisk in [b]) and papaverine infusion of M2 (arrow in [b]).

Vascular dissection

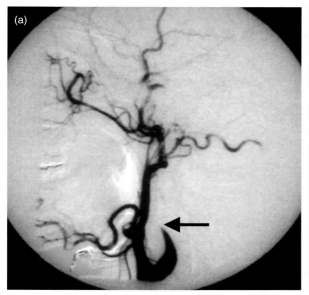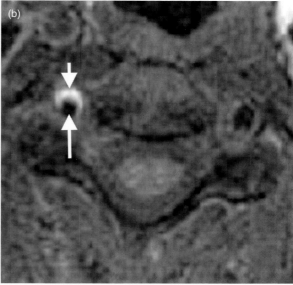

Figure 6.256 **Vascular dissection:** lateral common carotid artery angiogram (a) shows a tapered, complete occlusion of the proximal internal carotid artery (arrow) just above the carotid bulb. Fat suppressed non-contrast axial T1WI of the neck (b) in another patient shows an intramural hematoma (short arrow), eccentric to the flow void within the right vertebral artery (long arrow). *Source:* Figure 6.256b used with permission from Barrow Neurological Institute.

Fibromuscular dysplasia

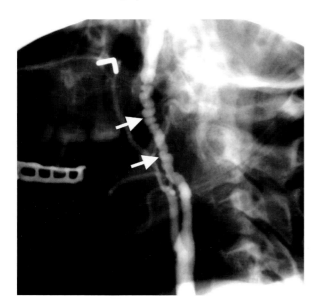

Figure 6.257 **Fibromuscular dysplasia:** lateral carotid angiogram of the neck shows the typical string-of-beads appearance of the medial form of fibromuscular dysplasia (arrows).

Vascular injury

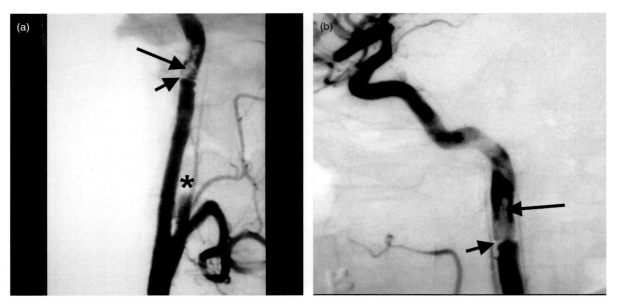

Figure 6.258 Traumatic vascular injury: anteroposterior oblique (a) and lateral (b) common carotid angiograms show focal injury to the vessel wall (short arrow), associated with an intraluminal thrombus (long arrow) propagating superiorly from the level of the vessel wall disruption. Note the transection of the external carotid artery (asterisk in [a]).

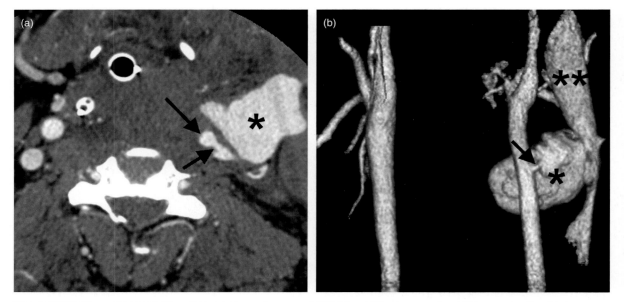

Figure 6.259 Traumatic vessel disruption: axial image from a neck CTA (a) and 3D volume rendered CTA reconstruction (b) show complete disruption of the posterolateral wall of the common carotid artery with extraluminal extravasation (short arrow in [a,b]), with a large pseudoaneurysm (single asterisk) and a carotid–jugular fistula (double asterisk in [b] indicated by jugular vein opacification). The long arrow in (a) indicates the common carotid artery.

PRES, hypertensive encephalopathy

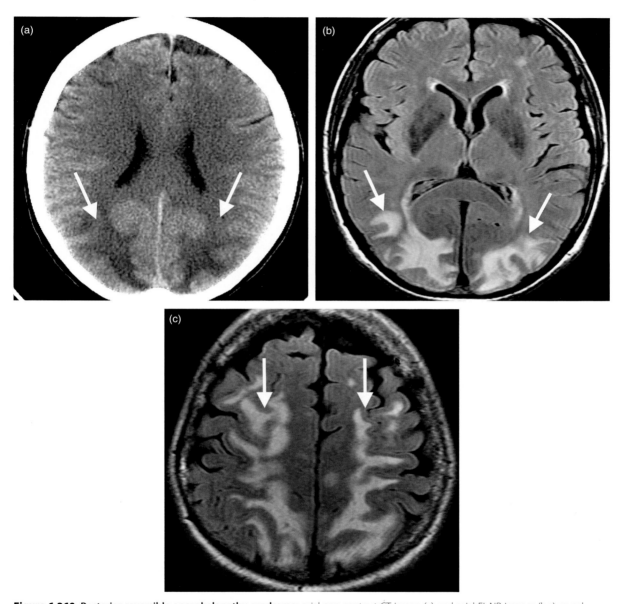

Figure 6.260 Posterior reversible encephalopathy syndrome: axial non-contrast CT image (a) and axial FLAIR images (b,c) reveal hypodensity (arrows in [a]) and increased signal intensity (arrows in [b,c]) in the subcortical white matter of the occipital and parietal lobes, with anterior extension into the frontal lobes in this patient with hypertensive encephalopathy. *Source:* Used with permission from Barrow Neurological Institute.

Neurodegenerative disorders (specific locations)

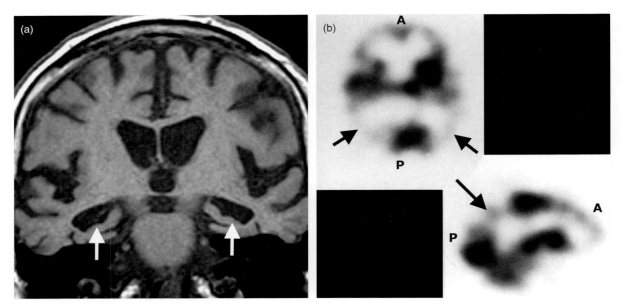

Figure 6.261 Alzheimer's dementia: non-contrast coronal T1WI (a) and representative images from a brain SPECT study (b) show severe bilateral hippocampal atrophy (arrows) in (a), and areas of decreased activity in the temporal (short arrows) and parietal (long arrow) regions on the SPECT study (b).

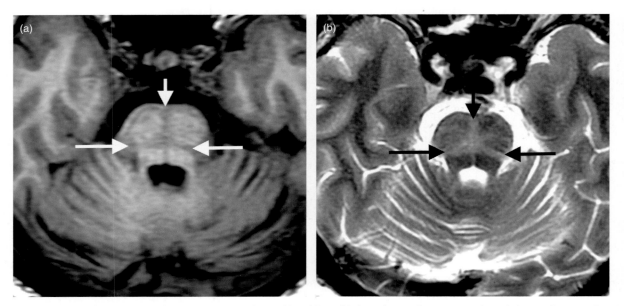

Figure 6.262 Multisystem atrophy: non-contrast axial T1WI (a) and T2WI (b) show the cruciform pattern of signal abnormality secondary to degeneration of the transverse pontocerebellar fibers and the pontine raphe (arrows). *Source:* Used with permission from Barrow Neurological Institute.

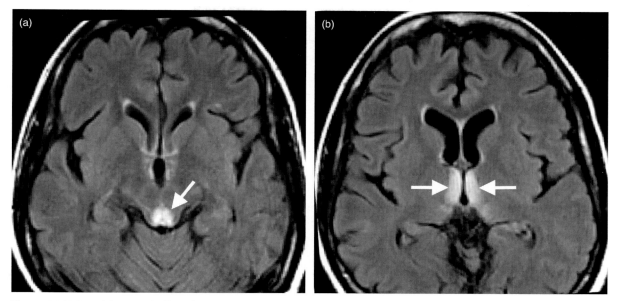

Figure 6.263 Wernicke–Korsakoff syndrome: axial FLAIR images (a,b) show abnormal increased signal in the periaqueductal gray matter (arrow in [a]) and medial thalami (arrows in [b]). The patient also had mammillary body atrophy (not shown).

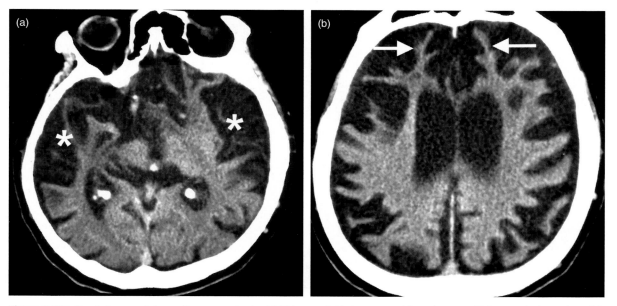

Figure 6.264 Frontotemporal dementia: non-contrast axial CT images (a,b) show severe bilateral temporal lobe atrophy (asterisks in [a]), and severe frontal lobe atrophy with the knife-blade atrophy of frontal gyri (arrows in [b]).

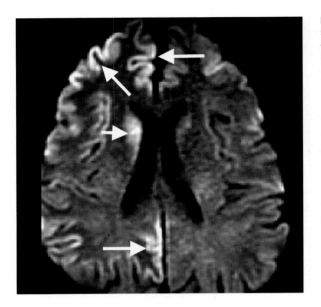

Figure 6.265 Creutzfeld-Jakob disease: diffusion trace image shows increased signal intensity along the cortical gyri (long arrows) and in the right caudate nucleus (short arrow). *Source:* Used with permission from Barrow Neurological Institute.

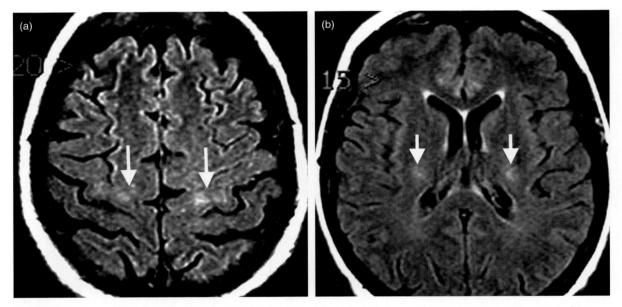

Figure 6.266 Amyotrophic lateral sclerosis: axial FLAIR images (a-d) show increased signal intensity beginning in the region of the precentral gyri (arrows in [a]), extending in a confluent fashion through the corona radiat (arrows in [b]), through the cerebral peduncles (arrows in [c]), into the ventral pons (arrows in [d]), along the course of the corticospinal tracts.

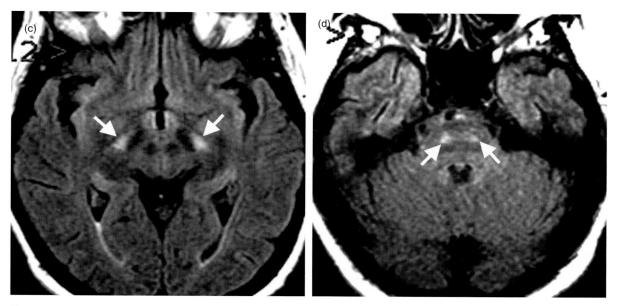

Figure 6.266 (*cont.*)

Miscellaneous disorders of the brain

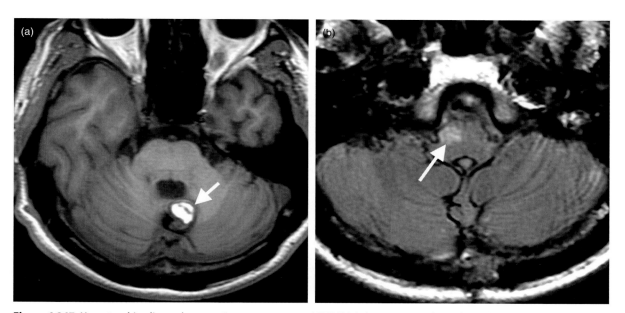

Figure 6.267 Hypertrophic olivary degeneration: non-contrast axial T1WI (a) shows an area of mixed signal intensity hemorrhage involving the left dentate nucleus (arrow) associated with mild enlargement and increased signal, on the axial FLAIR image (b), within the right inferior olivary nucleus (arrow). *Source:* Used with permission from Barrow Neurological Institute.

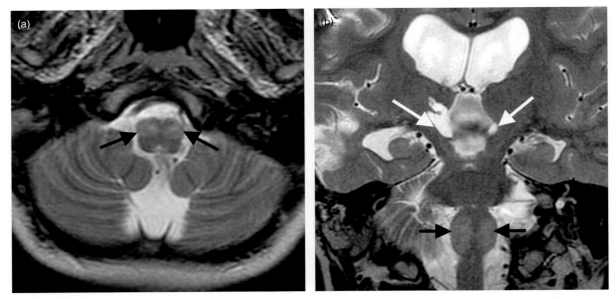

Figure 6.268 Bilateral hypertrophic olivary degeneration: axial (a) and coronal (b) T2WI show damage to the bilateral midbrain regions (right worse than left), indicated by the white arrows in (b) associated with enlargement and increased signal in both inferior olivary nuclei (shown by the black arrows in [a and b]). *Source:* Used with permission from Barrow Neurological Institute.

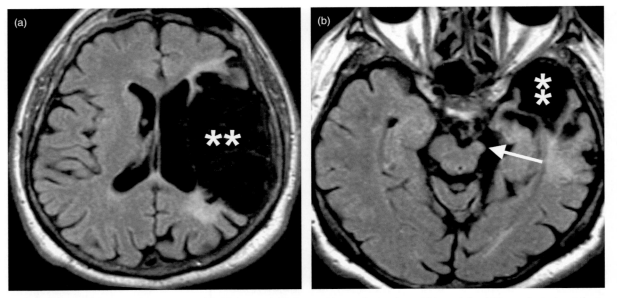

Figure 6.269 Wallerian degeneration: axial FLAIR images (a,b) show evidence of a previous old, large, left middle cerebral artery infarct (double asterisks) associated with atrophic changes of the left cerebral peduncle (arrow in [b]).

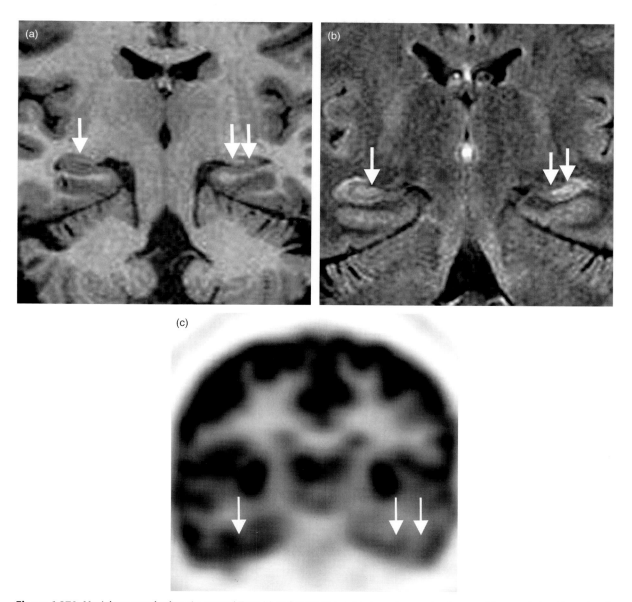

Figure 6.270 Mesial temporal sclerosis: coronal T1WI (a) and FLAIR image (b) show decreased volume and increased signal intensity of the left hippocampal body (double arrows), compared with the normal right side (single arrow). Coronal PET scan (c) shows asymmetric decreased metabolism in the left temporal lobe (double arrows).

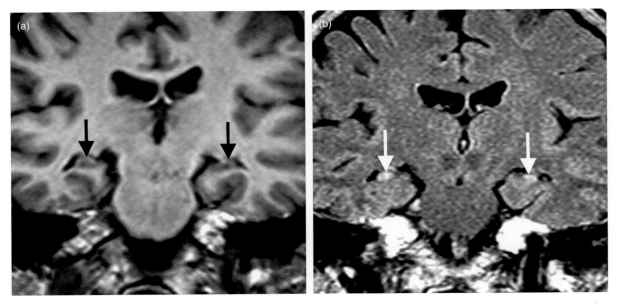

Figure 6.271 Bilateral mesial temporal sclerosis: coronal T1WI (a) and FLAIR image (b) show decreased volume and increased signal intensity in both the right and left hippocampal bodies (arrows).

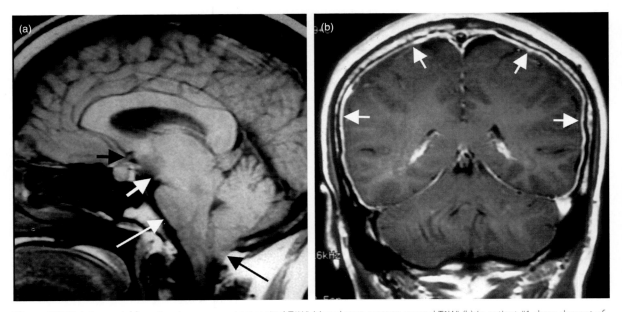

Figure 6.272 Intracranial hypotension: non-contrast sagittal T1WI (a) and post-contrast coronal T1WI (b) in patient #1 show descent of the posterior fossa contents with inferior tonsillar herniation (long black arrow in [a]), flattening of the ventral pons along the clivus (long white arrow in [a]), loss of the interpeduncular cistern (short white arrow in [a]), and loss of the suprasellar cistern (short black arrow in [a]). There is mild diffuse uniform dural thickening and enhancement (arrows in [b]). In patient #2 (c) similar findings are present on the non-contrast sagittal T1WI. *Source:* Figure 6.272c used with permission from Barrow Neurological Institute.

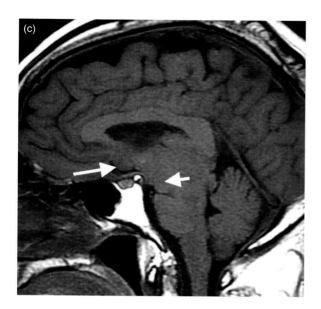

Figure 6.272 (cont.)

Hydrocephalus

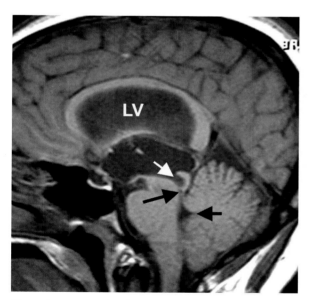

Figure 6.273 Aqueductal stenosis: non-contrast sagittal T1WI demonstrates benign stenosis of the posteroinferior aqueduct of Sylvius (long black arrow), with dilatation of the proximal aqueduct (short white arrow), a small fourth ventricle (short black arrow), and dilatation of the third and lateral (LV) ventricles.

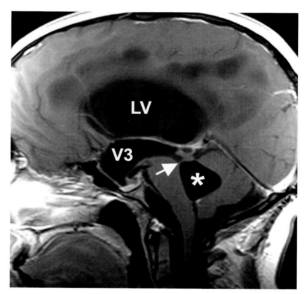

Figure 6.274 Aqueductal stenosis and trapped fourth ventricle: post-contrast sagittal T1WI shows benign stenosis of the posteroinferior aqueduct of Sylvius (white arrow), with prominent dilatation of the fourth ventricle (asterisk) in addition to dilatation of the third (V3) and lateral ventricles (LV).

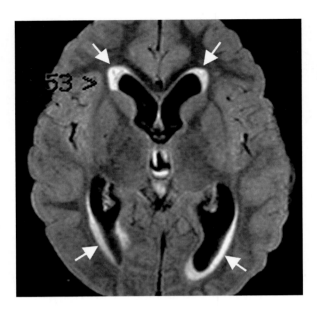

Figure 6.275 Transependymal resorption of CSF: axial FLAIR image shows dilatation of the third and lateral ventricles, with a confluent rind of increased signal intensity surrounding the lateral ventricles reflecting transependymal resorption of CSF in this case of obstructive hydrocephalus.

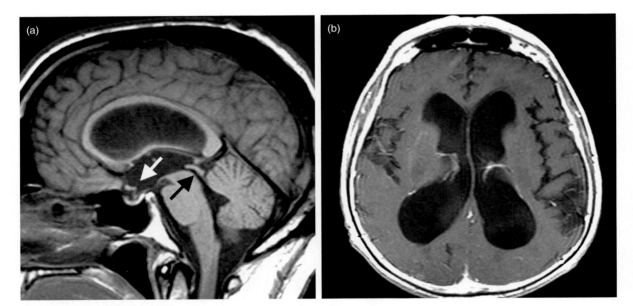

Figure 6.276 Communicating hydrocephalus: non-contrast sagittal T1WI (a) and post-contrast axial T1WI (b) show dilatation of the third and lateral ventricles out of proportion to the size of the sulci. There is accentuated flow void through the aqueduct of Sylvius (black arrow in [a]). The fourth ventricle is normal in size. The white arrow in (a) indicates dilatation of the infindibular and optic recesses of the third ventricle.

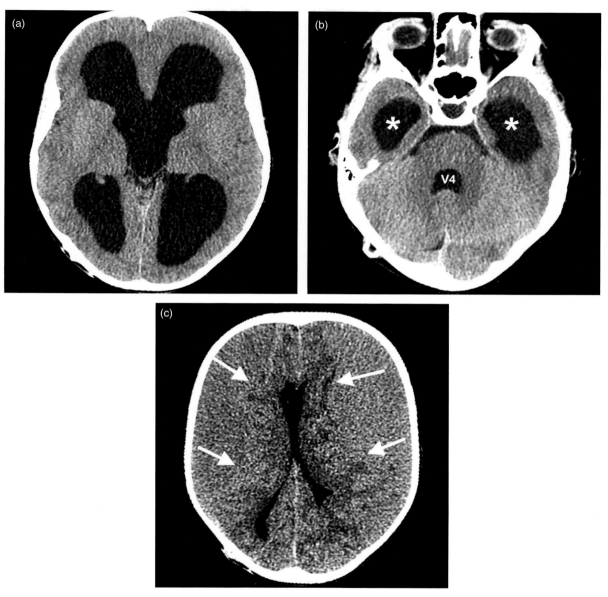

Figure 6.277 Communicating hydrocephalus: non-contrast axial CT images (a,b) show dilatation of the third and lateral ventricles with absent sulci. Note the enlarged temporal horns (asterisks in [b]). The fourth ventricle (V4) is normal to slightly prominent. Non-contrast axial CT image (c) shows massive bilateral isodense, subacute subdural hematomas (arrows), with marked compression of the cerebral hemispheres and lateral ventricles owing to overshunting.

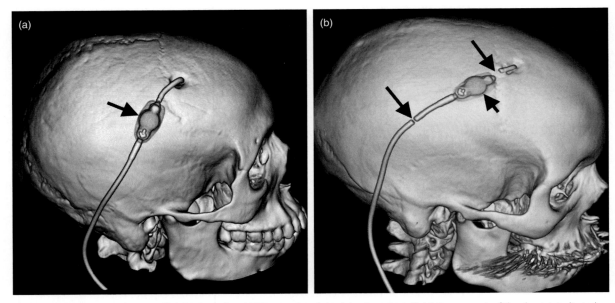

Figure 6.278 Shunt catheters: 3D volume rendered CT images in two patients. In patient #1 (a) the reservoir of the shunt is indicated by the black arrow. The visualized tubing of the shunt catheter is intact. In patient #2 (b) you can see two discrete breaks (long arrows) in the shunt catheter to either side of the reservoir (short black arrow).

Suggested reading

1. Arbour R. Intracranial hypertension monitoring and nursing assessment. *CriticalCareNurse* 2004; **24**(5): 19–32.

2. Barkovich AJ. Concepts of myelin and myelination in neuroradiology. *American Journal of Neuroradiology* 2000; **21**: 1099–1109.

3. Barkovich AJ, Moore KR, Grant E, et al. *Diagnostic Imaging: Pediatric Neuroradiology*. Salt Lake City, Utah: Amirsys, Inc., 2007.

4. Bourekas EC, Varakis K, Bruns D, et al. Lesions of the corpus callosum: MR imaging and differential considerations in adults and children. *American Journal of Roentgenology* 2002; **179**(1): 251–257.

5. Cheon JE, Kim IO, Hwang YS, et al. Leukodystrophy in children: a pictorial review of MR imaging features. *Radiographics* 2002; **22**: 461–476.

6. Duncan JS, guest ed. Epilepsy. *Neuroimaging Clinics of North America* 2004; **14**(3): xi.

7. Edwards-Brown MK & Barnes PD, guest eds. Pediatric neuroimaging. *Neuroimaging Clinics of North America* 1999; **9**(1): 1–226 [editorial].

8. Erdag N, Bhorade RM, Alberico RA, Yousuf N, & Patel MR. Primary lymphoma of the central nervous system: typical and atypical CT and MR imaging appearances. *American Journal of Radiology* 2001; **176**: 1319–1326.

9. George AE, guest ed. Neurodegenerative diseases: Alzheimer's disease and related disorders. *Neuroimaging Clinics of North America* 1995; **5**(1): 1–44 [editorial].

10. Glass RB, Fernbach SK, Norton KI, Choi PS, & Naidich TP. The infant skull: a vault of information. *Radiographics* 2004; **24**: 507–522.

11. Greenberg MS. *Handbook of Neurosurgery*. New York: Thieme, 2006.

12. Kolias SS, Ball WS, & Prenger EC. Cystic malformations of the posterior fossa: differential diagnosis clarified through embryologic analysis. *Radiographics* 1993; **13**: 1211–1231.

13. McRobbie DW, Moore EA, Graves MJ, & Prince MR. *MRI from Picture to Proton*. Cambridge: Cambridge University Press, 2008.

14. Mokri B. The Monro-Kellie hypothesis. *Neurology* 2001; **56**: 1746–1748.

15. Mukherji SK, consulting ed. Advanced imaging techniques in brain tumors. *Neuroimaging Clinics of North America* 2009; **19**(4): xi.

16. Osborn AG. *Diagnostic Neuroradiology*. St. Louis, Missouri: Mosby-Year Book, Inc., 1994.

17. Osborn AG, Saltzman KL, & Barkovich AJ. *Diagnostic Imaging: Brain*. Salt Lake City, Utah: Amirsys, Inc., 2004.

18. Parazzini C, Baldoli C, Scotti G, & Triulzi F. Terminal zones of myelination: MR evaluation of children aged 20–40 months. *American Journal of Neuroradiology* 2002; **23**: 1669–1673.

19. Ricci PE, guest ed. Brain tumors. *Neuroimaging Clinics of North America* 1999; **9**(4): 581–831 [editorial].

20. Ruzek KA, Campeau NG, & Miller GM. Early diagnosis of pontine myelinolysis with diffusion-weighted imaging. *American Journal of Neuroradiology* 2004; **25**: 210–213.

21. Schaefer PW & Gonzalez RG, eds. Imaging acute stroke and its consequences. *American Journal of Neuroradiology* 2008; **29**: 306 [editorial].

22. Scheid R, Preul C, Gruber O, Wiggins C, & von Cramon DY. Diffuse axonal injury associated with chronic traumatic brain injury: evidence from T2*-weighted gradient-echo imaging at 3 T. *American Journal of Neuroradiology* 2003; **24**: 1049–1056.

23. Ukisu R, Kushihashi T, Tanaka E, et al. Diffusion-weighted MR imaging of early-stage Creutzfeldt–Jakob disease: typical and atypical manifestations. *Radiographics* 2006; **226**: S191–S204.

24. Willing SJ. *Atlas of Neuroradiology*. Philadelphia, Pennsylvania: W. B. Saunders Company, 1995.

25. Yalçın O, Yildirim T, Kizilkiliç O, et al. CT and MRI findings in calvarial non-infectious lesions. *Diagnostic and Interventional Radiology* 2007; **13**: 68–74.

26. Young GS, Geschwind MD, Fischbein NJ, et al. Diffusion-weighted and fluid-attenuated inversion recovery imaging in Creutzfeldt–Jakob disease: high sensitivity and specificity for diagnosis. *American Journal of Neuroradiology* 2005; **26**: 1551–1562.

27. Zee CS & Go JL, guest eds. Intracranial infectious diseases. *Neuroimaging Clinics of North America* 2000; **10**(2): 297–464 [editorial].

Basic concepts and terminology

The principles of CT and MR imaging of the brain also apply to the spine. GM and WM within the cord appear the same on MRI as GM and WM within the brain namely, GM is hypointense with respect to WM on T1WI. The difference is that GM occupies an H-shaped central aspect of the cord while WM occupies the periphery of the cord, the reverse of the arrangement within the brain. On CT imaging, GM and WM cannot be differentiated. Even with intrathecal contrast, only cord, nerve root, and vessel contour are evaluated. With MRI, GM–WM differentiation is possible on T2WI, particularly with gradient recalled echo (GRE) images. GM and WM are poorly delineated with T1WI.

Vertebral marrow is best evaluated with non-contrasted T1WI, supplemented by FSE T2 and short tau inversion recovery (STIR) images. Vertebral marrow is predominantly composed of yellow (fatty) and red (hematopoietic) marrow. Hematopoietic marrow is relatively hypointense and fatty marrow relatively hyperintense on T1WI. Marrow infiltrative processes are characterized by hypointensity on T1WI images with respect to the intervertebral discs. By contrast, post-radiation changes within vertebral marrow are characterized by nearly uniform fatty marrow replacement, manifest as hyperintense signal on T1WI. Marrow edema is best evaluated with STIR images, a sequence that is highly sensitive to the presence of stationary water.

On CT imaging, evaluation of the intervertebral disc is limited to height, the presence of gas (i.e. vacuum disc), and the presence of calcification. Soft tissue and ligamentous anatomy can often be partially evaluated with good soft tissue windows. The structure of the intervertebral disc is best evaluated with MRI. The normal disc is composed of three components: the nucleus pulposus, inner annulus fibrosus, and outer annulus fibrosus. The nucleus pulposus and inner annulus are normally hyperintense on T2/STIR images owing to the presence of water and glycosaminoglycans. There is a small amount of collagen within the central portion of the nucleus pulposus that manifests as linear hypointense signal that parallels the endplates. The outer annulus is composed of radially arranged, concentric layers of collagen that are hypointense on all standard pulse sequences.

Ligamentous anatomy is best evaluated on FSE T2 and STIR images. The major ligaments of the spinal column, the ALL, PLL, ligamentum flavum, interspinous ligaments, and supraspinous ligaments are normally hypointense or black on all sequences. Ligamentous injury is characterized on MR T2/STIR imaging on a spectrum from linear or diffuse hyperintense signal within the ligament to frank disruption.

CSF within the spine is hypointense on T1WI and hyperintense on T2WI. Normal CSF pulsation can create special problems within the spinal subarachnoid spaces and can simulate hemorrhage, flow voids, and other pathology. The shorter echo time used in GRE T2 weighted sequences reduces pulsation artifacts and is a useful adjunctive sequence.

As is the case elsewhere in the body, cortical bone is seen as a thin, hypointense line on all pulse sequences. The cartilagenous surfaces of the facet joints display features of cartilage at other locations, namely uniform hyperintensity on T2WI. The epidural spaces are primarily fat-containing within the thoracic and lumbar spine and are hyperintense on T1 and FSE T2 images. There is very little epidural fat within the cervical spine.

Spaces and potential spaces

Epidural space: contains vessels, lymphatic tissue, loose connective tissue, and fat. The epidural space is a negative pressure space, with pressures reported between −1 and −7 cm H_2O. This space is a target for therapeutic injections of anesthetics, steroids, and autologous blood. Blood within this space generally displaces the dural sac away from adjacent bone.

Subdural space: a potential space between the dura and arachnoid layers. Hemorrhage within this space generally does not displace the dural sac and circumferentially narrows the subarachnoid space.

Subarachnoid space: the anatomic space located between the inner surface of the arachnoid and pia mater. The subarachnoid space is the target for lumbar punctures, intrathecal administration of medications, and the intrathecal administration of contrast agents for myelography and cisternography. Blood within this space generally layers dependently or in clumps along nerve roots.

Subpial space: a potential space only.

Cerebrospinal fluid

The normal CSF volume in an adult is 135–150 mL. Approximately 500 mL of CSF is produced daily. There is a net flow of CSF from the lateral and third ventricles into the aqueduct of Sylvius, and fourth ventricle. A small amount of CSF flows caudally into the central canal of the spinal cord via the obex of the fourth ventricle. The majority of CSF flows through the foramina of Magendie and Luschka into the ventral and dorsal subarachnoid spaces around the spinal cord and cerebral convexities. CSF flow is characteristically pulsatile and turbulent, particularly within the cervical spine. This pulsatility is thought to be transmitted from the cerebrovascular arterial system and is responsible for a variety of flow related artifacts on MRI. Normal CSF pressure is less than 20 cm CSF. Normal values for CSF constituents are as follows: protein 15–45 mg/dL, glucose 50–80 mg/dL, WBC <5 mm^3, RBC 0–5 mm^3, and opening pressure 5–20 cm H$_2$O. CSF should be clear and colorless.

Monroe–Kellie doctrine and the spine

The Monro–Kellie doctrine should be understood in order to avoid mischaracterizing pathologic processes within the spine. In the Monro–Kellie doctrine, the sum of the CSF, blood, and parenchymal volumes is assumed to remain constant. Alterations in one component result in compensation by the other components. In the case of CSF leak, the overall volume of CSF decreases and there is compensatory expansion of the blood component. This is manifested within the spine as increased dural enhancement, enlarged epidural venous plexuses, and engorgement of the spinal and pial venous plexuses. This pattern can generally be distinguished from that of a dural AVF by the lack of cord signal abnormality and epidural venous engorgement in cerebrospinal hypotension.

Compartments

Traditionally, the spinal column has been divided into three anatomic compartments. Thorough understanding of the boundaries of these compartments and proper placement of lesions within spinal compartments are essential in the development of a good differential diagnosis. The compartments of the spine are as follows:

Intramedullary compartment – includes the central spinal canal, spinal cord, and pia

Intradural extramedullary compartment – includes the inner surface of the dural sac, subarachnoid space, nerve roots, ligaments, cauda equina, and filum terminale

Extradural compartment – includes the outer surface of the dural sac, epidural spaces, vertebral bodies and posterior elements, intervertebral discs, and paraspinous soft tissues.

The Three Column Theory of the spine (Denis, 1984)

Anterior column – includes the ALL, anterior one half of the vertebral body, and the anterior one half of the intervertebral disc and annulus

Middle column – includes the posterior one half of the vertebral body, posterior half of the intervertebral disc and annulus, and PLL

Posterior column – includes the posterior elements, ligamentum flavum, interspinous and supraspinous ligaments

Instability of the spinal column is graded on the basis of the number of columns involved. In this model, instability is presumed when two contiguous columns or three columns are involved.

Basic approach to image interpretation

The interpretation of spine imaging studies requires a firm understanding of the basic anatomy and physiology of the spinal column. As is the case with brain imaging, accurate spine imaging interpretation requires synthesis of all available information, including clinical and demographic data, prior imaging studies, and determination of the morphology, location, and physiologic characteristics of the lesion in question.

The imaging appearance of various disease processes involving the spine can overlap significantly. However, the differential diagnosis in such cases can be made more manageable with the use of demographic data, knowledge of the patient's clinical presentation, and laboratory and physical examination findings. When combined with accurate lesion localization and basic epidemiologic data, the differential diagnosis can frequently be narrowed to a small number of possibilities.

You will quickly come to realize that there is a wide range of approaches to the interpretation of spine imaging studies, even among the most experienced neuroradiologists. You are encouraged to pay close attention to the habits and search patterns of the best spine imagers around you and to combine the best approaches into your own style. Developing your own rigorous and repeatable search pattern is essential. With the rise of voice recognition reporting systems, the use of structured reporting has become commonplace and, if used properly, will significantly reduce errors of omission. In the absence of voice recognition based structured reporting, a template structure can be internalized and reproduced with each dictation.

Computed tomography

Within the spine, CT is primarily used to assess bony anatomy and is the preferred modality in the evaluation of acute trauma. CT is also used in the setting of the postoperative spine, primarily to evaluate hardware and bony fusion. In addition, CT imaging is an integral component in the myelographic evaluation of the spine.

CT offers superior characterization of calcified and ossified spine lesions. For instance, ossification of the PLL and calcific tendonitis of the longus coli muscles can be difficult diagnoses with MRI, but may be easily diagnosed with CT imaging.

My approach to the interpretation of spine CT is similar to my approach to spine MRI. I always review the scout images first. It is important to keep in mind that the cross-sectional images are derived from reference points on the scout image. Invariably, the coverage area on the scout images is greater than that included on the subsequently obtained cross-sectional images. It is for this reason that the scout images should be carefully scrutinized as they may contain important information, incidental or otherwise.

Next I look at the sagittal reformatted images. The sagittal images allow a rapid assessment of curvature, vertebral body alignment, zygapophyseal joint alignment, fractures, vertebral body and disc space height, and spinal canal integrity. The coronal reformatted images provide optimal evaluation of the C0–C1 joints, the dens, and C1–C2 interrelationships.

The axial images are viewed in soft tissue and bony detail. In the setting of trauma, the optimal evaluation for fractures includes thin section (i.e. 0.6–1.0 mm) images with the use of a bone algorithm, rather than merely bone windows. Subtle fractures are often missed with the use of thicker sections (i.e. 3–4 mm) reviewed in standard bone windows.

Perhaps there is no other series of images that is more neglected than images of the spine processed in soft tissue algorithm or reviewed in soft tissue windows. For some reason, there is a general sense that the images in these series are low yield. I have not found this to be true. Acute hemorrhage within the compartments of the spine is often readily visualized. Disc disease, ligamentous hypertrophy, epidural processes, synovial cysts, multicompartmental masses, and a wide variety of other processes are visible with soft tissue windows.

Magnetic resonance imaging

I tend to view the MR images in the order they were obtained, starting with the localizer images. These images are often ignored, but valuable and potentially life-saving information is available on the localizer images. They are obtained with large fields of view and, as such, contain information outside of the standard narrow fields of view utilized for spine imaging. Incidental lesions are frequently encountered on the localizer images. In addition, scoliotic curves are easily viewed in the large field of view coronal localizer images, and are often the only coronal images that are obtained in most spine imaging studies. After reviewing the localizer series, I turn to the sagittal image sets.

The sagittal image sets are central to the imaging evaluation of the spine at all levels. Multilevel or diffuse processes are easily recognized on single images. Alignment, longitudinal ligamentous integrity, and vertebral body and disc space height are best evaluated on the sagittal image sets. STIR images are often acquired in the sagittal plane and are invaluable for the delineation of soft tissue, ligamentous, marrow, and cord edema.

Sagittal FSE T2 and STIR images are the workhorses of most spine imaging studies. The intervertebral discs are best evaluated on these images with disc degeneration manifest as loss of signal. Cord signal is best evaluated on the FSE and STIR sequences. The STIR sequence is exquisitely sensitive to marrow and ligamentous edema.

The sagittal T1WI, at first glance, seem to provide less information than the more visually appealing T2WI. However, with time one realizes that the T1WI provide information that can significantly impact the interpretation of each study. For instance, vertebral marrow is best evaluated with the T1WI. Second, the presence of intrinsic T1 hyperintensity can assist in the differential diagnosis. A short list of substances is intrinsically T1 hyperintense, including methemoglobin, fat, gadolinium, melanin, manganese, iron, certain concentrations of protein, and certain forms of calcium. Third, review of the pre-contrast T1WI is essential when gadolinium is administered. A hyperintense lesion on the post-contrast images must be compared to the pre-contrast images to ensure that the hyperintensity present on the post-contrast images is actually enhancement and not intrinsic T1 hyperintensity. In brief, T1WI are the friend you may not know you have.

Next are the axial FSE T2 or axial gradient images. Many PACS workstations allow users to label spinal levels in multiple planes. Such a practice is highly recommended to ensure accurate level by level reporting. Axial images allow a more complete assessment of the spinal canal, lateral recesses, and neural foramina. Localization within the various compartments of the spine is most often determined on the axial images. Disc herniations, syringohydromyelia, ligamentum flavum pathology, and cord signal abnormalities are examples of lesions that are more precisely evaluated on the axial images. Gradient recall echo (GRE) images are often a component of the axial evaluation of the spine. It is important to keep in mind that spinal canal and neuroforaminal stenoses will be overestimated on the GRE images owing to magnetic susceptibility artifact.

Finally, I complete a series of housekeeping steps, including returning to the clinical question to ensure that it has been satisfactorily answered. Assessment of the soft tissues of the neck, thorax, or retroperitoneum completes the examination.

Generalized categorization of diseases and location

Normal aging and degenerative disease of the spine
Normal aging and the spine

Changes in the appearance of the spine that occur normally in the process of aging should be differentiated from degenerative disease. While it is certain that there is overlap in the imaging appearance of the normal aging spine and degenerative disease, some general points of differentiation exist. There is a slight decrease in T2 signal intensity with age that is related to decreases in water content, a decrease in glycosaminoglycans content, and a relative increase in collagen content within the intervertebral disc. Concentric and transverse tears have also been reported within the peripheral annulus. A central transverse zone of hypointensity on T2WI is typical of the aging disc. Intervertebral disc space height and the relative T2 hyperintensity within the nucleus pulposus and inner annulus should be maintained in normal aging.

With increasing age, the proportion of red marrow declines and there is a proportionate increase in yellow marrow. A rough rule of thumb is that the percentage of red marrow is equal to 100 minus a person's age in years. For instance, a normal 70-year-old person would have approximately 30% hemopoietically active marrow. On T1WI, there is an increase in the heterogeneity of vertebral marrow and a relative increase in percentage of hyperintense (fatty) marrow with age.

There is progressive thinning of the cartilage at the surfaces of the articular facets or zygapophyseal joints, particularly within the cervical and lumbar spine. There is also near universal appearance of osteophytes at the margins of the aging facet joints. However, hypertrophy of the zygapophyseal or uncinate/enchancure interface are not considered to be a part of the normal aging process.

After the fifth decade, small anterior and lateral osteophytes are ubiquitous. Osteophytes tend to occur at stress points within the spine, specifically the mid- to lower cervical spine, the mid-thoracic spine, and the lower lumbar spine. Osteophytes in the thoracic spine are predominantly right sided, likely a direct result of aortic pulsations. In the ninth decade, large osteophytes should be considered normal.

Degenerative spondylolisthesis

Spondylolisthesis is a term that describes a change in the alignment of one vertebral body with reference to another vertebral body. By convention, the position of the more superiorly located segment is described with reference to the segment immediately below. For instance, if the posterior margin of the L4 vertebral body is displaced 3 mm anterior to the posterior margin of L5, this would be described as an anterolisthesis of L4 on L5. Spondylolisthesis is graded as follows: grade 1 (0%–25% of the width of the vertebral body), grade 2 (25%–50%), grade 3 (50%–75%), grade 4 (75%–100%), and grade 5 (>100% spondyloptosis). When reporting spondylolisthesis, these two descriptors are generally used together. Using the example above, the text of the report would read, "There is a grade 1 anterolisthesis of L4 on L5." Degenerative spondylolisthesis is most commonly grade 1 and related to osteophyte formation within the facet joints. Facet degenerative changes are often exacerbated by loss of intervertebral disc space height with resultant alteration in the orientation of the facet joints and subsequent proliferation of osteophytes.

Spondylolysis
(see Figure 11.1a,b, page 286)

Spondylolysis is a defect in the pars interarticularis (isthmus) that has an estimated prevalence of 8%–10% in the general population. Trauma is suspected as the mechanism, supported by an increased prevalence of spondylolysis in various athletes. There are similar rates of back pain in patients with spondylolysis and the general population. It most commonly occurs at L5 (80%) and is usually bilateral (80%). In cases of unilateral pars interarticularis defects, there can be hypertrophy and sclerosis of the contralateral pedicle. Approximately 15% of all cases progress to spondylolisthesis. Progressive facet hypertrophy and disc degeneration are commonly associated findings.

On plain x-ray films, spondylolysis is best seen on oblique images that show discontinuity of the "Scotty dog" neck. CT is the most sensitive modality and will show the isthmic defects on parasagittal images. On axial CT images there is characteristic anteroposterior elongation of the spinal canal. The isthmic defects may appear similar to facets and produce a double facet sign on axial images. Associated spinal canal and neuroforaminal stenosis is best evaluated with MRI. However, the sensitivity and specificity of MRI for identifying pars defects is significantly lower than CT imaging. Occasionally, marrow edema can be seen adjacent to pars defects.

Ligamentous ossification and interspinous arthrosis
(see Figures 11.2a,b, 11.3a,b, page 287)

OPLL is most common in the mid-cervical spine (C3–C6) and less common in the mid-thoracic spine. OPLL has been classified as: continuous (extending over several segments), segmental (one or multiple separate lesions located along the posterior surface of the vertebral body), mixed type, or circumscribed (occurring at the level of the intervertebral disc space). OPLL is generally asymptomatic. However, the ossified PLL can contribute to spinal canal stenosis and can be associated with a progressive myelopathy. Patients with OPLL are at a significantly increased risk of spinal cord injury in the setting of trauma.

Ossification of the ALL is more commonly referred to as diffuse idiopathic skeletal hyperostosis (DISH). DISH is defined as the presence of flowing anterior osteophytes extending over four or more contiguous vertebral levels and the relative absence of degenerative disc disease and zygapophyseal ankylosis. DISH is typically discovered incidentally on chest radiographs. It is associated with OPLL and increasing age, is generally asymptomatic, and can be associated with restricted range of movement

within the spine. It can be seen at all levels of the spine, but most commonly within the thoracic spine, followed by the cervical and lumbar spine in descending order of frequency.

Ossification of the ligamentum flavum is less commonly seen and is visualized as flowing calcification or ossification dorsal to the cord and can produce significant spinal canal stenosis. It can be seen at one segment or multiple segments and may be unilateral or bilateral.

On plain films and sagittal CT reconstructions, there is flowing ossification anterior (DISH) and posterior (OPLL) to the vertebral body. In the thoracic spine, the ossification in DISH predominantly occurs to the right of the midline as a function of aortic position. DISH is distinguished from spondylosis by the presence of ossified or calcified material at levels other than the disc level. On axial CT images, OPLL has the appearance of an inverted "T" that projects dorsally from the posterior margin of the vertebral body. The ossification may be contiguous or noncontiguous with the vertebral body. On MRI, OPLL, DISH, and ossification of the ligamentum flavum are generally hypointense on all pulse sequences. When fatty marrow is present, T1 signal will be iso- to hyperintense. In OPLL, axial images will also demonstrate the inverted "T" morphology. MRI best demonstrates the degree of spinal canal stenosis and the presence of cord edema.

Baastrup syndrome refers to a rare lumbar pain syndrome characterized by worsened pain with extension and relief with flexion. The process can range from inflammatory changes to bursa formation. The bursae can project into the epidural spaces and cause or contribute to spinal canal stenosis. On imaging, there is close approximation of the spinous processes of one or multiple levels along with associated osseous hypertrophy, eburnation, and flattening of the apposing surfaces. MRI best demonstrates bursa formation as T1 hypointense and T2 hyperintense signal in the interspinous space. Enhancement of the bursa can be seen. Epidural cyst formation and resultant canal stenosis is best evaluated with MRI (see Figure 11.4, page 288).

Spinal stenosis

Stenosis refers to narrowing of the spinal canal, subarticular recesses, or neural foramina of the spine. Stenosis can be congenital (in association with short pedicles) or acquired. Spinal canal stenosis can result from a variety of abnormalities that vary according to the spinal level.

Cervical stenosis

Spinal canal stenosis in the cervical spine can result from impingement by disc material, osteophytes, disc osteophyte complexes, uncovertebral joint hypertrophy, zygapophyseal joint hypertrophy, ligamentous hypertrophy, ligamentous ossification, or a combination of these. In the cervical spine, subarticular recess and neuroforaminal stenosis primarily result from uncovertebral joint hypertrophy and zygapophyseal joint hypertrophy. There are varying methods of determining spinal canal stenosis, both quantitative and qualitative. The Torg–Pavlov ratio has been used with plain films and CT images. It is the ratio of vertebral body width to cervical canal diameter on the lateral projection view or mid-sagittal slice on the CT image, and should equal 1.0. Ratios less than 0.80–0.85 indicate spinal canal stenosis. Other systems use the degree of effacement of the subarachnoid spaces or measurements of spinal canal diameter.

Thoracic stenosis

Symptomatic stenosis is less commonly encountered in the thoracic spine. Spondylosis in the thoracic spine is most common from T4–T5 to T7–T8. Anterior osteophytes increase in frequency with age and are more common to the right of the midline. Disc protrusions and posterior osteophytes may be seen in the thoracic spine, but are less commonly symptomatic than in the cervical and lumbar levels. Spinal canal stenosis, subarticular recess stenosis, and neuroforaminal stenosis are uncommon in the thoracic spine. This may be because of the greater structural stability provided by the thoracic cage.

Lumbar stenosis

Spondylosis in the lumbar spine is most common at the L4–L5 and L5–S1 levels. Congenital spinal stenosis results from short pedicles and is generally not symptomatic until middle age. With increasing age, acquired stenosis increases in frequency. Acquired spinal stenosis within the lumbar spine can result from impingement by disc material, disc osteophyte complexes, zygapophyseal joint hypertrophy, synovial cysts, ligamentum flavum hypertrophy, epidural lipomatosis, and high-grade spondylolisthesis. Symptomatic spinal canal stenosis is associated with dural sac

areas of less than $100\,mm^2$ and decreasing CSF to nerve root ratios. Lateral recess and neuroforaminal stenosis in the lumbar spine are associated with disc herniations, zygapophyseal joint arthropathy, synovial cysts, marginal osteophytes, and high-grade spondylolisthesis.

Degenerative disc disease
(see Figure 11.5a,b, page 288)

Degenerative disc disease on CT imaging is visualized as loss of disc space height, gas containing clefts within radial tears (i.e. vacuum discs), and occasionally calcification. On MRI, degenerative disc disease is typically characterized as a loss of signal on T2WI and STIR sequences and a loss of intervertebral disc space height. Vacuum discs may be visible as signal dropout on a background of a low-signal intervertebral disc on MRI. Calcification of the intervertebral discs is also occasionally visible on MRI. A strong correlation between the signal changes of degenerative disc disease on MRI and patient symptoms has not been convincingly established.

Nomenclature of disc contour abnormalities

In order to improve accuracy and consistency in the reporting of lumbar disc pathology, the combined task forces of the North American Spine Society, American Society of Neuroradiology, and the American Society of Spine Radiology have agreed to a set of recommendations on nomenclature (www.asnr.org/spine_nomenclature/).

Using this system, disc herniation is defined as displacement of disc material beyond the normal intervertebral disc space. Disc herniation is classified according to the percentage of the total disc material that is displaced and may be localized (<50%) or generalized (>50%). Localized disc material displacement can be further classified as focal (<25%) or broad-based (25%–50%). A disc bulge exists when there is displacement of disc material 50%–100% beyond the edges of the ring apophysis.

The location of the displaced disc is also important to convey and can be described in the axial plane as central, right/left central or paracentral, subarticular, foraminal and extraforaminal, or far lateral. In the sagittal plane, the location of the displaced disc can be described as discal or disc level, infrapedicular and suprapedicular.

The morphology of the displaced disc may also be further categorized as protruded or extruded. Disc material is considered protruded when the greatest measurement of the disc material beyond the disc space is less than or equal to the greatest measurement of the disc material at the base, in any imaging plane. Disc material is considered extruded when, in any one plane, the measurement between the margins of the disc material located beyond the disc exceeds the measurement of the margins of the base of the displaced disc material. Disc material is considered sequestered when there is no contact between the displaced disc material and the parent disc. Disc material is referred to as migrated when it is displaced from the site of the opening in the annulus through which it was extruded. Migration in this sense only refers to position, so disc material may displace and maintain contact with the parent disc (migrated, non-sequestered), or migrate and lose contact with the parent disc (migrated, sequestered).

The Schmorl node represents herniation of disc material through a defect in the vertebral endplate into the vertebral marrow. Schmorl nodes may be seen in the setting of multilevel loss of anterior vertebral body height and kyphotic deformity in teenagers and young adults, in a condition referred to as Scheuermann's disease (see Figure 11.6, page 289). Herniation of disc material between the non-fused ring apophysis and the adjacent vertebral body is referred to as a limbus vertebra.

Endplate marrow changes associated with degenerative disc disease
(see *Figure 11.7a,b, page 289*)

Marrow signal changes can be associated with degenerative disc disease and were first categorized by Modic and colleagues. Type 1 endplate changes are hypointense on T1, hyperintense on T2/STIR sequences, and can enhance following gadolinium administration. Type 2 changes are hyperintense on T1 and iso- to hyperintense on T2 images. Type 3 changes are the least common and consist of hypointense signal on T1 and T2 images. Type 1 changes are inflammatory in etiology, are most likely to indicate segmental instability, are more likely to be associated with active symptoms, and tend to predict a desirable outcome following lumbar fusion. Type 1 changes may be impossible to distinguish from early discitis osteomyelitis. Type 2 changes are the most common and tend to be the most stable over time. Type 3

changes tend to correspond to subchondral sclerosis on plain films or CT imaging. Conversion to different subtypes can occur over time and combinations are commonly encountered, particularly Type 1 changes superimposed on Type 2 changes.

Annular tears
(see *Figure 11.8,* page 290)

Radial and transverse annular tears are generally located within the dorsal annulus and can be seen on both sagittal and axial images. Annular tears are generally curvilinear in morphology, hyperintense on T2WI and STIR, and enhance following gadolinium administration. Only radial and transverse tears are visible on MRI. Radial tears extend from the periphery of the annulus to the nucleus pulposus. Transverse tears represent disruption of Sharpey fibers at the periphery of the annulus.

The significance of annular tears, as identified on MRI, is currently a matter of debate. Annular tears on MRI have been demonstrated to correlate with symptomatic levels at discography. However, annular tears are frequently seen in asymptomatic populations. Annular tears are more reliably identified on post-contrast T1WI. T2 signal abnormalities and contrast enhancement can persist for prolonged periods of time and should not be assumed to indicate acuity.

Spinal trauma

Acute injury to the spine occurs in approximately 5% of injury-related emergency department visits or approximately 150,000 cases per year in North America. Early and accurate diagnosis of spinal injury is essential as delayed diagnosis is strongly associated with worsened neurological outcome.

The use of CT imaging and MRI in the setting of trauma has increased significantly over the past two decades. CT imaging offers several advantages over plain films, including decreased need for meticulous patient positioning, significantly decreased imaging time, superior sensitivity and specificity, and multiplanar capabilities. MRI is the modality of choice for the identification of injuries to the spinal cord, spinal ligaments, intervertebral discs, and paraspinous soft tissues. Post-traumatic hemorrhages within the compartments of the spinal canal can often be visualized with CT imaging, but are best evaluated with MRI. The combination of myelography and CT myelography may offer improved evaluation of nerve root avulsions over MRI. CTA and MRA are indicated when vascular injury is suspected. CTA can be performed in a fraction of the time that it takes to perform MRA.

Cervical spine injuries

Injuries to the cervical spine represent approximately 60% of all spinal injuries. The cervical spine is commonly divided into the craniocervical (C0–C1 and C1–C2) and subaxial components. The subaxial cervical spine is fractured more commonly (65%) than the craniocervical spine (35%).

Craniocervical injuries

Injuries at the craniocervical junction are associated with significant morbidity and mortality and are notoriously difficult to detect, estimated to be missed on initial inspection up to 50% of the time. Of those cases missed initially, neurological deterioration occurs in approximately one-third of cases. The most common injuries of the upper cervical spine include occipital condyle fractures, atlanto-occipital subluxation, atlantoaxial subluxation, C1 ring fractures, odontoid fractures, and hangman fractures.

Occipital condyle fractures

These are classified as follows: the type I fracture is a comminuted impaction fracture (stable), the type II fracture is an occipital bone fracture that extends into the occipital condyle (stable), the type III fracture represents an alar avulsion fracture (usually unstable). Occipital condylar fractures are often missed on plain films and are largely diagnosed with CT imaging.

Atlanto-occipital subluxation

This injury is associated with significant morbidity and mortality and is most commonly observed in association with type III occipital–condyle fractures, disruption of the tectorial membrane, and C0–C1 ligamentous disruption. This type of injury is up to ten times more common in the first decade and the resulting mortality is higher in this age group. The general mechanism is that of extension and distraction. On plain films and CT images, C0–C1 subluxation should be suspected when the basion–dens interval is greater than 12 mm. The basion–posterior axial line interval is more reliable in children under thirteen years of age and should not exceed 12 mm anterior or 4 mm posterior to the posterior axial line. The Powers ratio can be normal with pure distraction and is not recommended. On CT

images, subluxation is seen as widening of one or both C0–C1 joints and displacement of the C1 lateral masses with respect to the occipital condyles. On MRI, STIR images best demonstrate abnormal hyperintense signal (fluid) within the C0–C1 joints. In subtle cases, there may be increased STIR signal without abnormal basion–dens and basion–posterior dens intervals. Commonly associated cervicomedullary, ligamentous, and soft tissue injuries are best demonstrated with MRI. Commonly associated vascular injuries include vasospasm and dissection, best evaluated with CTA, MRA, or traditional angiography (see Figure 11.9, page 290).

Atlantoaxial subluxation

This results from injury to the C1–C2 joint capsules, alar ligaments, tectorial membrane, and transverse ligament. This injury is up to ten times more common in the first decade of life. The mechanism of injury and associated morbidity and mortality are similar to that of C0–C1 subluxation. The imaging findings are similar to those of C0–C1 subluxation. GRE is the ideal sequence employed to evaluate the integrity of the transverse ligament (see Figure 11.9, page 290).

C1 ring fractures

These fractures represent approximately 6% of all vertebral injuries and include disruption of the anterior arch, posterior arch, combined anterior and posterior arch (Jefferson fracture), lateral masses, and transverse processes. Anterior arch and transverse process fractures at C1 are most commonly avulsion fractures. All of the above fractures are considered stable except for a Jefferson fracture with an associated transverse ligament avulsion fracture. An isolated fracture of the C1 arch is exceedingly rare. Jefferson fractures are classically four-part fractures, but three-part and two-part fractures can be seen. The presence of a Jefferson fracture should raise the interpreting physician's suspicion for fractures at other vertebral levels, seen in approximately 25%–50% of cases. The general mechanism is that of axial loading and hyperextension. Incomplete osseous fusion across the C1 synchondroses can potentially be confused with a fracture (see Figure 11.10, page 290).

Odontoid fractures

These types of fractures represent approximately 10%–20% of all cervical fractures and are classified as follows: alar ligament avulsion fracture at the odontoid tip (type I; 2%), fracture of the odontoid base (type II; 50%–75%), and fracture of the C2 body at the union of the C2 body and dens (type III; 15%–25%). All three fracture subtypes may be mechanically unstable. Type II fractures are most likely to progress to nonunion (30%–50%). The general mechanism can be hyperflexion or hyperextension. Odontoid fractures are the most common cervical spine fractures in the elderly and can occur as an isolated injury. The role of MRI is to evaluate for cord or ligamentous injury and to evaluate the spinal canal. Marrow edema is visualized as hyperintense T2/STIR signal along the fracture lines. Lateral extension of a fracture line into a transverse foramen should raise suspicion of an associated vertebral artery injury, best evaluated with CTA, MRA, or traditional angiography (see Figure 11.11, page 291).

Hangman fracture

The hangman fracture represents approximately 5% of all cervical spine fractures and is characterized as a disruption of both C2 pedicles (or pars interarticularis) and associated traumatic spondylolisthesis of C2 on C3. These fractures are generally classified in accordance with the presence of angulation and the degree of distraction of the fragments. Fractures at other spinal levels are seen in one-third of cases. The general mechanism is that of sudden hyperextension with axial loading or forced hyperflexion. As with odontoid fractures, extension of a fracture line into a transverse foramen should raise suspicion for coexistent vertebral artery vasospasm or dissection. CTA, MRA, or traditional angiography may be indicated in these instances (see Figure 11.12, page 291).

Subaxial cervical spine injuries

The subaxial cervical spine includes the C3 to C7 segments. Injuries at these segments have a bimodal distribution with the first mode in the late teens and early twenties and a second mode in the middle of the sixth decade. Injuries are typically the result of high impact trauma in the former group and low impact trauma in the latter group.

Most subaxial cervical spinal injury classification systems are based on morphologic descriptions of fracture patterns and presumed mechanisms of trauma. These classification systems do not emphasize ligamentous injury, associated neurologic injury, or other clinical parameters. As a result, the older classification systems tend to have limited clinical relevance. A promising new system attempts to incorporate clinical status, fracture morphology, and information regarding the integrity of the discs and ligamentous structures into a classification system that appears to provide more relevant clinical information and predictive value. This system may also assist in clinical management (Vaccaro AR, et al., 2007) (see Figure 11.13a,b, page 292).

Common patterns of subaxial cervical spine injuries include: simple compression fractures, burst fractures, flexion teardrop fractures, distraction injuries, and rotation/translation injuries. In general, these fracture patterns are listed from the most stable to the most unstable injuries.

Simple compression fractures

This injury includes fractures of the endplates with associated loss of vertebral body height resulting in a wedge shaped vertebral body. There is no extension into the posterior elements and no evidence of disc or ligamentous injury. The posterior wall of the vertebral body remains intact. Simple compression fractures of the subaxial cervical spine are stable. MRI will demonstrate normal signal within the posterior ligamentous structures in simple compression fractures. Loss of anterior vertebral height greater than 25% and increased interspinous distance are suggestive of associated posterior ligamentous injury and instability. Complicated compression fractures will demonstrate T2/STIR hyperintense signal within the vertebral marrow and abnormal hyperintense T2/STIR signal within the posterior ligamentous structures. The predominant vector of force is presumed to be flexion.

The clay shoveler's fracture

This is a vertical or oblique avulsion fracture of the spinous process that can occur from C6–T3, but most commonly at C7. The mechanism is that of direct trauma or forcible hyperflexion. It is one of the most stable fractures. Schmitt disease is the childhood analogue of this injury and is characterized by avulsion of the secondary ossification center at the spinous process tip.

Burst fractures

These are comminuted, vertically oriented fractures of the vertebral body extending through the superior and inferior endplates and often with associated anterior height loss. There is frequently retropulsion of fracture fragments into the spinal canal that can result in spinal cord and/or nerve root compression. The fracture lines do not extend into the posterior elements. Posterior ligamentous injury may be observed, but is not a dominant component of this injury. The overall vector of force is presumed to be flexion and axial loading.

Distraction injuries

These injuries have in common disruption of vertical stabilizing elements of the spine. Bilateral perched facets, facet subluxation, and anterior column injuries such as disruption of the ALL and anterior intervertebral disc are all examples of distraction injuries. As such, both flexion and extension vectors of force can contribute to distraction injuries.

Translation/rotation injuries

The most severe subaxial cervical spine injuries involve components of translation and/or rotation. Translation is movement of one vertebral segment in relation to another vertebral segment and should normally not exceed 3.5 mm. Rotation increases the probability of injury to the intervertebral disc and is associated with greater degrees of spinal instability. The flexion teardrop fracture is the most severe example within this category and includes a sagittally oriented triangular avulsion fracture of the antero-inferior vertebral body, anterior compression fracture, ALL and posterior ligamentous disruption. Frequently, the teardrop fragment maintains continuity with the anterior spinal line. The posterior fragment often displaces into the spinal canal and may compress the cord. The PLL is variably disrupted. Evidence of posterior ligamentous injury includes widening of the interspinous and interlaminar spaces on plain films and CT imaging and abnormal hyperintense signal within or disruption of the posterior ligaments on MRI. Cord injury (usually anterior) is commonly associated with this injury complex and manifests as hyperintense T2/STIR signal. Cord hemorrhage is best evaluated with axial GRE images. Other fracture patterns in this category include bilateral facet dislocations (or fracture dislocations), bilateral pedicle or pars interarticularis fractures with segmental translation, and unilateral pedicle and lamina fractures (floating lateral mass).

Thoracic and lumbar spine injuries

Thoracolumbar injuries are present in approximately 4%–6% of all blunt traumas. The thoracolumbar junction is the most common location, likely the result of a transition from the relatively immobile thoracic segments to the mobile lumbar segments, effectively creating a fulcrum. A significant percentage (40%) of patients with injuries at one level have additional injuries at two or more levels. Lumbar injuries occurring below L1 (typical conus level) carry a better prognosis. Thoracolumbar spine fractures are rare in children. However, there is a higher incidence of spinal cord injury without radiographic abnormality (SCIWORA), presumably owing to the differential elasticity of the spinal column and cord, the cord being the more inelastic structure of the two.

Several thoracolumbar fracture classification systems have been proposed, none of which has become dominant. The systems vary somewhat in the terminology used, the number of spinal columns (two or three), incorporation of discoligamentous injuries, and use of clinical parameters (Sethi MK, et al., 2009). Wherever possible, concepts that are common to all or most of these classification systems will be employed in this section.

The most commonly encountered fractures in the thoracolumbar spine are compression fractures, burst fractures, Chance fractures, translational-rotational injuries, flexion-distraction injuries, and hyperextension injuries.

Compression fractures

These are the most commonly observed fractures in the thoracolumbar spine in adults and children. Endplate fractures produce anterior vertebral body height loss (<15% in simple compression fractures). There is no extension into the posterior elements or evidence of posterior ligamentous disruption. The posterior vertebral wall remains intact. There may be a single level of involvement or multiple levels of contiguous or non-contiguous involvement. Simple thoracolumbar compression fractures are stable. The primary vectors of force are axial loading and flexion. Plain films and CT imaging best demonstrate the fracture lines. MRI will demonstrate T2/STIR hyperintense marrow signal adjacent to the fracture, and the fracture line itself is occasionally visible as a hypointense line (see Figure 11.14a,b, page 292).

Burst fractures

These are comminuted, vertically oriented vertebral body fractures that traverse the superior and inferior endplates. The posterior fragment can displace into the spinal canal and compress the cord. The primary vector of force is axial loading (i.e. falling from a height), but there may be a flexion component that produces anterior wedging. Thoracolumbar burst fractures most commonly occur in the mid- to upper thoracic spine and upper lumbar spine. Burst fractures that occur below the conus have a lower incidence of neurologic morbidity. There is variable involvement of the posterior ligamentous complex and posterior elements. Ligamentous injury may be implied by widened interspinous and interlaminar spaces on plain films/CT images or directly visualized with STIR images. CT imaging best defines the bony fragments. MRI is optimal in evaluating for cord injury, posterior ligamentous integrity, and spinal compartmental hemorrhage. Cord hemorrhage is best identified with GRE (see Figure 11.15a,b, page 293).

Chance fracture

The Chance fracture was originally described as a horizontally oriented fracture involving the posterior vertebral body, neural foramen, neural arch, and spinous process. As originally described, this injury does not involve translation (horizontal displacement of one segment over another), distraction (vertical dissociation), or cord injury. The primary vectors of force are flexion and distraction. Chance fractures, in their pure form, are very rare.

Translational-rotational injuries

These injuries result from a combination of flexion-distraction, rotational, and shearing forces. The combination of these forces can result in vertebral compression, anterior or lateral translation, anterior disc disruption, posterior ligamentous disruption, and facet capsular dislocations, fractures or fracture dislocations. Often, a combination of CT imaging and MRI is required to fully characterize these injuries.

Flexion-distraction injuries

These Chance variants are similar to the Chance fracture but are associated with variable injuries to the intervertebral disc and ligamentous structures with resultant translation and distraction. As a result, flexion-distraction injuries are considered unstable. A pure ligamentous Chance variant has also been described. On plain films and CT images, the anterior wedging can be subtle and posterior ligamentous injury may be implied by an increased interspinous distance, widened interlaminar spaces, or facet subluxation.

Ligamentous injury can be evaluated with supervised flexion and extension views or MRI. On MRI, the ALL is typically intact. Disruption of the PLL and abnormal STIR signal within the interspinous ligaments may be seen. Cord contusion can be present and is manifest as hyperintense T2/STIR signal. Coexistent injuries to the mesentery and bowel are present in approximately 40% of patients (see Figure 11.16a,b, page 293).

Hyperextension injuries

Hyperextension injuries are uncommon, representing approximately 0.2% of all thoracolumbar injuries. A substantial percentage of the cases that have been reported occur after minor falls in patients with diffuse idiopathic skeletal hyperostosis or ankylosing spondylitis. The pattern of injury is the reverse of the flexion mechanism with fractures of the posterior elements, posterior vertebral body compression deformities, and variable disruption of the ALL and intervertebral disc. Of the cases reported, there is a high incidence of associated cord injury (see Figure 11.2, page 287).

Imaging of neurovascular injuries
Spinal cord trauma

Traumatic spinal cord injury is a significant cause of morbidity. There are approximately 12,000 new cases of spinal cord injury per year in the United States, the great majority of which are individuals under the age of 50 years. As discussed above, spinal cord injuries in children can occur without evidence of spinal column fractures, an entity called SCIWORA. With preexisting spinal canal stenosis, even seemingly trivial trauma can lead to significant cord contusion. MR is the imaging modality of choice. Cord contusion (edema) is visualized as an increase in cord caliber and hyperintense signal on T2, STIR, and GRE sequences at the levels of injury. Cord transection is best evaluated on T1 sequences and is visualized as ill-defined, irregular cord margins. Cord transection is probably overestimated on MRI. MRI is ideal for evaluating the degree of canal stenosis and cord compression. CT imaging is often used in conjunction with MRI to separate bony fragments from cord and hemorrhage. MR findings associated with a poor clinical outcome include cord hemorrhage, cord transection, long segment cord involvement, and greater degrees of cord compression.

Spinal cord infarcts secondary to arterial injury in the setting of trauma are rare. The mechanisms are likely systemic hypoperfusion and reduced cardiac output. MR is the imaging modality of choice and demonstrates hyperintense T2/STIR signal in the central GM ("owl's eyes") and cord expansion over multiple levels. With increasingly extensive ischemia, GM and WM involvement can be seen. The anterior spinal artery territory is more commonly involved than the posterior spinal artery (see Figure 11.17a,b, page 294).

Intraspinal hemorrhage
(see images on page 304–320)

Intraspinal hemorrhage includes bleeding into the epidural, subdural, subarachnoid, and intramedullary spaces. It is uncommon in the setting of spinal trauma. When hemorrhage does occur, it is most likely to be found in the epidural space. While intraspinal hematomas may cause or contribute to spinal canal stenosis in trauma, they can mostly be managed conservatively.

Epidural hematomas

Epidural hematomas occur in the potential space between the vertebral periostium and the dural sac. The epidural space is continuous from the foramen magnum to the sacrum. Trauma is an uncommon etiology of epidural hemorrhage. On imaging, traumatic spinal epidural hematomas are most commonly located in the dorsal epidural space and may extend multiple levels from the site of injury. They tend to be lentiform in shape, contiguous with bony structures, and displace epidural fat and the dural sac, unlike subdural hematomas. Multiple septations may be present. On CT images, acute hemorrhage appears hyperdense. On MRI, the imaging appearance varies over time. Acute hematomas tend to be iso- to hypointense on T1, heterogeneously hyperintense on T2, and hypointense on GRE images (deoxyhemoglobin). If there is a significant component of oxyhemoglobin, hyperintense signal will be seen on GRE images. Subacute hematomas (3–10 days) will begin to demonstrate T1 hyperintense signal (extracellular methemoglobin). There may be dural enhancement corresponding to reactive dural hyperemia. Focal contrast collections may indicate the presence of extravasation (see Figure 11.18a,b, page 294).

Subdural hematomas

Subdural hematomas occur in the space between the arachnoid mater and the dural sac. They are very rare in the setting of trauma. On imaging, subdural hematomas are intradural, are outlined by epidural fat, and are not contiguous with bony structures. Subdural hematomas can either outline or compress the cord. Multilevel involvement is common. CT images can be less confusing than MRI and will demonstrate hyperdensity within the subdural space. Signal characteristics on MRI vary according to the presence of various hemoglobin species, similar to hemorrhage in other spaces.

Subarachnoid hemorrhage

Trauma is the most common cause of subarachnoid hemorrhage (>50% of cases). However, most of these cases are attributable to procedures (e.g. lumbar puncture). On imaging, spinal subarachnoid hemorrhage can have a nodular, globular, or mass-like appearance, or may present as a fluid–fluid level. Because this hemorrhage is within the subarachnoid space, it can interdigitate with the cauda equina. On CT images, acute hemorrhage is hyperdense. On MRI, signal characteristics of subarachnoid hemorrhage are similar to hemorrhage in other spaces. Following contrast administration, there can be reactive never root enhancement.

Intramedullary hemorrhage

Intramedullary hemorrhage or hematomyelia is rare, seen in approximately 0.8% of patients with spine trauma. The presence of hemorrhage within the cord substance is a reliable indicator of poor neurologic outcome. Hematomyelia can be difficult to identify on CT images. On MRI, intramedullary hemorrhage generally appears as focal hypointense signal on T2WI and GRE images. GRE is the most sensitive MR sequence.

Vascular injuries

Extracranial vascular injuries associated with blunt trauma are rare. The most commonly encountered injuries are dissection, pseudoaneurysm, and vasospasm.

Dissection

This refers to a hematoma that collects within the arterial media and enters through a tear in the intima. A dissection that continues to the adventitia is called a dissecting aneurysm. Vertebral artery dissection is more common than internal carotid artery dissection. The cervical internal carotid artery distal to the carotid bulb and proximal to the proximal petrous segment is the most common location in the carotid arteries. The V2 (cervical) and V3 (suboccipital) segments are the most common locations in the vertebral arteries. Catheter angiography is still considered the gold standard, but has largely been supplanted by CTA and MRA. Imaging findings include: long tapered eccentric and irregular stenosis, increased external vessel diameter, crescentic mural thickening, dual lumen, intimal flap, and dissecting aneurysm. The intramural hematoma can be seen as crescentic hyperdensity on non-contrasted CT images and variable signal on MRI, depending on the age of the blood products. Vertebral artery dissections are not as well evaluated with MRI (see Figure 11.19a–c, page 295).

Pseudoaneurysm

A pseudoaneurysm refers to a focal outpouching from the vessel lumen with no surrounding normal vessel components. There is discontinuity of the vessel wall and the so-called wall of the pseudoaneurysm is composed of contoured thrombus. Pseudoaneurysms can be central (fusiform) or eccentric (saccular). In the fusiform type, there is central contrast enhancement along with focal luminal caliber enlargement and irregularity that is outlined by thrombus. In the saccular type, there is contrast enhancement within a lumen that is eccentric to the parent vessel lumen and surrounded by thrombus. On CT images, the thrombus is hypodense and may partially or completely fill the lumen of the pseudoaneurysm. On MRI, flow voids and complex flow signal may be seen in the residual pseudoaneurysm. There may be significant magnetic susceptibility artifact within the thrombus on GRE images (see Figure 11.20, page 296).

Vasospasm

Vasospasm tends to occur at the site of blunt trauma and is visualized on CT imaging, MRI, and catheter angiography as focal or multifocal smooth luminal narrowing. Differentiation from dissection may not be possible with static imaging modalities.

Infectious, inflammatory, and metabolic diseases of the spine

Spinal infections

Discitis/osteomyelitis

These conditions nearly always occur together and are most commonly associated with infection. In adults, the source is usually a recent procedure, surgery, or systemic infection. In children, the source is usually hematogenous. The most common organisms are

Staphylococcus aureus (50%–60%), streptococcus, and Gram negatives (intravenous drug abuse). More than 80% of patients have elevations in the ESR (erythrocyte sedimentation rate) and CRP (C-reactive protein). Plain films and CT images are insensitive in the early stages. In later stages, endplate erosions and loss of disc space height will be seen. Compression fractures may also be visible. MRI is the modality of choice. Typical findings include T1 hypointensity and the T2 hyperintensity of adjacent vertebral bodies and intervening disc. The most sensitive MR findings include: paraspinal or epidural inflammation, hyperintense disc signal on T2, disc enhancement, and endplate erosions. Early discitis/osteomyelitis may look identical to type 1 endplate marrow changes (see Figure 11.21a–d, page 297).

Non-pyogenic etiologies of discitis/osteomyelitis include mycobacteria, fungi, and brucellosis. Tuberculous spondylitis (Pott's disease) is most common in immunosuppressed patients. Brucellosis is uncommon in the United States. MRI with contrast is the best imaging modality. Findings suggestive of TB include: multilevel thoracic (skip) involvement, disc sparing, paraspinous abscesses (especially calcified), and vertebral destruction with Gibbus deformity. Brucellosis tends to involve the lower lumbar spine and sacroiliac joints. Vertebral destruction and paraspinous abscesses are less common. Fungal discitis/osteomyelitis may be indistinguishable from other non-pyogenic etiologies (see Figure 11.22a–c, page 298).

Epidural abscess

This type of abscess is a suppurative fluid collection in the space between the dura and the periostium. *S. aureus* (including MRSA) is the most common organism (65%). Patients often have predisposing conditions (e.g. diabetes, HIV), have contiguous infections, and have undergone various spinal procedures or surgeries. Epidural abscesses can produce progressive cord, conus, and cauda equina compression or ischemia. MRI is the optimal modality and will demonstrate T1 hypointensity, T2 hyperintensity, central diffusion restriction, and peripheral enhancement (abscess) or hetero- to homogeneous enhancement (phlegmon) (see Figure 11.21a–d, page 297).

Leptomeningitis

Leptomeningitis refers to inflammation of the leptomeninges (pia and arachnoid) and pachymeningitis is inflammation of the dura. The most common causes of acute meningitis are streptococci (neonates), *Hemophilus influenzae* (infants and children), and streptococci (adults). Depending on the patient population and region, a variety of fungal, mycobacterial, and/or opportunistic etiologic agents may be encountered. Lumbar puncture should be performed in all cases, unless contraindicated. The imaging appearance may overlap with carcinomatous meningitis, sarcoidosis, acute or chronic disseminated inflammatory polyradiculoneuropathy, and sterile arachnoiditis. In the early stages, imaging may be negative. MRI is the imaging modality of choice and may show smooth or nodular nerve root enhancement, dural enhancement, CSF enhancement, and nerve root clumping (see Figure 11.23a,b, page 299).

Infectious myelitis

Infectious myelitis is most commonly caused by viral or bacterial agents. Common viral causes include Epstein–Barr virus (EBV), CMV, herpes zoster, HIV, human T-cell leukemia virus – type 1 (HTLV-1), and enteroviruses. Causes of bacterial myelitis include staphylococcus, streptococcus, mycoplasma, borrelia, and treponema. MRI is the diagnostic modality of choice and may be negative in the early stages. The imaging findings are nonspecific and include multisegmental cord expansion, diffuse T2/STIR hyperintense signal within the involved segments, and variable enhancement (see Figure 11.24, page 299).

Spinal cord abscesses

Spinal cord These abscesses are very rare and characterized by T1 hypointensity, T2 hyperintensity, peripheral enhancement, and central diffusion restriction.

Inflammatory and autoimmune diseases of the spine
(see images on page 199)
Multiple sclerosis

MS is an autoimmune process directed at myelin. Cord lesions without intracranial lesions are seen in 10% of cases. MRI is the most sensitive and specific modality and will demonstrate well-delineated T2 hyperintense lesions that are most commonly seen in the cervical cord, are commonly posterolaterally located, and are less than two segments in length. STIR is more sensitive than FSE T2 imaging for identifying MS lesions. Acute or subacute lesions may enhance. Cord atrophy may be seen with a large lesion burden. Diffusion restriction can occasionally be seen in active plaques (see Figure 11.25a,b, page 300).

Acute disseminated encephalomyelitis

ADEM is typically a monophasic inflammatory demyelinating disease that arises in the setting of recent viral infection or vaccination and affects children or young adults. Multiphasic disease is rare and can mimic MS clinically. New lesions should not be seen after six months in ADEM. MR is the best imaging modality and demonstrates punctate or fluffy T2/STIR lesions that predominantly involve the dorsal WM, but can involve GM. Enhancement is variable, depends upon the stage of disease, and may be peripheral or central. The presence of cranial nerve enhancement suggests ADEM (see Figure 11.26, page 300).

Neuromyelitis optica

NMO or Devic's disease is a monophasic or relapsing demyelinating disease that has a predilection for the optic nerves and cervical cord. Features that help distinguish NMO from MS include: involvement of more than three contiguous segments of the cord, normal or nondiagnostic initial brain MRI, and NMO-IgG positivity. MRI displays multisegment (more than two) cord expansion and central cord T2/STIR hyperintensity and variable enhancement that more commonly occurs in the late subacute to chronic stages.

Radiation myelitis

Radiation myelitis is very rare and tends to occur when total doses of radiation exceed 5000 cGy. Clinical symptoms often precede imaging findings. When imaging is performed within eight months, MRI demonstrates long segment T1 hypointensity and T2 hyperintensity with cord expansion and variable enhancement within the radiation port. When imaged after more than three years post-radiation, cord atrophy can be seen.

Subacute combined degeneration

This form of degeneration can result from B12 deficiency through a variety of mechanisms including pernicious anemia, gastrectomy, inadequate intake, Crohn's disease, and others. The characteristic MRI findings include T2/STIR hyperintensity that is restricted to the dorsal columns, and occasional enhancement. The imaging appearance may be indistinguishable from infectious myelitis (see Figure 11.27a,b, page 301).

Sarcoidosis

Sarcoidosis affecting the spine is rare, but deserves special mention owing to its variable appearance on imaging. Any compartment can be involved, including enhancing cord lesions, smooth and nodular leptomeningeal enhancement, nerve root enhancement, epidural enhancing lesions, lytic vertebral lesions, and paraspinous masses. CT imaging best demonstrates lytic vertebral lesions. MRI best demonstrates cord, leptomeningeal, nerve root, and epidural lesions.

Rheumatic diseases affecting the spine
Seronegative spondyloarthropathies

The seronegative spondyloarthropathies include ankylosing spondylitis, reactive arthritis, psoriatic arthritis, spondyloarthropathy associated with inflammatory bowel disease, and undifferentiated spondyloarthropathy. Patients are seronegative for rheumatoid factor and positive for HLA-B27. As opposed to rheumatoid arthritis, there is involvement of the entheses (ligamentous attachments). MRI is the most sensitive for early involvement, which may be manifest as marrow edema (T1 hypointense, T2/STIR hyperintense) and enhancement along the anterior and posterior endplates, corresponding to the attachment sites of ALL and PLL. This has been referred to as shiny corners. As the disease progresses, these changes may be visualized as erosions on CT images. Aseptic spondylodiscitis may be present and is indistinguishable from infectious discitis/osteomyelitis. Facetitis and eventual ankylosis can be seen early on MRI and late on CT images. Late in the disease process, ossification of the entheses results in formation of syndesmophytes. Ankylosis can occur via syndesmophytes, through the disc, across facets, costovertebral, and costotransverse joints. Extra care should be taken when evaluating patients with ankylosis in the setting of trauma. Even minor trauma can be associated with significant spinal injury. CT imaging and MRI are the best modalities in this regard. Sacroiliac involvement is characteristic (see Figure 11.28, page 301).

Rheumatoid arthritis

RA commonly involves the cervical spine (80%–90%). The spine is virtually never involved if there is no evidence of disease in the hands or feet. RA is a disease of synovial joints, with involvement of the C0-C1 and C1-C2 articulations, uncovertebral and facet joints. The most common presentation is atlantoaxial subluxation, best seen with flexion and extension plain films, CT imaging, or MRI. Disruption of the transverse ligament is best demonstrated on axial FSE T2 or GRE images. Erosion of the dens secondary to pannus formation is a common pattern and can be associated with cord compression. Erosions and ankylosis are best seen on CT images. Pannus is hypointense on T1, heterogeneous on T2, and enhances avidly (see Figure 11.29, page 301).

Other rheumatic diseases affecting the spine and/or paraspinous soft tissues include juvenile idiopathic arthritis, gout, SLE, polymyositis-dermatomyositis, Sjogren's syndrome, and systemic sclerosis (scleroderma).

Spinal tumors
Spinal compartments

A useful way to organize your thought processes when it comes to the spine is to break it into compartments. The most widely used categorization system divides the spine into three main compartments: intramedullary (i.e. within the substance of the cord), intradural extramedullary (i.e. outside of the substance of the cord, but within the thecal sac), and extradural (i.e. located outside of the thecal sac). This system is simple and aids greatly in the development of differential diagnoses.

Intramedullary tumors

Tumors arising from the substance of the spinal cord are rare. They represent approximately 4%–10% of tumors of the CNS. The incidence of spinal cord tumors is lowest in children and peaks in the eighth and ninth decades. The vast majority of spinal cord tumors are gliomas, are malignant, and occur most commonly in the cervical spine. The most common histologic types are ependymoma (60%) and astrocytoma (30%). Hemangioblastomas are the third most common spinal cord neoplasm.

Astrocytomas/ependymomas

There is significant overlap in the imaging appearance of astrocytomas and ependymomas and differentiation by imaging may not always be possible. Certain imaging features can aid in differentiation. Astrocytomas tend to be located eccentrically within the cord, have indistinct margins, involve long segments, and enhance variably. Ependymomas tend to be more centrally located, are more circumscribed, enhance more avidly, are more likely to hemorrhage, and form necrotic cavities. Both astrocytomas and ependymomas expand the cord and dilate the central canal of the cord at the rostral and caudal margins of the tumor, referred to as satellite or polar cysts. Astrocytomas occur with greater frequency in the setting of NF-1. Ependymomas tend to occur with greater frequency in the setting of NF-2 (see Figure 11.30a,b, page 302).

Hemangioblastomas and paragangliomas

Hemangioblastomas occur most commonly in the thoracic cord and tend to be solitary lesions. They tend to expand the cord, enhance homogeneously, dorsally located, intramedullary (75%) may have peritumoral flow voids, hemorrhage, and cause syringohydromyelia. Hemangioblastomatosis occurs in the setting of von Hippel–Lindau disease. Paragangliomas of the cord are less common and may be indistinguishable from hemangioblastomas by imaging (see Figure 11.31a,b, page 303).

Myxopapillary ependymomas

These tumors are the most common neoplasm found within the conus medullaris, filum terminale, or cauda equina and represent approximately eight out of 10 neoplasms found in these locations. When these tumors arise from the filum and cauda equina, they are better characterized as intradural extramedullary. The imaging features are less specific than the location of the lesion, but include: intense enhancement, sausage shape, T2 hyperintensity, and susceptibility artifact from hemosiderin deposition. T1 signal is variable and reflects variable mucin concentration.

Other intramedullary tumors

All of the other intramedullary tumors are very uncommon. Lymphoma confined to the cord is very rare, making up far less than one percent of all cases of lymphoma within the body. Unlike other CNS lymphomas, intramedullary lymphomas tend to be hyperintense on T2WI and enhance heterogeneously. Intramedullary metastases are also very uncommon. They tend to present as homogeneously enhancing masses with prominent peritumoral edema and cord expansion. There are case reports of intramedullary gangliogliomas, oligodendrogliomas, meningiomas, schwannomas, sarcomas, and PNETs.

Intradural extramedullary tumors

Tumors located within the dural sac but outside of the substance of the cord represent approximately 80% of intraspinal tumors in adults and 65%–70% of intraspinal tumors in children. The most common neoplasms arising within the extramedullary intradural space are schwannomas, meningiomas, and neurofibromas. The incidence of neurofibromas is increased in the setting of NF-1. There is a greater incidence of schwannomas in the setting of NF-2. Less common extramedullary intradural tumors include paragangliomas, metastases, and lymphoma.

Schwannomas

These are the most common spinal neoplasms and the most common tumor to occur within the extramedullary intradural compartment (30%). They are benign neoplasms that arise from a single nerve fascicle, generally from dorsal spinal nerve roots. Schwannomas are largely sporadic and solitary, but can occur in the setting of NF-2, schwannomatosis, and the Carney complex. On CT imaging, findings include bony remodeling and erosions, including neural foraminal expansion and remodeling. On MRI, schwannomas are iso- to hypointense on T1WI, hyperintense on T2WI, are more commonly cystic than neurofibromas, and enhance either homogeneously or peripherally. Hyperintense signal on T1 images may indicate hemorrhage or a melanotic component. There may be intradural and extradural components, creating a dumbbell shape with the handle of the dumbbell representing the intraforaminal component of the mass. Schwannomas and neurofibromas are generally not distinguishable by imaging. However, the presence of cystic changes and hemorrhage are suggestive of a schwannoma (see Figure 11.32a,b, page 304).

Meningiomas

Meningiomas are the second most common extramedullary intradural tumor (25%). They are slow growing, benign neoplasms that originate from the dura mater and are most commonly solitary and sporadic. They most commonly arise in the thoracic spine (80%). Meningiomas are typically extramedullary and intradural and are rarely intramedullary (<1%) or extradural (5%–10%). A single lesion can have intradural and extradural components, producing a dumbbell shape. On CT images, meningiomas tend to be hyperdense and avidly enhance. Indirect findings on CT imaging may include hyperostosis and neural foraminal expansion. On MRI, meningiomas tend to be isointense on T1WI and T2WI, enhance avidly following gadolinium administration, and may have a dural tail. Differentiation from a schwannoma may not be possible by imaging. Imaging features that suggest meningioma include: isointense signal on T2WI (schwannomas tend to be hyperintense on T2WI), calcification (rare in schwannomas), the presence of a dural tail, and dorsal location (ventrolateral in schwannomas) (see Figure 11.32a,b, page 304).

Neurofibromas

Neurofibromas are benign nerve sheath tumors that are overwhelmingly sporadic and solitary (90%). There are two main types of neurofibromas, solitary (i.e. localized) and plexiform. Plexiform neurofibromas are pathognomonic for NF-1 and are characterized by multilevel, bulky nerve enlargement in the background of infiltrating soft tissue mass. Individuals with NF-1 have a 5%–8% lifetime risk of malignant degeneration. Rapid growth suggests malignant degeneration. The imaging appearance of solitary neurofibromas is indistinguishable from that of the schwannoma on CT images and MRI. Occasionally, neurofibromas display a rim of hyperintensity peripherally and low signal centrally on T2WI, the so-called target sign. Plexiform neurofibromas are characteristically aggressive appearing, multilevel masses that are isointense on T1WI and hyperintense on T2WI, and enhance heterogeneously.

Other intradural extramedullary tumors

Extramedullary intradural metastases are uncommon and have been described in approximately 5% of patients diagnosed with malignancies at autopsy. The most common primaries are breast, lung, and gastrointestinal malignancies, and lymphoma. Seeding of the subarachnoid spaces with metastatic deposits from a primary intracranial malignancy is more common and is referred to as drop metastasis. Drop metastases are most frequently associated with medulloblastomas, ependymomas, germinomas, astrocytomas (including glioblastoma multiforme), choroid plexus papillomas, and choroid plexus carcinomas. There are three characteristic patterns of leptomeningeal seeding: multiple enhancing nodules within the subarachnoid spaces (particularly in association with the cauda equina and nerve roots), smooth and diffuse leptomeningeal enhancement (i.e. sugar coating or Zuckerguss), and blunting of the caudal-most portion of the thecal sac by enhancing soft tissue (see Figure 11.33, page 304).

Other neoplasms rarely located within the extramedullary intradural compartment include paragangliomas, lymphomas, lipomas, and leukemias.

Extradural tumors
(see images on page 315)

There is a long list of extradural tumors of the spine and paraspinous soft tissues. Primary tumors of the spine are very rare and comprise less than 5% of all spinal neoplasms. Primary benign neoplasms, as a group, are more common than primary malignant neoplasms.

Benign primary extradural neoplasms
(see images on page 315)

The most common primary benign neoplasms include vertebral hemangioma, osteoid osteoma, osteoblastoma, Langerhans cell histiocytosis, giant cell tumor, and aneurysmal bone cyst.

Hemangiomas

Hemangiomas are the most common primary benign tumor of the spinal column and are seen in 10%–15% of adults. They contain vascular stroma and fat, are typically found incidentally, and are rarely symptomatic. On plain films and CT images, hemangiomas are well-circumscribed lesions that are typically located within the vertebral body, rarely within the posterior elements, with characteristic coarsened vertical trabeculae (corduroy or polka-dot appearance). On MRI, hemangiomas are hyperintense on T1 and T2, partially suppress on STIR images, and avidly enhance. An uncommon variant is the so-called aggressive hemangioma, which can mimic malignancy and present as destructive lesions with an epidural soft tissue component that can produce spinal canal and neural foraminal stenosis (see Figure 11.34a-d, page 305).

Osteoid osteomas/osteoblastomas

Osteoid osteomas are common, representing 10%–12% of all benign skeletal neoplasms. Osteoblastomas are less common (3% of all benign skeletal neoplasms). These entities are histologically identical, but are clinically distinct. Pain associated with osteoid osteomas is heightened at night, relieved with NSAIDs, and pain stabilizes or abates with time. Osteoblastomas tend to progress over time and recur. Osteoblastomas are larger in size (>1.5 cm) than osteoid osteomas (<1.5 cm) with a predilection for the posterior elements (75%–90%). On CT images, osteoid osteomas typically have a well-defined radiolucent central nidus, and a surrounding zone of reactive sclerosis. MRI of osteoid osteomas can often be confusing. The nidus is iso- to hypointense on T1 and iso- to hyperintense on T2 sequences, and there is a T2 hyperintense reactive zone at the periphery of the lesion. Osteoblastomas are variable in appearance on both CT images and MRI, but characteristically are located within the posterior elements, are expansile and well-marginated, and often extend into the vertebral body. On CT images, there is a narrow zone of transition, sclerotic rim, and variable matrix that can be indistinguishable from chondrosarcoma. On MRI, osteoblastomas are typically iso- to hypointense on T1WI and iso- to hyperintense on T2WI, with variable enhancement. There can be an associated aneurysmal bone cyst component (see Figure 11.35, page 306).

Langerhans cell histiocytosis

LCH is a disease of unknown etiology that is characterized by a monoclonal proliferation of Langerhans cells. Vertebral involvement is rare in LCH. The thoracic spine (54%) is most commonly involved, with a strong predilection for the vertebral body. The characteristic appearance on CT imaging is a lytic lesion that may or may not be associated with uniform collapse (vertebra plana) with preservation of the adjacent intervertebral discs. On MRI, the lesions are typically hypointense on T1 and hyperintense on T2 sequences, with a paraspinous or epidural enhancing soft tissue component. Vertebral body height of the involved segments can be restored or nearly restored with healing.

Giant cell tumors

GCTs represent approximately 5% of all primary bone tumors. They tend to occur in the second to fourth decades. The sacrum is by far the most common location of spinal GCTs. Those that occur in the rest of the spine tend to arise within the vertebral body. They are locally aggressive and tend to recur. Sarcomatous transformation has been reported in approximately 5%–10% of cases, often related to prior radiation treatment. The typical imaging features on CT images include an expansile, lytic lesion with internal soft tissue density that has a narrow zone of transition and no visible matrix. On MRI, GCTs are typically iso- to hypointense on T1 and iso- to hypointense on T2 images. Fluid–fluid levels can be seen in conjunction with an aneurysmal bone cyst component.

Aneurysmal bone cysts

Aneurysmal bone cysts represent approximately 1%–2% of primary bone tumors. They most commonly arise in the posterior elements and most often extend into the vertebral body (80%–90%). Aneurysmal bone cysts can arise de novo or secondary to other tumors, such as osteoblastomas, GCTs, sarcomas, and fibrous dysplasia. On CT images, aneurysmal bone cysts are expansile lesions with a sharp zone of transition and multiple, thin, bony septations that create a bubbly or multicystic appearance. Characteristically, fluid–fluid levels are encountered within the cystic spaces that can have variable density on CT images and variable signal on MRI. Enhancement is typically at the margins of the tumor and within the septae. Extension into the epidural space is common (see Figure 11.36a-c, page 307).

Malignant primary extradural neoplasms (see images on page 315)

Multiple myeloma

Multiple myeloma is a monoclonal proliferation of malignant plasma cells and is the most common primary malignant neoplasm of the spine. The median age at diagnosis is 65 years. CT imaging is the most sensitive modality early in the disease process, but plain films are still commonly used. The typical pattern on plain films and CT images is multifocal and/or confluent lytic lesions with multilevel endplate fractures and kyphosis. There may be an associated epidural or paraspinous soft tissue component. There are two main patterns observed on MRI, diffuse and heterogeneous. In the diffuse pattern, marrow signal is diffusely low on T1, hyperintense on T2 and STIR sequences, and there is diffuse enhancement on postcontrast T1WI. The heterogeneous pattern is best visualized on STIR and fat suppressed gadolinium enhanced T1WI (see Figure 11.37a-c, pages 308–309).

Lymphoma

This tumor can be found in any of the spinal compartments, but is discussed in this section because it is most commonly found within the extradural compartment. The great majority of lymphoma cases identified within the spine occur in the setting of diffuse disease. Primary lymphoma within the spine is a very rare entity, representing approximately 3%–4% of all malignant bone tumors. Whether primary or secondary, spinal lymphomas are overwhelmingly non-Hodgkins (80%–90%) and of B-cell origin (80%–90%). Extradural compartment involvement is the most common, followed by the intradural extramedullary and intramedullary compartments. Regardless of the compartment, lymphomas tend to be iso- to hyperdense on CT images, iso- to hypointense on T1, iso- to hyperintense on T2/STIR sequences, and display uniform intense enhancement following gadolinium administration. The most common extradural manifestations of lymphoma include osseous vertebral erosions, multisegment enhancing epidural mass and, rarely, vertebra plana and the ivory or densely sclerotic vertebral body (see Figure 11.38a-f, pages 310–311).

Chordomas

Chordomas arise from notochordal remnants and are the most common primary non-lymphoproliferative tumor of the spine. The most frequent locations are sacrococcygeal (50%), spheno-occipital (35%), and vertebral (10%). They are slow growing malignant tumors and are generally not discovered until they are large. On CT images, chordomas are midline, lobulated, destructive, low density soft tissue masses that often contain dysmorphic calcifications. On MRI, chordomas display heterogeneous low signal on T1WI and enhance modestly. On T2WI, the lesions are hyperintense and may have multiple hypointense septi. Calcifications may be seen as susceptibility artifact on GRE images.

Chondrosarcomas

Chondrosarcomas are the second most common primary non-lymphoproliferative tumor of the spine. The mean age at diagnosis is 45 years. Chondrosarcomas can arise de novo or secondary to sarcomatous transformation of an osteochondroma or enchondroma (rare). The incidence of sarcomatous transformation is increased in the setting of hereditary multiple exostoses (osteochondroma) and Ollier disease (enchondroma). Chondrosarcomas characteristically arise at the midline and are most commonly found in the thoracic spine. On CT images, chondrosarcomas are typically large destructive lesions with a soft tissue component that often displays a chondroid matrix (rings-and-arcs). On MRI, chondroid matrix is visualized as signal void. Lesions are typically iso- to hypointense on T1, hyperintense on T2 and STIR images, and enhance heterogeneously.

Osteosarcomas

Osteosarcomas of the spine are rare. They can arise de novo or as secondary lesions developing from previously irradiated bone, Paget's lesions, or bone infarcts. They characteristically arise in the thoracolumbar spine, involve the vertebral body eccentrically, secondarily involve the posterior elements, and have a soft tissue component that invades the spinal canal. The most common appearance on plain films and CT images is that of permeative lesions that produce an osteoid matrix and have a wide zone of transition. The ivory vertebral body appearance has also been described. Owing to the osteoid matrix, osteosarcomas are typically iso- to hypointense on T1WI and T2WI. The presence of fluid–fluid levels suggests telangectatic osteosarcoma.

Plasmacytoma

Plasmacytoma are monoclonal proliferations of malignant plasma cells and are regarded as a precursor to multiple myeloma. Plasmacytoma may exist as a solitary lesion for years without evidence of multiple myeloma. The most common presentation is a single collapsed vertebral body. On CT imaging, plasmacytomas are predominantly lytic and expansile. The characteristic mini-brain appearance is produced by preferential destruction of trabecular bone, relative preservation of cortical bone, and the presence of thickened cortical struts. On MRI, plasmacytomas are hypointense on T1, hyperintense on T2/STIR images, and enhance diffusely. Thickened cortical struts appear as hypointense bands on T1 and T2 sequences. There may be an enhancing soft tissue component with paraspinous or epidural involvement.

Ewing sarcoma

Ewing sarcoma is the most common non-lymphoproliferative primary malignant tumor in childhood. The sacrum is more commonly involved than the spine. On plain films and CT images, the lesions are characteristically lytic, permeative, involve the vertebral body, and have a wide zone of transition. Cortical thinning is frequently observed without destruction or breakthrough. There is a non-calcified paraspinous soft tissue mass observed in half of all cases. CT imaging and MRI best demonstrate the intramedullary location of the lesions. On MRI, lesions are hypointense on T1 and hyperintense on T2/STIR images in comparison to surrounding marrow. Post-contrast T1WI demonstrate heterogeneous enhancement with regions of necrosis.

Secondary extradural neoplasms

Metastases represent more than 90% of all spinal tumors. The most common primary neoplasms to metastasize to the spine are lung (31%), breast (24%), gastrointestinal tract (9%), prostate (8%), and melanoma (4%). Osteolytic metastases (70%) are more common than osteoblastic (15%) and mixed metastases (10%). Renal, gastrointestinal, and thyroid metastases are typically osteolytic. Prostate, genitourinary malignancies, and carcinoid tumors are typically osteoblastic. Breast and lung metastases are the most common primaries associated with mixed metastases. Osteolytic lesions with an expansile component suggest renal cell or thyroid carcinoma.

Osteolytic metastases

Osteolytic metastases nearly always involve the posterior aspect of the vertebral body, involve the anterior aspect of the vertebral body in 75% of all cases, and in just over half of all cases involve the pedicle. Fewer than 25% of lytic metastases there is involvement of the lamina or spinous processes. Most lesions involve the trabecular bone. Involvement of the cortical bone is more unusual and suggests a lung or breast primary. On CT images, osteolytic lesions are typically ill-defined and permeative, and may be solitary or multiple. On MRI, osteolytic metastases tend to be hypointense on T1WI, hyperintense on T2WI, and variably enhance. MRI is the imaging modality of choice for the identification and characterization of epidural and paraspinal extension. STIR is the most sensitive MR sequence (see Figure 11.39d–f, pages 312–313).

Osteoblastic metastases

Osteoblastic metastases on CT imaging are most commonly observed as heterogeneous increased density with indistinct margins that primarily involve spongiform bone and often incite a periosteal reaction. Cortical bone is rarely involved and epidural and paraspinous soft tissue masses are unusual. On MRI, osteoblastic lesions are most commonly hypointense on T1, T2, and STIR sequences. Osteoblastic lesions are less likely to enhance. Diffuse osteoblastic metastases can also be observed as diffusely low marrow signal on T1WI and T2WI (see Figure 11.39a–c, page 312).

Benign versus malignant compression fractures

Insufficiency fractures result from normal stress on bone that has diminished elastic resistance. A pathologic fracture occurs in an area of bone that is compromised by another lesion. Imaging findings that suggest metastatic fractures include a convex posterior vertebral body border, involvement of the posterior elements, epidural or paraspinous mass, or the presence of multiple lesions. Findings that suggest benign insufficiency fractures include the presence of a retropulsed fracture fragment, the presence of a transverse hypointense band on T1WI and T2WI, sparing of normal marrow signal within the vertebral body, and a single lesion. On CT imaging, metastatic compression fractures often display round or ovoid areas of trabecular or cortical destruction. DWI has not been shown to effectively discriminate between pathologic and nonpathologic compression fractures.

Spinal cysts, cyst-like lesions, and spinal vascular disorders
Meningeal cysts

Spinal meningeal (arachnoid) cysts are outpouchings of the arachnoid that communicate with the subarachnoid space. They represent approximately 1%–3% of all spinal masses. The most common location is the thoracic spine (65%). They are typically located in the dorsal aspect of the canal. The most commonly used classification system of meningeal cysts was published by Nabors et al. (1988) and includes: extradural cysts without nerve fibers (type I), extradural cysts with nerve fibers (type II), and intradural cysts (type III).

Type I cysts

Type I meningeal cysts cysts are subdivided into extradural arachnoid cysts (type IA) and sacral meningoceles (type IB). Type IA and IB cysts are diverticula of the arachnoid through a defect in the dura. Growth over time is most likely via a ball valve-like mechanism. Supporting this notion is that symptoms can worsen with valsalva's maneuver or vigorous activity. Typical imaging findings include multilevel involvement, dorsal location, and bony scalloping. Neural foraminal expansion may be seen. CT myelography will demonstrate the communication with the subarachnoid space by immediate or delayed (3–12 hours) filling of the cyst with intrathecal contrast. On MRI, type I meningeal cysts follow CSF signal on all pulse sequences and there is no enhancement. The communication with the subarachnoid space may not be identified with MRI (see Figure 11.40a,b, page 314).

Type II cysts

Type II meningeal cysts contain nerve tissue of some kind, typically nerve roots. Rarely, the spinal cord can herniate through a dural defect. The usual location is distal to the dorsal root ganglion within the neural foramen. The most common location is the lower spine, but type II cysts can be found at any spinal level. Type II cysts occurring within the sacral spine are also known as Tarlov cysts. They are generally found incidentally and are largely asymptomatic, but can cause low back or perineal pain. Spontaneous rupture can cause a CSF leak and intracranial hypotension. CT myelography will demonstrate early or delayed filling of the cyst with intrathecal contrast. On MRI, the cysts are hypointense on T1 and hyperintense on T2 images, and do not enhance. Nerve roots are often seen within the central or peripheral portions of the cyst. Tarlov cysts have the propensity to remodel the sacral foramina and canal (see Figure 11.40c, page 314).

Type III cysts

These cysts are lined by arachnoid, are intradural extramedullary, may communicate with the subarachnoid space through a small caliber pedicle, and can be congenital or acquired. They are most commonly located dorsal to the cord and are frequently associated with cord compression. The mid-thoracic spine is the most common location. CT myelography may demonstrate communication with the subarachnoid space on immediate or delayed images. MRI displays a thin walled cyst that is hypointense on T1WI, hyperintense on T2WI, and does not enhance. There may be flow related artifact within the cyst on T2 and variable T1 signal owing to proteinaceous cyst contents (see Figure 11.40d, page 314).

Dermoids and epidermoids

Dermoids are inclusion cysts that contain sebaceous glands, sweat glands, hair, and sloughed sqamuous epithelium. They are contained within an ectodermal lining. Epidermoids are also lined by ectoderm, but contain only sloughed squamous epithelium. They represent less than 1% of all spinal tumors and are predominantly congenital lesions. A small percentage of cases arise from displacement of viable dermal or epidermal rests through trauma, lumbar puncture (particularly neonates), or various surgical procedures. They are slow growing tumors that can be intramedullary (40%), extramedullary intradural (60%), or rarely extradural. The imaging appearance of dermoids and epidermoids is similar to other locations. The reader is referred to the brain imaging section for a detailed description.

Neurenteric cysts

Neurenteric cysts are very rare endoderm lined cysts, representing less than 1% of all spinal tumors. They are thought to be remnants of the embryonic canal of Kovalevsky. The lesions are largely intradural extramedullary (85%) and located ventral to the cord. They are most commonly located in the thoracic (40%) and cervical (30%) spine, but can be seen in the lumbar and sacral spine. Vertebral anomalies may coexist and include clefts, hemivertebrae, butterfly vertebrae, anterior and posterior spina bifida, midline tubular vertebral body defect (classic, but uncommon), and others. Split cord anomalies have also been described. Characteristic imaging findings include an intradural extramedullary multilevel ovoid or lobulated mass within the ventral subarachnoid space with associated cord displacement or compression. These lesions have variable signal on T1 (protein content), are hyperintense on T2 sequences, and do not enhance. Vertebral anomalies (~50%) are best demonstrated on CT imaging.

Juxta-articular cysts

This category includes synovial cysts and ganglion cysts. Synovial cysts have a synovial lining and often communicate with the facet joint. Ganglion cysts arise from the periarticular soft tissues and do not have a synovial lining. Both types of cysts are rare within the spine. They most commonly occur at L4–L5 (80%) and approximately 10% of cases occur in the cervical and thoracic spine. They are most often unilateral. The typical location is adjacent to the facet joint in the posterolateral aspect of the spinal canal, but may be subarticular, foraminal, extraforaminal, and extending from the spinal canal into the neural foramen. When foraminal or extraforaminal, there may or may not be a connection with the joint. Synovial cysts can change in size with body position and can spontaneously regress without treatment.

MR is the imaging modality of choice and shows a rounded, extradural mass adjacent to the facet in the posterolateral canal that is typically hypointense on T1WI and hyperintense on T2WI and does not enhance. Hemorrhage within synovial cysts can result in T1 hyperintensity (methemoglobin) or T2 hypointensity (hemosiderin or calcification). Variable protein content within ganglion cysts can result in variable T1 signal, depending on the protein content. There can be a thin rim of contrast enhancement or more significant enhancement of the cyst and/or the adjacent facet, implying active inflammation or infection. Juxta-articular cysts can be easily overlooked on CT images, owing to their typical CSF density. Hemorrhage and calcification can assist in identifying this lesion (see Figure 11.41a,b, page 315).

Traumatic pseudomeningoceles

Pseudomeningoceles are extradural fluid collections that result from tears in the dura and arachnoid of the root sleeve that generally occur in the context of forcible separation of the head and shoulder with lateral flexion of the cervical vertebrae. As a result of this force, nerve roots may be severed at their cord insertion or more distally. There may be nerve root retraction into the neural foramen or distally. Identifying the injury as pre- or post-ganglionic has treatment implications as post-ganglionic injuries are much more amenable to repair. Pseudomeningoceles can occur without nerve root avulsion and vice versa. Traumatic nerve root avulsions are most common at C5 and C6. Fat saturated T2WI is the optimal sequence for the identification of the extradural CSF collections, and is probably superior to myelography in this regard. Identifying the retracted nerve root and nerve root stumps may be more difficult with MRI. Myelography and CT myelography remain the gold standards to demonstrate dilated, empty nerve root sleeves, leakage into the extradural tissues, identification of fistulas, and locating the avulsed nerve root or stump (see Figure 11.42, page 315).

Syringohydromyelia

Hydromyelia is dilatation of the central part of the cord and the lining is that of the ependyma. Syringomyelia is a cystic fluid collection that dissects through the ependyma into the cord parenchyma and is not lined by ependyma. Syringohydromyelia is an all-encompassing term used to describe a cystic dilatation within the cord as the two entities often cannot be differentiated on imaging. Common etiologies include Chiari malformations (I and II), tethered cord, arachnoiditis, trauma, intramedullary tumors, leptomeningeal carcinomatosis, and a long list of other conditions. In severe cases, there can be extension into the brainstem (syringobulbia) and cerebral peduncles or brain parenchyma (syringocephaly).

MR is the optimal imaging modality and will demonstrate cord diameter expansion by a fusiform or saccular cavity. Sagittal images will best demonstrate the craniocaudal extent of the cavity. On axial images, the cavity may be central or eccentric. With larger cavities, cord parenchyma may be atrophic or compressed. The fluid contained within follows CSF signal. On FSE T2, there may be irregular signal associated with complex flow-related artifacts. Enhancement of the cavity should raise suspicion of infectious, inflammatory, or neoplastic processes. MRI is usually the ideal modality for evaluating the causative lesions. On CT images, the cord diameter is expanded with an associated CSF density fusiform central component. Septations may be readily visualized. CT myelography may demonstrate thin adhesions that may not be visible on MRI (see Figure 11.43, page 316).

Ventriculus terminalis

The ventriculus terminalis or the so-called fifth ventricle is a fusiform dilatation of the central canal of the cord at the level of the conus. It is lined by normal ependyma, rarely exceeds 4 mm in diameter, and is considered a normal variant. The conus is located in the normal location and the filum terminale is normal in appearance. On CT images, the fluid within the ventriculus terminalis is isodense to CSF. On MRI, the fluid within the cavity follows CSF on all pulse sequences and there is no enhancement.

Congenital anomalies of the spine
(see images on pages 316–318)

Understanding spinal malformations is best achieved with a basic understanding of CNS embryology. In the second or third week of embryonic development, the bilaminar embryonic disc is converted to a trilaminar disc that is composed of ectoderm, mesoderm, and endoderm (gastrulation). During the third to fourth week of embryonic development, the neural plate is formed at the interface of the notocord and the ectoderm. The neural plate then folds and seals simultaneously in the craniocaudal and caudocranial directions along its dorsal aspect (primary neurulation). At five to six weeks, the conus tip and filum are formed from a solid epithelial cord that eventually cavitates (secondary neurulation).

In order to understand spinal dysraphisms, it is also important to understand the concept of the neural placode. While most classifications include descriptions of the neural placode, the definition of the neural placode is often not included. The neural placode is a mass of neural tissue that is formed by the unfolded portion of the neural tube. The position of the neural placode, and the tissues with which it interfaces, is the basis of most classification systems.

Spinal dysraphism refers to incomplete closure of the neural tube. Spinal dysraphisms have been broadly categorized as either open (spina bifida apperta) or closed (spina bifida occulta). Open spinal dysraphisms are characterized by defects in the posterior elements and skin with exposure of neural tissue to the external environment. Open spinal dysraphic defects include myelomeningocele and myelocele. Closed spinal dysraphisms are characterized by skin overlying the neural tissue. Closed spinal dysraphisms with a subcutaneous mass include meningoceles, myelocystoceles, lipomyeloceles, and lipomyelocystoceles. Closed spinal dysraphisms without a subcutaneous mass include dermal sinus, lipoma of the filum terminale, tight filum terminale, and intradural lipoma. Also included in this category are caudal regression, neurenteric cyst, and diastematomyelia.

Open spinal dysraphisms

Myeloceles are characterized by contiguity of the neural placode with the cutaneous ectoderm. The mesoderm destined to form the posterior elements is displaced laterally, resulting in a large dorsal defect (spina bifida). The cord is invariably tethered. Early surgical intervention is required.

Myelomeningoceles are similar to myeloceles in that the neural placode is located in contiguity with the skin surface, but there is expansion of the adjacent subarachnoid space that results in protrusion of the neural placode and CSF expanded meninges beyond the normal skin plane. The cord is tethered.

Myelomeningoceles comprise approximately 98% of open spinal dysraphisms. They are most frequently diagnosed with the use of prenatal ultrasound and are readily identifiable on clinical examination. As such, myelomeningoceles are rarely imaged postnatally. Early surgical intervention, including fetal surgical intervention, is the current standard of care.

Myeloceles and myelomeningoceles are associated with diastematomyelia in 8%–45% of cases. Open dysraphisms are invariably present in the setting of the Chiari II malformation. Myelomeningoceles are more common than myeloceles in the setting of Chiari II malformations.

Closed spinal dysraphisms (subcutaneous mass)

In the meningocele, there is herniation of a CSF filled, dura lined sac through a defect in the bony elements of the spine. Meningoceles are most commonly located in the lumbosacral spine. Most meningoceles are posteriorly located, herniating through defects in the posterior elements. Less commonly, the CSF containing dural sac herniates through an anteriorly located defect. Anterior herniation most commonly occurs in the sacral spine (anterior sacral meningocele). By definition, neural tissue is not present within the sac. Meningoceles are very rare.

In the lipomyelocele, there is contiguity of the neural placode with a subcutaneous lipoma through a defect in the posterior elements. If there is corresponding enlargement of the subarachnoid space, a lipomyelomeningocele exists. The cord is tethered in both entities (see Figure 11.44a,b, 5.45, pages 316–317).

A myelocystocele is a herniation of a syrinx (syringohydromyelia) through a defect in the posterior elements. Myelocystoceles are most common within the cervical spine. A myelocystocele is referred to as a terminal myelocystocele when a terminal syrinx (syringohydromyelia of the distal central canal) herniates through a defect in the posterior elements. Myelocystoceles and terminal myelocystoceles are very rare.

Closed spinal dysraphisms (no subcutaneous mass)

The dorsal dermal sinus is a stratified squamous epithelium lined tract of variable length that extends from the skin surface to the paraspinal fascia, meninges, or spinal cord. It is thought to arise from adhesion of the neural tube to the dermis. Not surprisingly, epidermoid and dermoid cysts are commonly associated with dorsal dermal sinuses (30%–50%). On MRI, the dorsal dermal sinus is hypointense on a background of hyperintense subcutaneous fat. Coccygeal pits originate below the superior margin of the gluteal crease and require no imaging workup or clinical follow-up.

Intradural lipomas are thought to result from premature dysjunction of the neural ectoderm from the surface ectoderm. They occur most commonly in the thoracic spine (30%), are predominantly dorsally located (75%), are contained by the thecal sac, and may or may not be associated with posterior element defects. Intradural lipomas constitute 4% of all spinal lipomas. On CT images, intradural lipomas are lobulated, fat density masses with or without associated bony dysraphic defects. On MRI, they present as intrinsically hyperintense masses on FSE T1 and T2, decreased signal on STIR sequences, and do not enhance (see Figure 11.46a,b, page 317).

The fibrolipoma of the filum terminale, on MRI, is seen as linear hyperintense T1 signal within the filum. The filum terminale is not thickened <2 mm and the conus is normally located (above the L2 inferior endplate). Patients are generally asymptomatic (see Figure 11.47, page 318).

Tight filum terminale is defined as a thickened filum (>2 mm) and low position of the conus (below the L2 inferior endplate). This can be associated with a fibrolipoma of the filum terminale or a terminal lipoma. The tethered cord syndrome is a clinical diagnosis that is comprised of low back and leg pain (exacerbated by exertion) and urinary bladder dysfunction in 70% of adults and 20%–30% of children.

Complex closed spinal dysraphisms include diastematomyelia and caudal regression syndrome. Neurenteric cysts were discussed previously in this chapter. Diastematomyelia refers to a sagittal split in the spinal cord. There is a strong association with vertebral anomalies. Approximately 85% occur between T9 and S1. The spinal cord above and below the diastematomyelia is generally normal. There may be one or two thecal sacs. Each cord has its own central canal, and dorsal and ventral horns. Diastematomyelia is classified by the presence of an osseous/fibrous spur and duplicated thecal sacs (Pang I) or no osseous/fibrous spur and a single thecal sac (Pang II) (see Figure 11.48, page 318).

Caudal regression is a rare disorder of the caudal cell mass that is associated with sacrococcygeal vertebral dysgenesis/agenesis and cord anomalies. When these anomalies occur in the setting of multiorgan system anomalies, particularly renal and gastrointestinal anomalies, it is referred to as the caudal regression syndrome. This syndrome is associated with maternal diabetes in 16% of cases. There is a wide spectrum of imaging appearances, ranging from coccygeal dysgenesis/agenesis to lumbosacral agenesis. Patients with caudal regression have been classified into one of two groups, based upon the conus position and the severity of caudal dysgenesis. Group 1 displays a characteristically blunted, high riding conus (above L1) and more severe caudal dysgenesis. Group 2 displays a low lying, tethered cord in association with a variety of open or closed dysraphic defects. Caudal dysplasia is less severe in Group 2 (see Figure 11.49, page 318).

Spinal vascular disorders
Spinal arteriovenous malformations

For the sake of brevity, the Anson and Spetzler (1992) classification system of spinal vascular lesions will be described in this text. The interested reader is referred to the more complex revision of the original Spetzler classification scheme (Spetzler et al., 2002). The original scheme included four types of lesions: dural AVF, spinal cord AVM, juvenile AVM, and perimedullary AVF.

Dural AVFs (type I)

Type I AVFs is the most common spinal vascular malformation (up to 85%). They are acquired, occur in an older patient group, and result in a progressive radiculomyelopathy. They are most commonly found in the thoracic spine. The type I AVF is a fistulous communication between dorsal radiculomedullary arteries and the corresponding radiculomedullary vein/coronal sinus that occurs within the dural nerve root sleeve. Spinal angiography is the gold standard and will precisely define the anatomy of the shunt. Spinal CTA or MRA may assist in defining the level of involvement in preparation for catheter angiography. T2WI display multilevel abnormal hyperintense central cord signal, cord enlargement, and serpentine perimedullary flow voids that are more commonly found dorsal to the cord. Subtle dilatation of the perimedullary veins may be better visualized on post-contrast T1WI. There is no intramedullary nidus of vessels (see Figure 11.50a,b, page 319).

Spinal cord AVMs (type II)

Type I AVM's are characterized by an intramedullary nidus that is supplied by the anterior spinal artery, posterior spinal artery, or both. Venous drainage is into the coronal venous plexus. The age at presentation is younger (mean age, 24 years) and the clinical course is that of fluctuation and progression. Aneurysms occur in 20%–40% of cases and are associated with an increased risk of hemorrhage. Spinal catheter angiography is the gold standard, precisely defining the anatomy of the lesion. T2/STIR images will demonstrate hyperintense cord signal with or without cord expansion. The intramedullary nidus can be seen as flow voids on T2WI and serpentine enhancement on post-contrast T1WI. Enlarged perimedullary veins can be seen. Hemorrhage is best seen as hypointense signal/blooming on GRE images (see Figure 11.51, page 320).

Juvenile AVMs (type III)

This type is a very rare lesion that primarily occurs in adolescents and young adults and has a very poor prognosis. The AVMs are complex lesions that have multiple arterial feeders at multiple levels. Involvement of an entire metamere is seen in the Cobb syndrome. The imaging appearance is similar to that of intramedullary AVMs, but with extramedullary and even extradural components.

Perimedullary AVFs (type IV)

Type IV AVFs are very rare and have a propensity to occur near the conus. The feeder is a spinal artery and drainage is into the coronal venous plexus. Catheter angiography is the gold standard. Spinal MRA or CTA can assist for catheter angiography. It may be difficult to distinguish type IV from type I lesions on MRI. The conspicuity of subtle lesions may be increased with phase contrast or dynamic enhanced MRI. Multilevel central cord hyperintensity is seen on T2/STIR images. Prominent flow voids can compress the cord and/or conus. Hemorrhage is best seen as hypointense signal/blooming on GRE images.

Spinal cord infarction
(see images on page 294)

Spinal cord infarction is rare, estimated to represent 1% of all strokes. The most commonly reported etiologies are aortic atherosclerotic plaque and abdominal aortic aneurysm repair. Other etiologies include embolic disease, aortic dissection, systemic hypotension, spinal vascular malformations, trauma, vasculitis, and many other entities. Most cases of cord infarction are a result of arterial events and the anterior spinal artery is more commonly involved than the posterior spinal arteries. Venous infarctions are rare and related to sepsis, vascular malformations (Foix–Alajounanine syndrome), and malignancy.

MRI is the modality of choice and will display multilevel cord expansion and hyperintense signal on T2WI. The hyperintense signal can be diffuse, but tends to be centrally located owing to the greater susceptibility of GM to ischemia. Coalescence of T2 hyperintense signal on axial images within the ventral horns of the GM in the setting of cord infarction is referred to as the owl's eyes pattern. The imaging appearance of cord infarction can overlap with inflammatory and demyelinating diseases. Findings that suggest cord infarction include: anterior location (anterior spinal artery territory), associated T2/STIR hyperintense vertebral marrow signal (vertebral infarction), diffusion restriction, and delayed central cord enhancement (see Figure 11.17a,b, page 294).

Spinal cavernous malformations

Cavernous malformations within the spinal cord represent approximately 3%–5% of all CNS cavernous malformations and 5%–12% of all spinal vascular disorders. Lesions within the spine are histologically identical to cavernous malformations elsewhere in the CNS. Most cavernous malformations are likely congenital, but there are reports of lesions arising de novo or following radiation treatment. Familial forms have been reported. MR is the imaging modality of choice and demonstrates a well-delineated lesion with a stippled appearance on T1 and T2 (hemorrhages of varying ages) and characteristic pattern of peripheral magnetic susceptibility artifact on FSE T2 and GRE (hemosiderin staining of the adjacent parenchyma) images. There may be faint enhancement. Occasionally, the lesions may have an exophytic component (see Figure 11.52, page 320).

Metabolic disorders affecting the spine
(see images on pages 297–321)

There is a multitude of metabolic disorders that affect the spine. Only vertebral Paget's disease, renal osteodystrophy, and osteopetrosis will be discussed for the sake of brevity. Osteoporosis is discussed in the context of discriminating benign versus malignant compression fractures.

Paget's disease

This is a common disease of unknown cause, affecting approximately 3%–4% of individuals over the age of 40 years. It is found within the spine in approximately 30%–75% of all cases. There are three phases of disease: lytic, mixed lytic-blastic, and blastic. Elevated hydroxyproline can be seen in the lytic phase. Elevated alkaline phosphatase is often seen in the mixed and blastic phases. Most cases will be encountered in the mixed phase. Plain films, CT images, and MRI obtained during the mixed phase of vertebral Paget's disease can demonstrate cortical and trabecular thickening. On lateral or sagittal images, the pattern of vertebral cortical thickening has been described as resembling a picture frame. Cortical thickening results in overall enlargement of the involved vertebral segment. During the blastic phase, diffuse sclerosis may be present, sometimes called the ivory vertebra. The posterior elements are more commonly involved in the blastic phase. Pagetic bone is susceptible to fracture and there is a 1% risk of sarcomatous degeneration, manifest as cortical destruction and a soft tissue mass (see Figure 11.53a,b, page 321).

Renal osteodystrophy

This condition occurs in the clinical setting of chronic renal failure and secondary hyperparathyroidism. The classic imaging appearance of renal osteodystrophy is the rugger jersey spine on plain films and CT images. While classic, this appearance is not specific. The rugger jersey appearance results from sclerotic bands paralleling the superior and inferior endplates and relative lucency within the central portion of the vertebral body. Paraspinous soft tissue calcifications may also be present (see Figure 11.54, page 321).

Osteopetrosis

Osteopetrosis is a collection of genetic diseases that have in common deficient osteoclastic resorption with resultant increased bone density, cortical thickening, and diminished marrow cavities. On plain films and CT images, diffuse sclerosis and cortical thickening are seen. The rugger jersey pattern may be seen. On MRI, diffuse sclerosis is demonstrated as marrow signal that is low on T1WI and T2WI. Extramedullary hematopoiesis may be visualized as soft tissue paraspinous masses on CT images or iso- to hypointense signal paraspinous masses on T1WI and T2WI (see Figure 11.55a,b, page 322).

Chapter

10

Differential diagnosis by lesion location and morphology

Intramedullary T2/STIR hyperintense signal without mass

Contusion

MS/ADEM/neuromyelitis optica

Infectious myelitis (EBV, CMV, herpes zoster, HIV, HTLV-1, enteroviruses, staphylococcus, streptococcus, mycoplasma, borrelia, treponema)

Infarction

Radiation myelitis

AVM/dural AVF

Intramedullary T2/STIR hyperintense signal – dorsal

MS (posterolateral, multifocal)

Subacute combined degeneration – dorsal columns

Posterior spinal artery infarcts

HIV

Neurosarcoidosis

Wallerian degeneration

Intramedullary T2/STIR hyperintense signal – central

Syringohydromyelia – central or paracentral

MS/ADEM – patchy, discontinuous

Contusion (central cord syndrome)

Infectious myelitis

Cord infarcts ("owl's eyes")

Radiation myelitis

Intramedullary mass-like lesions

Inflammatory (MS, ADEM)

Infectious (EBV, CMV, herpes zoster, HIV, HTLV-1, enteroviruses, staphylococcus, streptococcus, mycoplasma, borrelia, treponema)

Ependymoma

Astrocytoma

Hemangioblastoma

Cord hemorrhage

Rare etiologies (AVM, metastases, lymphoma, sarcoid, cavernous malformations)

Intramedullary lesion with flow voids

Type 2 AVM

Type 3 AVM

Hemangioblastoma

Hypervascular metastases

Paraganglioma

Intradural extramedullary flow voids – no mass

Artifact from pulsatile CSF flow (indistinct margins compared to vessels)

Type 1 dAVF

Type 4 dAVF

Venous obstruction

Intradural extramedullary lesion – fat containing

Fibrolipoma of the filum terminale

Dermoid

Intradural lipoma (coexisting intramedullary component is typical)

Terminal lipoma

Lipomyelomeningocele

Intradural extramedullary lesion – cystic

Arachnoid cyst (type III meningeal cyst)

Neurocysticercosis

Epidermoid

Dermoid

Neuroenteric cyst (ventral)
Echinococcus
Cystic schwannoma/meningioma (cystic solid)

Intradural extramedullary lesions (solitary)

Schwannoma
Meningioma
Neurofibroma
Myxopapillary ependymoma

Intradural extramedullary (nodular leptomeningeal enhancement)

Drop metastases
Metastases
Infectious meningitis (bacterial, mycobacterial, fungal)
Leukemia
Lymphoma
Hemangioblastoma
NF-1
Arachnoiditis
Sarcoidosis

Intradural extramedullary (smooth leptomeningeal enhancement)

Drop metastases
Metastases
Acute/chronic inflammatory demyelinating polyradiculoneuropathy (AIDP/CIDP)
Infectious meningitis
Aseptic meningitis
Arachnoiditis

Enlarged, enhancing nerve roots

AIDP
CIDP
Nerve sheath tumors (neurofibroma, schwannoma)
HIV neuropathy
CMV
Charcot–Marie–Tooth
Dejerine–Sottas
Retracted, avulsed nerve root

Intradural extradural (dumbbell-shaped) mass

Schwannoma
Neurofibroma
Meningioma
Malignant lesions (metastases, lymphoma, neuroblastoma)
Infectious
Meningeal cyst

Epidural mass – predominantly ventral

Intervertebral disc herniation
Disc osteophyte complex
Uncovertebral joint hypertrophy
Postoperative fibrosis
OPLL
Malignant or benign neoplasms with epidural component (e.g. metastases, multiple myeloma, plasmacytoma, chordoma, lymphoma/leukemia, GCT, aggressive hemangioma, sarcomas)
Phlegmon/abscess
Hematoma
Engorged epidural venous plexus
Pseudomeningocele

Epidural mass – predominantly dorsal

Ligamentum flavum hypertrophy/buckling/ossification
Facet hypertrophy
Epidural lipomatosis
Synovial cyst/ganglion

Type Ia meningeal cyst
Malignant or benign neoplasms (e.g. metastases, multiple myeloma, plasmacytoma, lymphoma/leukemia, ABC, osteoblastoma, sarcomas)
Hematoma
Phlegmon/abscess
Postoperative epidural fibrosis
Engorged epidural venous plexus

Erosion of the dens

Rheumatoid arthritis
Juvenile idiopathic arthritis

Metastases
Multiple myeloma
Osteomyelitis
Hyperparathyroidism
Calcium pyrophosphate dihydrate deposition
Gout

Extradural lesions with fluid–fluid levels

Aneurysmal bone cyst (de novo)
Aneurysmal bone cyst (as a component of GCT, osteoblastoma, fibrous dysplasia)
Telangectatic osteosarcoma
Synovial cyst
Hematoma
Abscess
Necrotic/hemorrhagic metastases
Vascular/lymphatic malformations

Lytic metastases

Breast
Lung
Renal
Gastrointestinal malignancies
Thyroid

Lytic expansile masses

Metastases (especially lung, RCC, thyroid)
Multiple myeloma/plasmacytoma
LCH
ABC/GCT/osteoblastoma
Aggressive hemangioma
Chordoma
Sarcomas

Blastic metastases

Prostate
Medulloblastoma
Genitourinary malignancies
Carcinoid

Sources of drop metastases

Medulloblastoma
Ependymoma
Astrocytoma
Choroid plexus papilloma

Choroid plexus carcinoma
Germinoma
Pineoblastoma

T1/T2 hypointense marrow – diffuse

Hyperplastic marrow (chronic anemias, chronic hypoxemia)
Metastases – osteoblastic
Multiple myeloma – diffuse pattern
Lymphoma/leukemia
Myeloproliferative disorders
HIV
Osteopetrosis

T1 hyperintense marrow – diffuse

Normal yellow marrow
Post-radiation – often see margins of the radiation port
Osteoporosis – often coexists with biconvex vertebral contour and compression fractures

Endplate marrow STIR signal hyperintensity

Endplate fracture (with or without compression)
Type 1 reactive endplate changes
Infectious osteomyelitis
Seronegative spondyloarthropathies (shiny corners)
ALL/PLL avulsion fractures
Postoperative/post-procedural

Ivory vertebra

Osteoblastic metastases
Paget's disease
Lymphoma
Chordoma
Tuberculosis

Vertebral trabecular thickening

Hemangioma (no cortical thickening)
Osteoporosis
Paget's disease (more pronounced thickening than hemangioma, cortical thickening)
Metastases – blastic
Plasmacytoma (trabecular thickening in the mini-brain pattern)

Rugger jersey spine

Renal osteodystrophy
Myelofibrosis
Fluorosis
Osteopetrosis

Neuroforaminal enlargement

Nerve sheath tumors (schwannoma,
   neurofibroma)
Types Ia, Ib, II meningeal cysts
Pedicle fracture
Pseudomeningocele
Destructive lesions (metastases, primary vertebral
   neoplasms, malignant peripheral nerve sheath
   tumors, neuroblastoma)
Lateral meningocele

Sacral mass lesion

Metastases
Multiple myeloma
Chordoma
GCT/ABC

Lymphoma
Meningocele
Sarcoma (primary or secondary)

T2/STIR hyperintensity – intervertebral disc

Degenerative disc disease
Annular degeneration/tear/fissure (usually dorsal)
Infectious discitis
Traumatic disc disruption
Postoperative (discectomy)
Post-procedural (discography)
Non-infectious discitis (e.g. seronegative
   spondyloarthropathies)

Diffusion restricting lesions

Cord infarct
Epidural abscess
Cord abscess
Bone metastases
Epidermoid
Bone infarct

Image gallery

Normal aging and degenerative disease of the spine

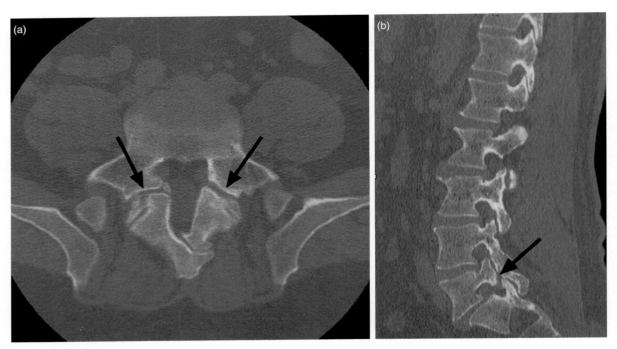

Figure 11.1 Spondylolysis: axial CT image (a) demonstrates L5 pars interarticularis defects bilaterally (black arrows) and anteroposterior elongation of the spinal canal. Sagittal CT image (b) shows the L5 pars interarticularis defect (arrow) and a grade 1/grade 2 anterolisthesis of L5 on S1.

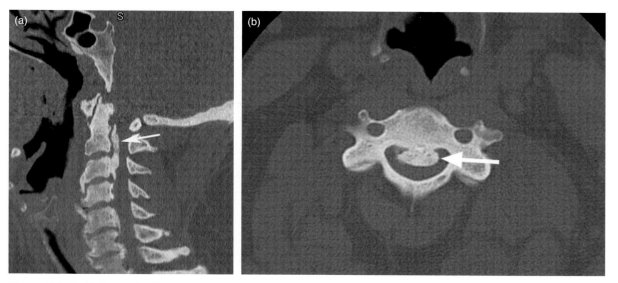

Figure 11.2 Ossified posterior ligamentous structures: sagittal CT image (a) shows segmental ossification of the posterior longitudinal ligament (arrow). Axial CT image (b) displays the characteristic mushroom shape of the ossified ligament with severe spinal canal stenosis (arrow).

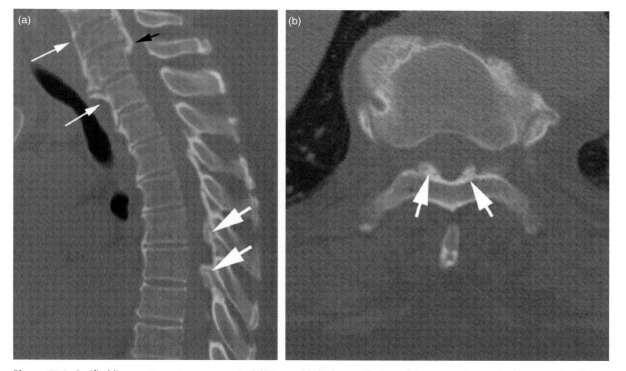

Figure 11.3 Ossified ligamentous structures: sagittal CT image (a) displays ossification of the anterior longitudinal ligament (small thin white arrows), ossification of the posterior longitudinal ligament (small black arrow), and multilevel ossification of the ligamentum flavum (large white arrows). Axial CT image (b) shows ossification of the ligamentum flavum (arrows).

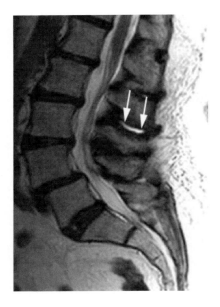

Figure 11.4 Baastrup syndrome: sagittal FSE T2 image of the lumbar spine demonstrates close apposition of the spinous processes at multiple levels, interspinous arthrosis, and interspinous bursa formation at L2-L3 (arrows).

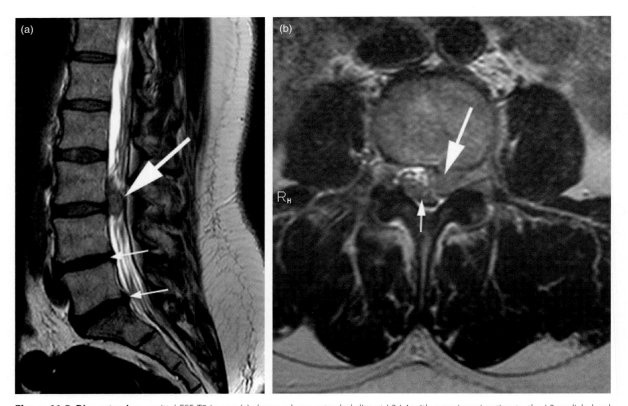

Figure 11.5 Disc extrusion: sagittal FSE T2 image (a) shows a large extruded disc at L3-L4 with superior migration to the L3 pedicle level (large arrow). Degenerative disc disease is present from L4-L5 and L5-S1 as manifest by low signal and loss of disc height (small arrows). Axial FSE T2 image (b) displays a left paracentral/subarticular disc extrusion that extends into the left neural foramen (large arrow) and displaces the dural sac to the right (small arrow). The exiting left L3 nerve root is compressed and the transiting left L4 nerve root is displaced posteriorly (not shown).

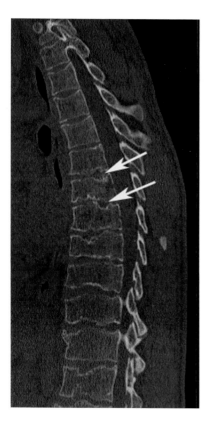

Figure 11.6 **Scheuermann's disease:** sagittal CT image of the thoracic spine showing multilevel Schmorl nodes (arrows), anterior vertebral wedging, and kyphotic deformity. *Source:* Used with permission from Barrow Neurological Institute.

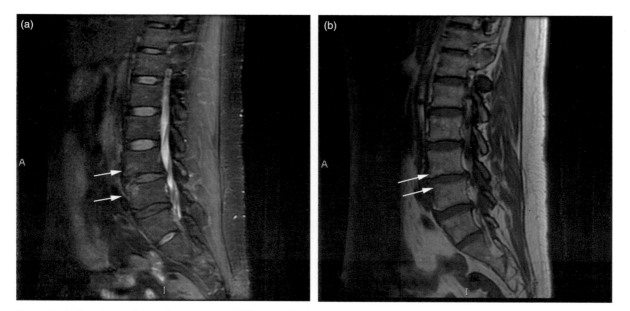

Figure 11.7 **Reactive endplate changes:** sagittal STIR image (a) shows hyperintense signal within the L3-L4 endplate marrow (arrows), consistent with type I changes. Sagittal T1WI (b) displays hyperintense signal within the endplate marrow at the same level (arrows), consistent with type II changes.

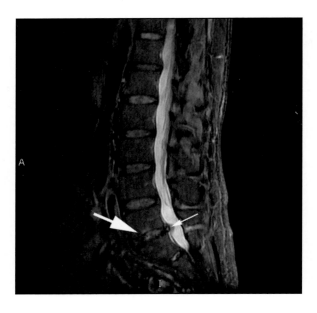

Figure 11.8 Annular tear: hyperintense signal is present within the dorsal aspect of the L5-S1 annulus (small arrow) on sagittal STIR. The L5-S1 disc displays mixed signal intensity (large arrow), with both hypointense and hyperintense signal, in the range of signal changes that can occur within degenerated discs.

Spinal trauma

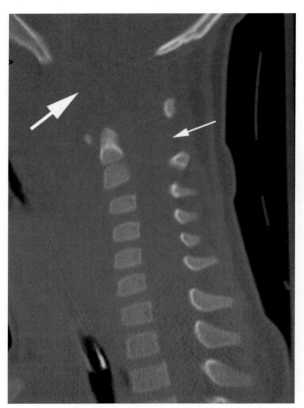

Figure 11.9 Craniocervical and atlantoaxial distraction injuries: sagittal CT image reveals an abnormal basion to dens interval (large arrow) and evidence of C1-C2 vertical distraction (small arrow).

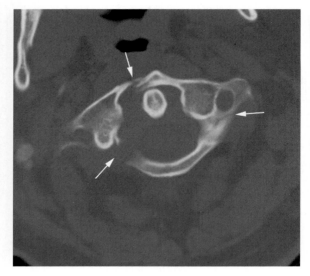

Figure 11.10 Jefferson fracture: axial CT image demonstrates a four-part fracture of C1 (arrows).

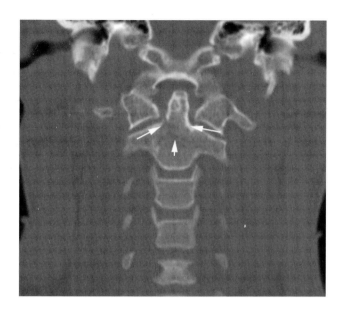

Figure 11.11 Odontoid fracture: coronal reformatted CT image displays a non-displaced fracture line extending through the base of the dens and C2 body (arrows), a type III odontoid fracture.

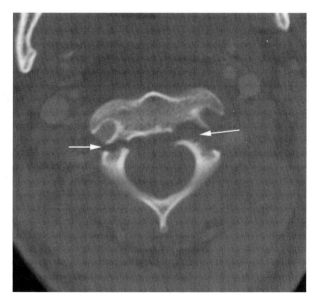

Figure 11.12 Hangman fracture: axial CT image shows mildly distracted fractures of the C2 pars interarticularis bilaterally (arrows).

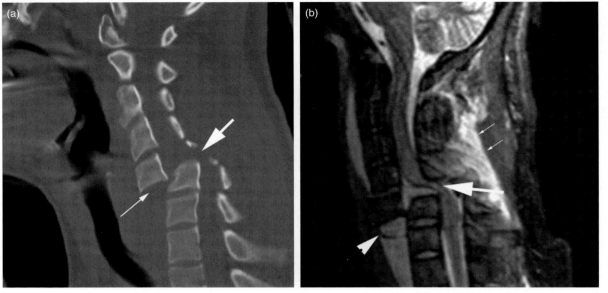

Figure 11.13 Subaxial translation injury: sagittal reformatted CT image (a) shows a severe translation injury at C5-C6 (large arrow). Three-column involvement is evident as a grade V anterolisthesis of C5 on C6 (small arrow). Sagittal FSE T2 image (b) displays a stripping and irregularity of the anterior longitudinal ligament within a large prevertebral hematoma (arrowhead). There is disruption of the C5-C6 disc, posterior longitudinal ligament, and ligamentum flavum. Severe translation results in cord compression and contusion (large arrow). Interspinous ligamentous injury is also seen (small arrows).

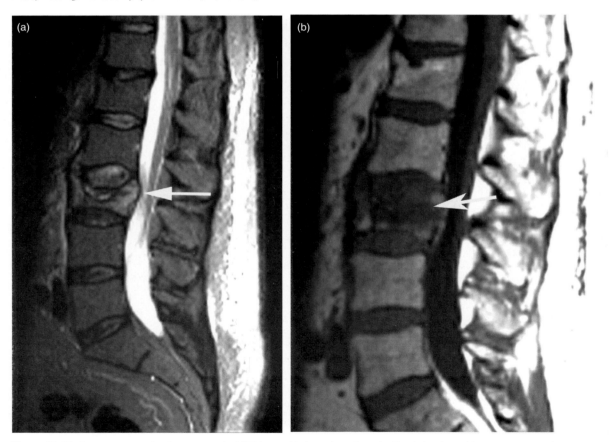

Figure 11.14 Acute compression fracture: sagittal STIR image (a) shows loss of vertebral body height and hyperintense signal representing edema at L3 (arrow). Sagittal T1WI (b) shows low signal in the compressed L3 vertebral body (arrow). There is mild retropulsion into the spinal canal. There is no associated paraspinous or epidural mass.

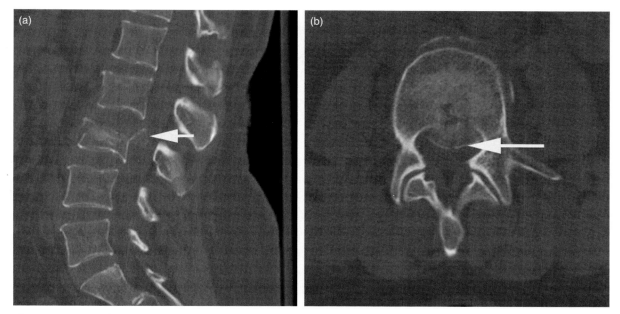

Figure 11.15 Burst fracture: reformatted sagittal (a) and axial (b) CT images show a burst type fracture at L3 with multiple fragments. There is dorsal displacement of fracture fragments that encroach upon the spinal canal (arrows).

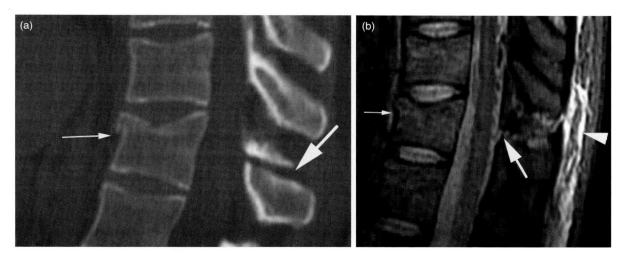

Figure 11.16 Chance fracture variant: sagittal reformatted CT image (a) shows a horizontally oriented fracture line extending through the T11 vertebral body (small arrow), pedicles, lamina, and spinous process (large arrow). Sagittal STIR image (b) shows minimal marrow edema within the T11 vertebral body (small arrow), and irregularity and/or disruption of the ligamentum flavum (large arrow). There is also evidence of interspinous ligamentous injury and paraspinous soft tissue edema (arrowhead).

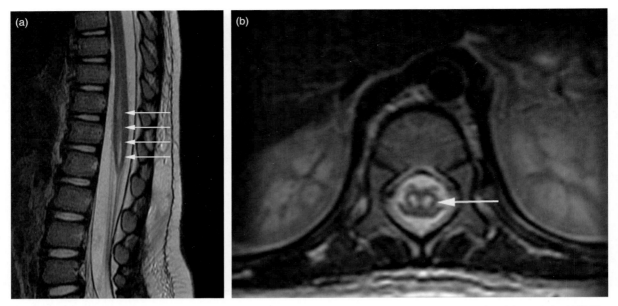

Figure 11.17 Cord infarct: sagittal FSE T2 image (a) displays abnormal hyperintense signal within the central cord (arrows). Axial FSE T2 image (b) reveals abnormal hyperintense signal within the central gray matter in the owl's eyes pattern (arrow). *Source:* Used with permission from Barrow Neurological Institute.

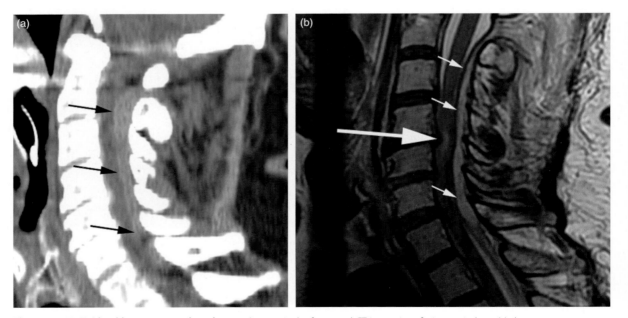

Figure 11.18 Epidural hematoma and cord contusion: sagittal reformatted CT image in soft tissue windows (a) demonstrates a hyperdense dorsal epidural fluid collection (arrows) that narrows the spinal canal. Sagittal FSE T2 image (b) better characterizes the extent of the dorsal epidural hematoma (small arrows) and the degree of spinal canal stenosis. In addition, MR shows a short segment cord contusion and a disc extrusion at C4-C5 (large arrow) that contributes to canal stenosis.

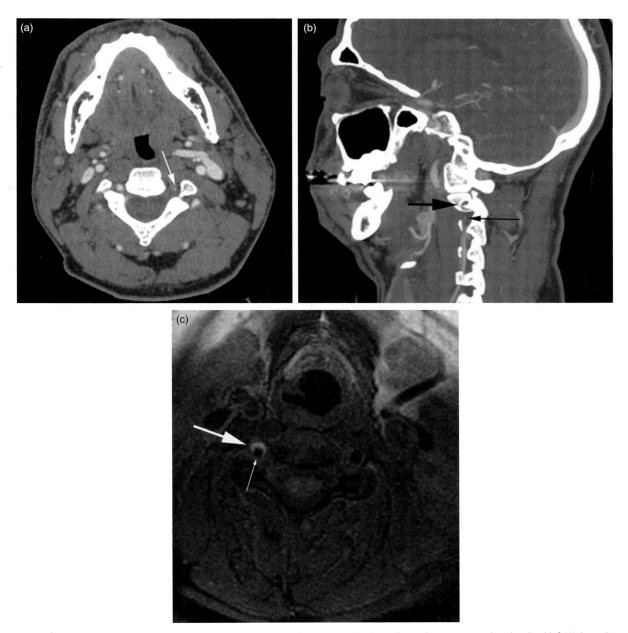

Figure 11.19 Traumatic vertebral artery (VA) dissection: axial CTA image (a) shows luminal narrowing within the distal left V2 (arrow). Sagittal reformat (b) from the same CTA shows irregular luminal narrowing of the distal left V2 (small arrow) and occlusion at the level of a transforaminal fracture (large arrow). Fat saturated T1WI (c) of a different patient delineates a methemoglobin-containing thrombus within the false lumen (large arrow) from the narrowed but patent true lumen (small arrow) of the right V2 segment. *Source:* Used with permission from Barrow Neurological Institute.

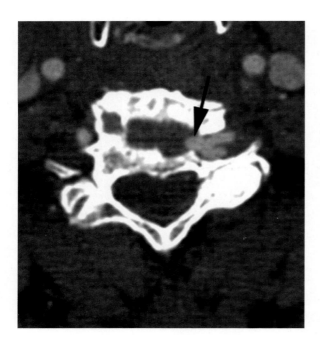

Figure 11.20 Post-traumatic vertebral artery pseudoaneurysm: axial image from a neck CTA shows a post-traumatic pseudoaneurysm projecting medially (arrow).

Infectious, inflammatory, and metabolic diseases of the spine

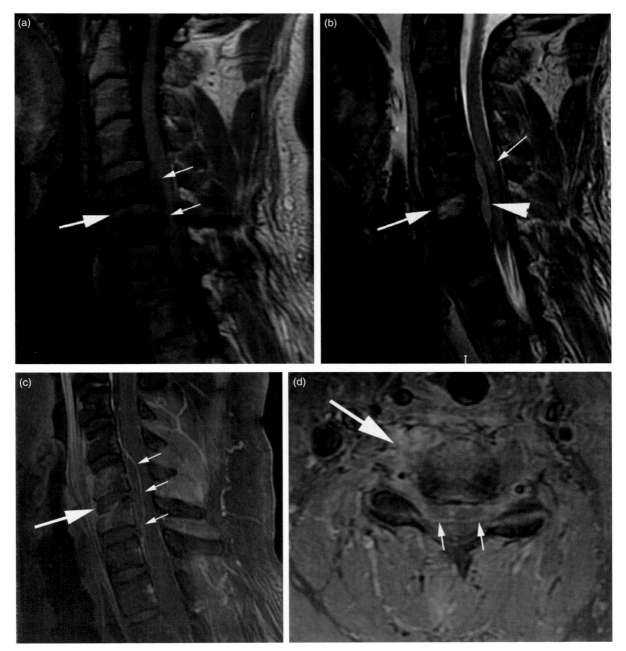

Figure 11.21 Discitis osteomyelitis and epidural abscess: pre-contrast sagittal T1WI (a) shows hypointense marrow and disc signal (large arrow) at C5-C6 and ventral epidural hypointensity (small arrows) that corresponds to hyperintense signal (large arrow and arrowhead in [b]) on sagittal FSE T2 image (b). There is evidence of cord contusion at the C5 level (small arrow). Post-contrast sagittal T1WI (c) demonstrates a peripherally enhancing ventral fluid collection extending from C4-C5 to C6-C7 (small arrows) with enhancement of the C5-C6 disc and adjacent marrow (large arrow). Axial post-contrast T1WI (d) shows the extent of canal stenosis (small arrows) and the extent of paraspinous phlegmon (large arrow).

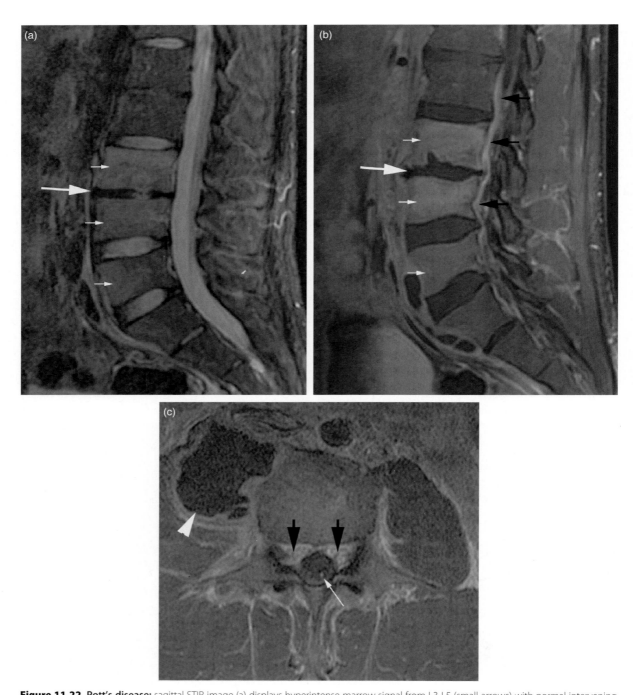

Figure 11.22 **Pott's disease:** sagittal STIR image (a) displays hyperintense marrow signal from L3-L5 (small arrows) with normal intervening discs at L4-L5 and L5-S1, and loss of disc signal and height at L3-L4 (large arrow). Sagittal post-contrast image (b) better demonstrates endplate irregularity and loss of disc space height at L3-L4 (large white arrow). There is marrow enhancement from L3-L5 (small white arrows) and ventral epidural phlegmon (black arrows). Axial post-contrast image (c) shows a large right psoas abscess (white arrowhead), ventral epidural phlegmon (black arrows), and nerve root enhancement (small white arrow).

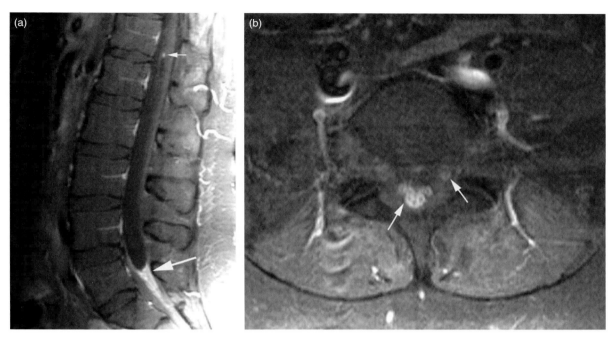

Figure 11.23 **Pyogenic leptomeningitis:** sagittal post-contrast T1WI (a) shows enhancement within the distal thecal sac (large arrow) and nodular cauda equina enhancement (small arrow). Axial post-contrast image (b) shows diffuse nerve root enhancement (arrows). *Source:* Used with permission from Barrow Neurological Institute.

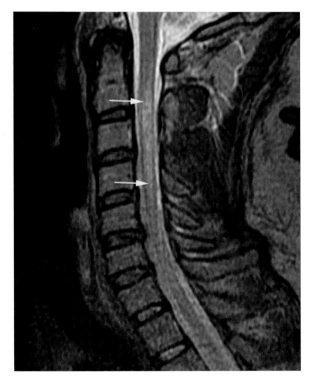

Figure 11.24 **Infectious myelitis:** sagittal STIR image displays multilevel cord expansion and central hyperintensity (arrows). There was no enhancement following contrast administration (not shown).

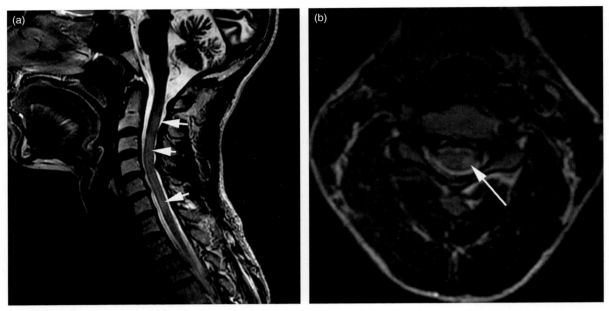

Figure 11.25 Multiple sclerosis: sagittal FSE T2 image (a) shows multiple foci of hyperintense signal, many of which are posteriorly located (white arrows). There is also a plaque within the medulla (black arrow). Axial T2WI (b) shows focal hyperintense signal in the posterolateral cord on the left (arrow), a characteristic location for MS lesions.

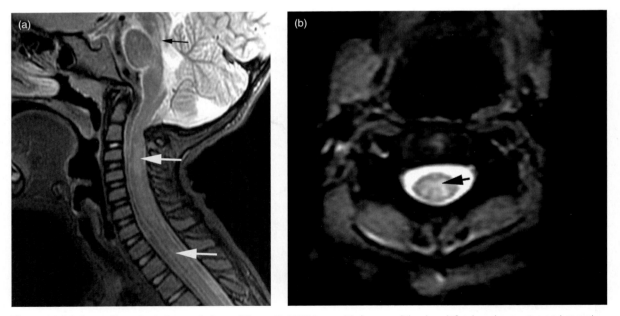

Figure 11.26 Acute disseminated encephalomyelitis: sagittal STIR image (a) shows multilevel, multifocal cord expansion and central hyperintense signal within the cervical cord (white arrows) and brainstem (black arrow). Axial GRE image (b) displays central gray matter hyperintensity (arrow).

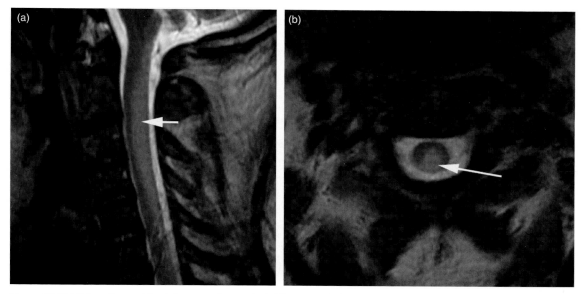

Figure 11.27 Subacute combined degeneration: sagittal STIR image (a) demonstrates multilevel dorsal hyperintense signal (arrow). Axial FSE T2 image (b) shows hyperintense signal isolated to the dorsal columns (arrow).

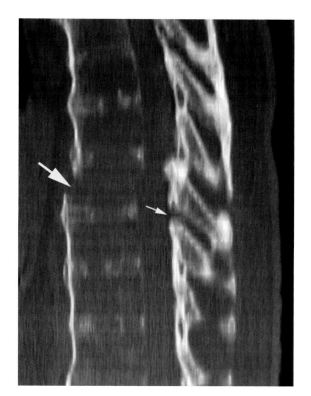

Figure 11.28 Ankylosing spondylitis: sagittal reformatted CT image obtained following minor trauma shows horizontally oriented fractures through a mid-thoracic vertebral body (large arrow) and posterior elements (small arrow) in the setting of diffuse syndesmophytes and ankylosis.

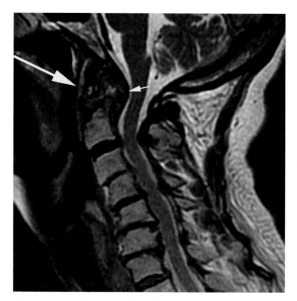

Figure 11.29 Rheumatoid arthritis: sagittal FSE T2 image displays erosion of the dens, pannus formation (small arrow), and widening of the atlantal dental interval (large arrow). *Source:* Used with permission from Barrow Neurological Institute.

Spinal tumors

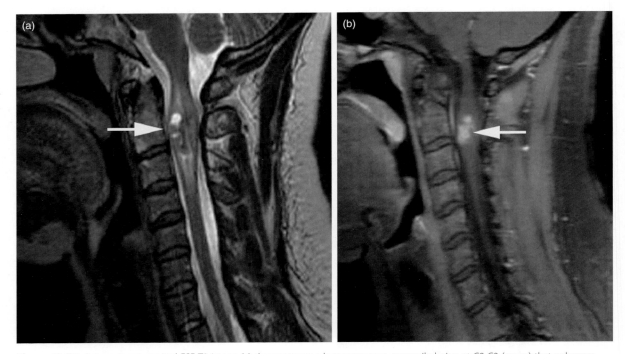

Figure 11.30 **Astrocytoma:** sagittal FSE T2 image (a) demonstrates a heterogeneous, expansile lesion at C2-C3 (arrow) that enhances heterogeneously (b) following gadolinium administration (arrow). *Source:* Used with permission from Barrow Neurological Institute.

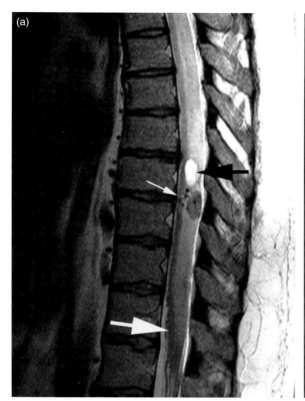
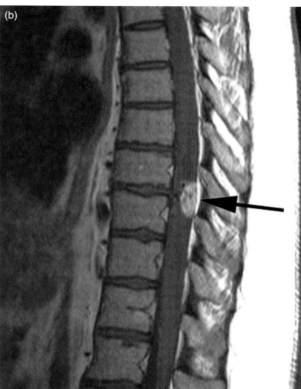

Figure 11.31 **Hemangioblastoma:** sagittal FSE T2 image (a) shows a solid and cystic (black arrow) lesion with flow voids (small white arrow), and evidence of previous hemorrhage (large white arrow). Following contrast administration (b), there is a prominently enhancing dorsal component (large arrow). *Source:* Used with permission from Barrow Neurological Institute.

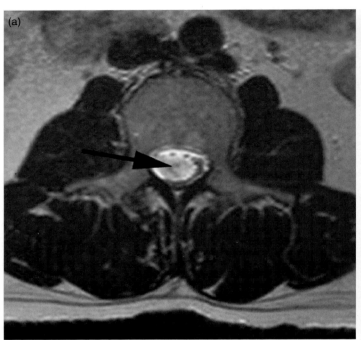

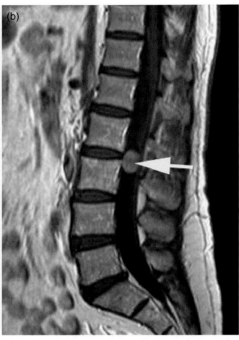

Figure 11.32 Intradural, extramedullary schwannoma: axial FSE T2 image (a) displaying a hyperintense intradural, extramedullary lesion (arrow) that compresses and displaces the thecal sac to the left. Post-contrast T1WI (b) shows homogeneous enhancement (arrow). Meningioma may have an identical appearance. *Source:* Used with permission from Barrow Neurological Institute.

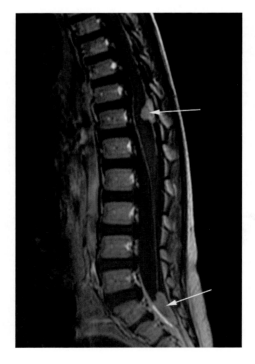

Figure 11.33 Drop metastases: sagittal post-contrast T1WI showing solidly enhancing nodular masses (arrows), as well as more diffuse smooth and nodular enhancement of the leptomeninges in a patient with posterior fossa ependymoma (not shown). *Source:* Used with permission from Barrow Neurological Institute.

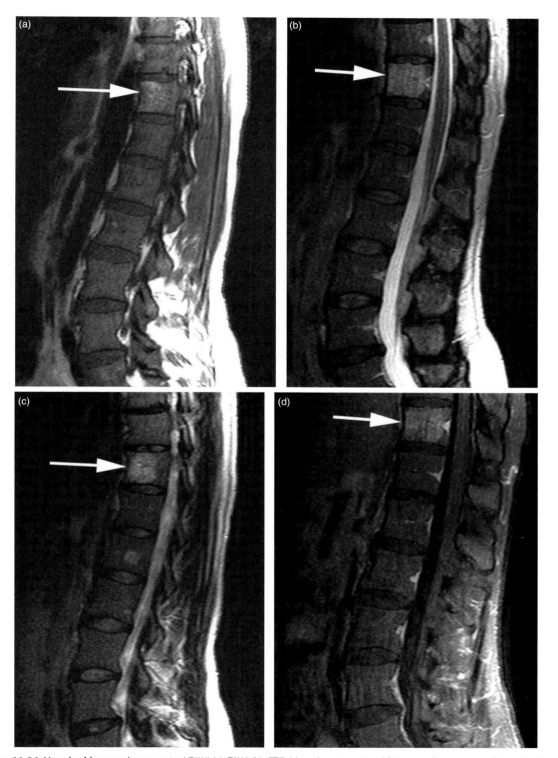

Figure 11.34 Vertebral hemangioma: sagittal T1WI (a), T2WI (b), STIR (c), and post-contrast (d) images demonstrate a lesion that is hyperintense on all pulse sequences (arrow). Note that there is partial suppression of the fatty elements on the STIR image.

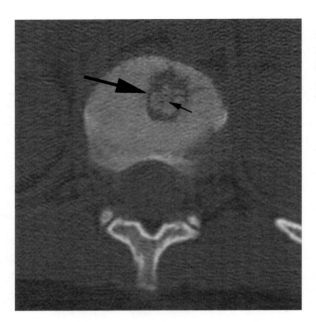

Figure 11.35 Osteoid osteoma: axial CT image demonstrating a well-defined radiolucent central nidus (large arrow), surrounding zone of reactive sclerosis that occupies most of the vertebral body, and a central matrix (small arrow). This is a typical appearance of an osteoid osteoma in an atypical location, usually found in the posterior elements. *Source:* Used with permission from Barrow Neurological Institute.

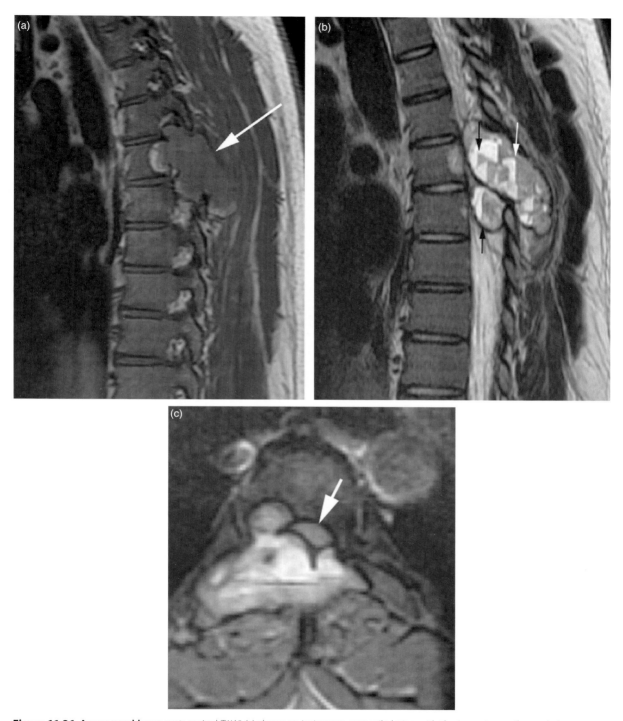

Figure 11.36 Aneurysmal bone cyst: sagittal T1WI (a) shows an isointense, expansile lesion with the isocenter on the posterior elements (white arrow). Fluid-fluid levels (arrows) are revealed on the sagittal FSE T2 image (b). Axial FSE T2 WI (c) confirms the posterior location and best characterizes the degree of encroachment upon the spinal canal (arrow). *Source:* Used with permission from Barrow Neurological Institute.

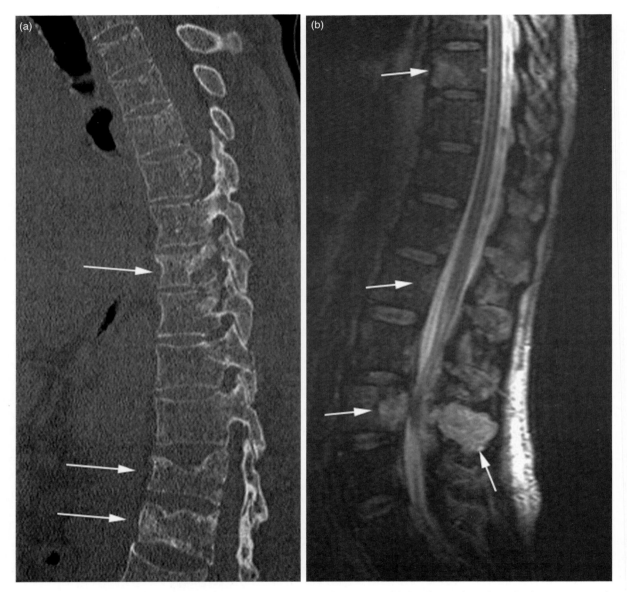

Figure 11.37 Multiple myeloma: sagittal reformatted CT image (a) displays innumerable lytic lesions throughout the thoracic spine and multiple compression fractures (arrows). Sagittal FSE T2 image (b) and post-contrast image (c) from a different patient display multiple T2 hyperintense, enhancing lesions (arrows). There is also an enhancing dorsal and ventral epidural component extending from L1-L5 (small arrows in [c]) and an enhancing mass engulfing the L3 posterior elements (large arrow in [c]).

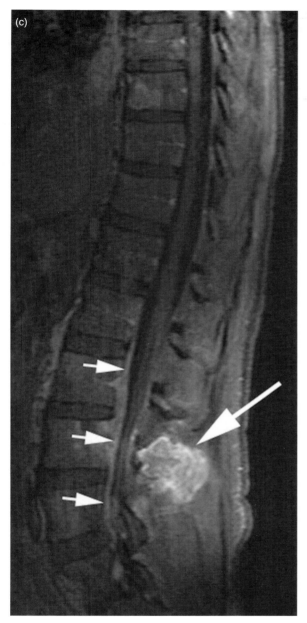

Figure 11.37 (*cont.*)

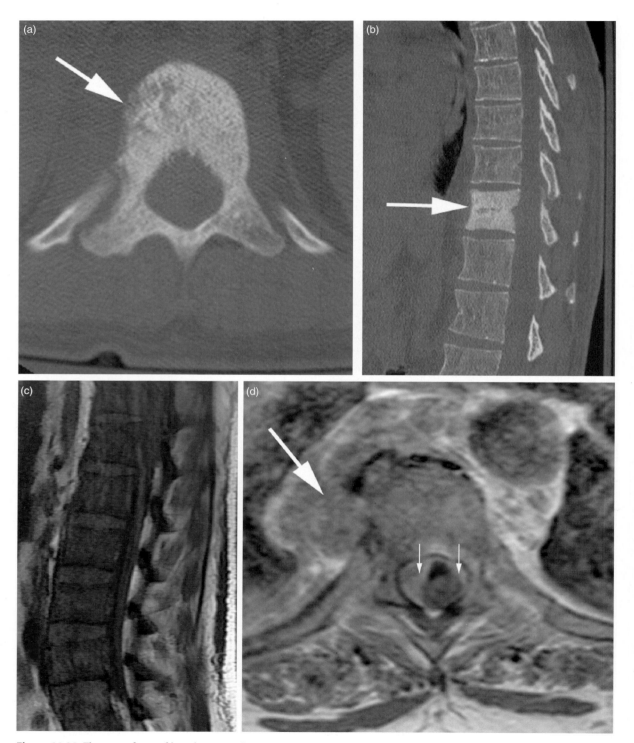

Figure 11.38 The many faces of lymphoma: axial (a) and sagittal (b) CT images display a sclerotic, non-enlarged vertebra (arrow). Sagittal T1WI (c) shows diffusely low marrow signal, lower than the adjacent intervertebral discs. Axial post-contrast MR image (d) shows enhancing epidural (small arrows) and paraspinous (large arrow) soft tissue. Sagittal post-contrast MR image (e) shows lymphomatous infiltration of the leptomeninges (arrows). Intramedullary lymphoma (arrow) is shown on a sagittal post-contrast T1WI (f).

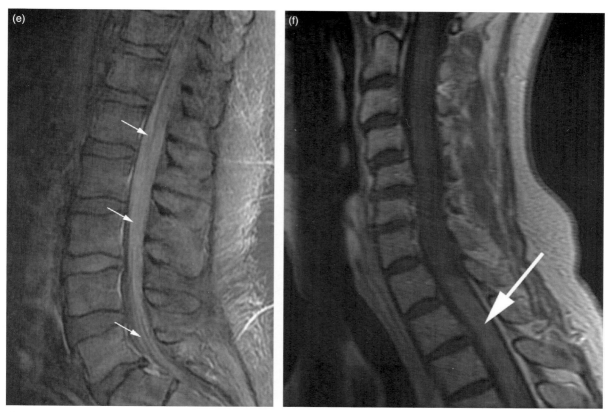

Figure 11.38 (*cont.*)

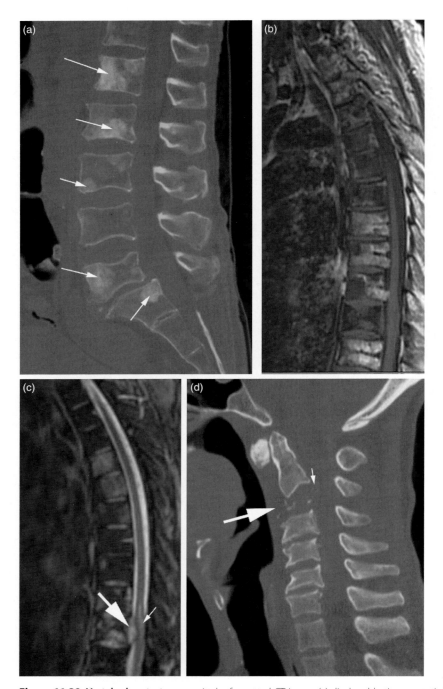

Figure 11.39 Vertebral metastases: sagittal reformatted CT image (a) displays blastic metastatic lesions throughout the lumbar spine (arrows). Sagittal T1WI (b) and STIR images (c) from a different patient show diffuse blastic lesions at all vertebral levels. Cord compression by ventral epidural extension (large arrow) produces cord signal abnormality (small arrow), best characterized on the STIR image (c). Sagittal reformatted CT image (d) shows near complete destruction of the C3 vertebral body (large arrow) and evidence of ventral epidural extension (small arrow). Sagittal T1WI (e) shows a pattern of marrow replacement within the T12 and L2 vertebral bodies (arrows). Sagittal STIR image (f) shows an irregular mixed signal mass within T12 (large arrow) and subtle hyperintense signal at L2 (small arrow).

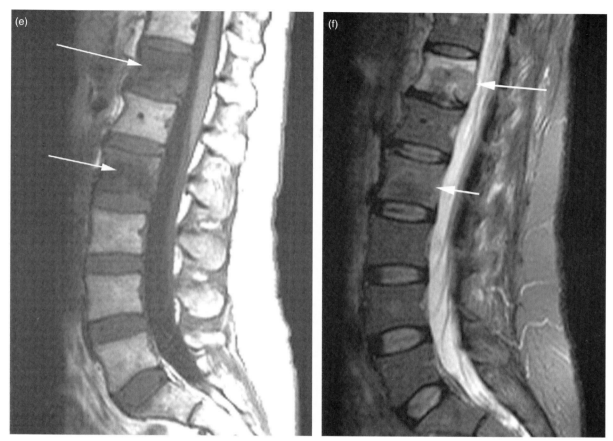

Figure 11.39 *(cont.)*

Spinal cysts, cyst-like lesions, and spinal vascular disorders

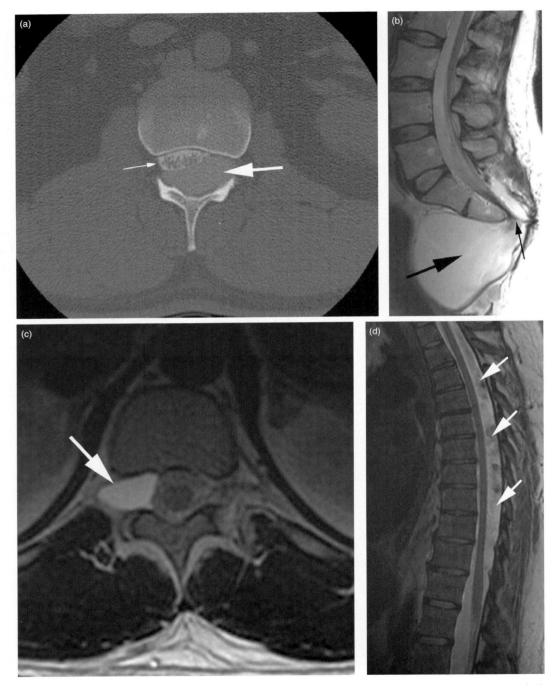

Figure 11.40 **Meningeal cysts:** axial CT myelogram (a) shows late filling of a type IA meningeal cyst (large arrow) and anterior displacement of the thecal sac (small arrow). Sagittal FSE T2 image (b) shows a type IB meningeal cyst (large arrow) projecting through a ventral sacral defect (small arrow). Axial FSE T2 image (c) demonstrates a type II meningeal cyst expanding the right neural foramen (arrow); the exiting nerve root is visible within the cyst on the sagittal images (not shown). Sagittal FSE T2 image (d) demonstrates a CSF signal intensity mass/type III meningeal cyst that displaces the cord anteriorly (arrows). Complex signal within the cyst represents CSF flow. *Source:* Used with permission from Barrow Neurological Institute.

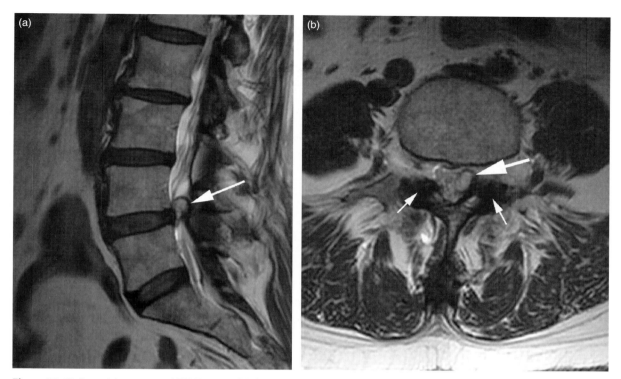

Figure 11.41 **Synovial cyst:** sagittal FSE T2 image (a) displays an extradural mixed signal intensity lesion with peripheral hemosiderin deposition (arrow). Axial FSE T2 image (b) shows facet degeneration (small arrows) and the close association of the cystic lesion with the left facet joint (large arrow). *Source:* Used with permission from Barrow Neurological Institute.

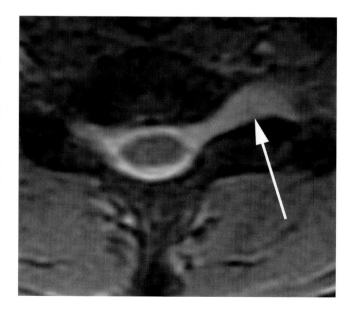

Figure 11.42 **Traumatic pseudomeningocele:** axial GRE image demonstrates a dilated, empty nerve root sleeve on the left (arrow).

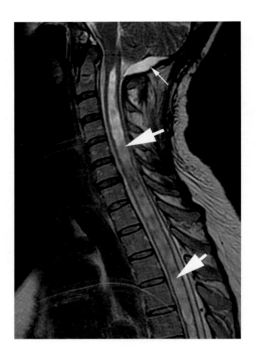

Figure 11.43 Syringohydromyelia: sagittal FSE T2 image shows a large caliber syringohydromyelia extending from the C1 level into the thoracic cord (large arrows). This patient has had a Chiari I decompression (small arrow).

Congenital anomalies of the spine

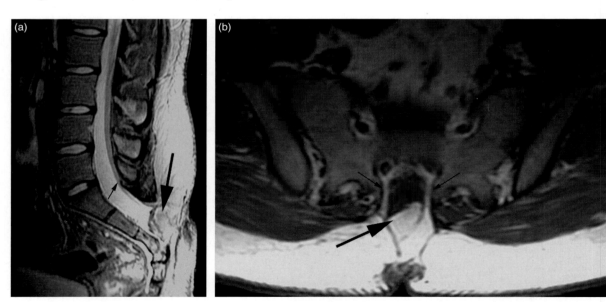

Figure 11.44 Lipomyelocele: sagittal FSE T2 image (a) demonstrates continuity of the neural placode with a dorsally located lipoma (large arrow). The cord is tethered (small arrow). Axial T1WI (b) shows the dorsal lipoma (large arrow) and a large sacral dysraphic defect (small arrows).

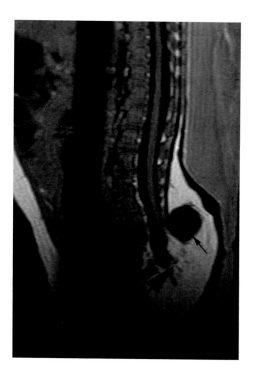

Figure 11.45 Lipomyelomeningocele: sagittal T1WI shows cord tethering to a large dorsal lipoma through a dorsal sacral defect (large arrow) and expansion of the subarachnoid space (small arrow).

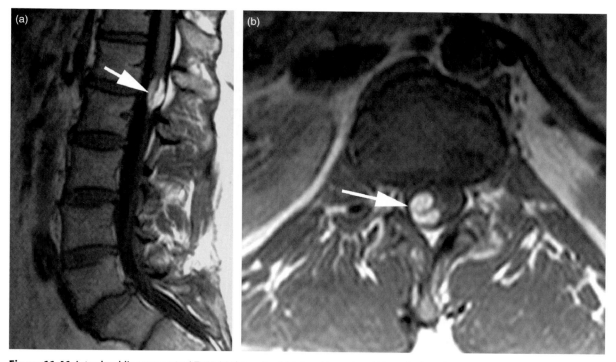

Figure 11.46 Intradural lipoma: sagittal T1WI (a) shows focal fat signal intensity within a distal cord/conus mass (arrow). Axial T1WI (b) confirms the intradural location of the eccentrically located fat signal mass (arrow). Signal within the mass is suppressed on STIR imaging (not shown). *Source:* Used with permission from Barrow Neurological Institute.

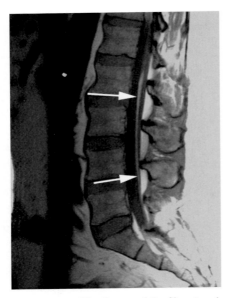

Figure 11.47 Fibrolipoma of the filum terminale: sagittal T1WI shows linear hyperintense signal that follows the course of the filum (arrows). This signal is suppressed on STIR imaging (not shown).

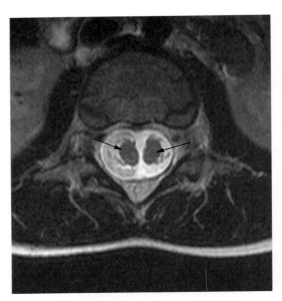

Figure 11.48 Diastematomyelia: axial FSE T2 image demonstrates a split cord (arrows). There is no evidence of a bony or cartilagenous septum. *Source:* Used with permission from Barrow Neurological Institute.

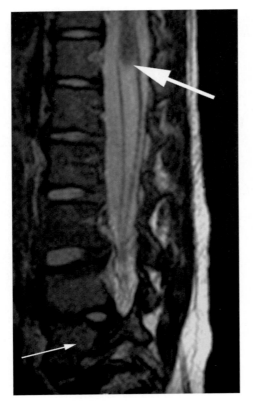

Figure 11.49 Caudal regression: sagittal T2WI shows multiple sacral anomalies (small arrow) and characteristic blunting of the conus (large arrow).

Spinal vascular disorders

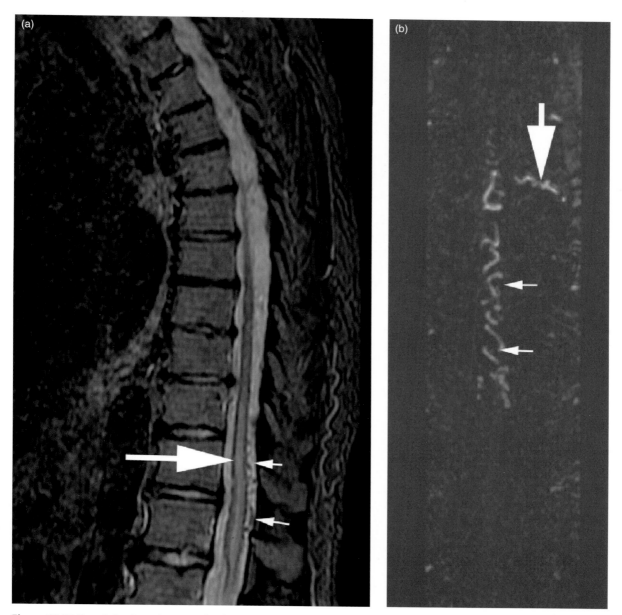

Figure 11.50 **Type I dural arteriovenous fistula:** sagittal FSE T2 image (a) shows hyperintense cord signal within the distal cord/conus (large arrow) and dorsally located serpentine perimedullary flow voids (small arrows). Spinal MRA (b) assists in planning for catheter angiography by showing a dilated radiculomedullary vein (large arrow) and a dilated coronal venous plexus (small arrows). *Source:* Used with permission from Barrow Neurological Institute.

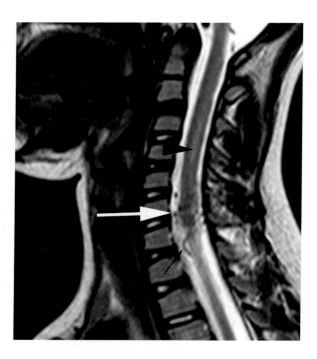

Figure 11.51 Type II arteriovenous malformation: sagittal FSE T2 image shows an intramedullary nidus (large white arrow) and numerous perimedullary flow voids (small black arrow). Cord signal abnormality is present centrally, cranial to the nidus (black arrowhead). *Source:* Used with permission from Barrow Neurological Institute.

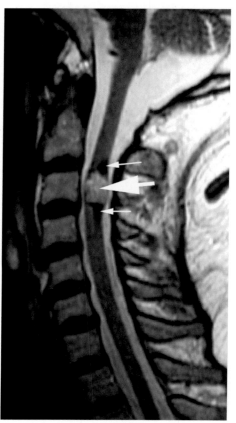

Figure 11.52 Cavernous malformation: sagittal FSE T2 image displays a heterogeneously hyperintense intramedullary lesion at C3 (large arrow). There is magnetic susceptibility artifact at the superior and inferior poles of the lesion, most likely hemosiderin from prior hemorrhage (small arrows). *Source:* Used with permission from Barrow Neurological Institute.

Metabolic diseases affecting the spine

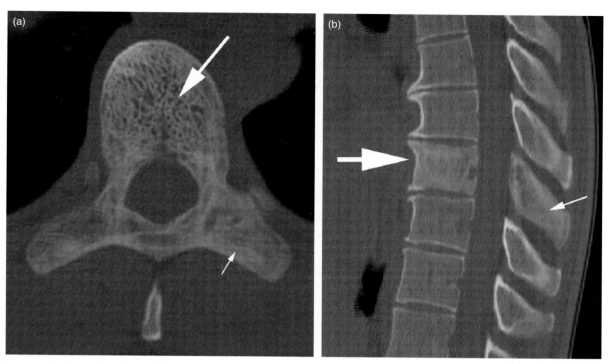

Figure 11.53 Vertebral Paget's disease: axial CT image (a) shows characteristic cortical (small arrow) and trabecular (large arrow) thickening. Sagittal reformatted CT image (b) shows relative enlargement of the involved vertebral body (large arrow) and posterior elements (small arrow) when compared to adjacent segments.

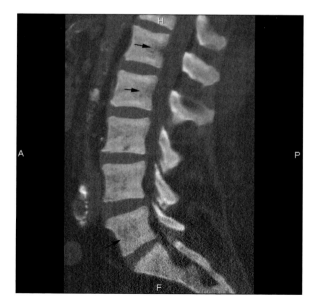

Figure 11.54 Renal osteodystrophy: sagittal reformatted CT image demonstrates diffuse osteosclerosis with relative radiolucency between the vertebral endplates (small black arrows).

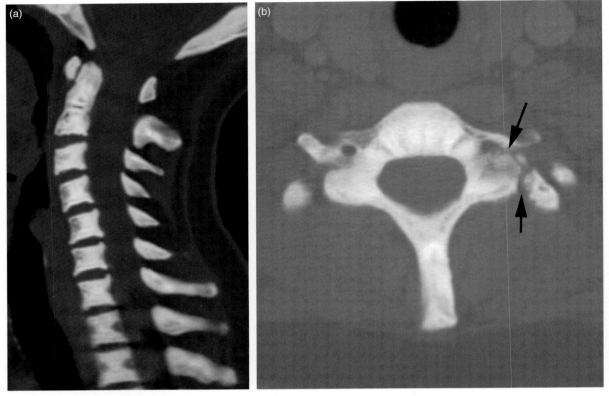

Figure 11.55 Vertebral osteopetrosis: sagittal reformatted CT image (a) shows diffuse osteosclerosis. Axial CT image (b) again shows diffuse osteosclerosis, but also demonstrates healing fractures (arrows). There were multiple healing fractures at various levels of the cervical and thoracic spine, reflecting the increased fracture risk in this patient population.

Suggested reading

1. Abul-Kasim K, Thurnher MM, McKeever P, & Sundgren PC. Intradural spinal tumors: current classification and MRI features. *Neuroradiology* 2008; **50**: 301–314.

2. Anderson PA & Montesano PX. Morphology and treatment of occipital condyle fractures. *Spine* 1988; **13**: 731–736.

3. Angtuaco EJC, Fassas AB, Walker R, Sethi R, & Barlogie B. Multiple myeloma: clinical review and diagnostic imaging. *Radiographics* 2004; **231**: 11–23.

4. Anson JA & Spetzler RF. Classification of spinal arteriovenous malformations and implications for treatment. *BNI Quarterly* 1992; **8**: 2–8.

5. Banks KP. The target sign: extremity. *Radiology* 2005; **234**: 899–900.

6. Bernstein MP, Mirvis SE, & Shanmuganathan K. Chance-type fractures of the thoracolumbar spine: imaging analysis in 53 patients. *American Journal of Radiology* 2006; **187**: 859–868.

7. Berquist TH. Imaging of adult cervical spine trauma. *Radiographics* 1988; **8**(4): 667–694.

8. Brooks BK, Southam SL, Logan J, & Rosett M. Lumbar spine spondylolysis in the adult population: using computed tomography to evaluate the possibility of adult onset lumbar spondylosis as a cause of back pain. *Skeletal Radiology* 2010; **39**(7): 669–673.

9. Coleman LT, Zimmerman RA, & Rorke LB. Ventriculus terminalis of the conus medullaris: MR findings in children. *American Journal of Neuroradiology* 1995; **16**: 1421–1426.

10. Deliganis AV, Baxter AB, Hanson AJ, et al. Radiologic spectrum of craniocervical distraction injuries. *Radiographics* 2000; **20**: 237–250.

11. Donkelaar HJ, Lammens M, & Hori A. *Clinical Neuroembryology: Development and Developmental Disorders of the Human Central Nervous System*. Berlin: Springer-Verlag, 2006.

12. Evans DG, Baser ME, McGaughran J, et al. Malignant peripheral nerve sheath tumours in neurofibromatosis 1. *Journal of Medical Genetics* 2002; **39**(5): 311–314.

13. Faris JC & Crowe JE. The split notocord syndrome. *Journal of Pediatric Surgery* 1975; **10**: 467–472.

14. Farsad K, Kattapuram SV, Sacknoff R, Ono J, & Nielsen GP. Best cases from the AFIP: sacral chordoma. *Radiographics* 2009; **29**: 1525–1530.

15. Grenier N, Kressel HY, Schiebler ML, & Grossman RI. Isthmic spondylolysis of the lumbar spine: MR imaging at 1.5T. *Radiology* 1989; **170**: 489–493.

16. Gunel M, Awad IA, Anson J, et al. Mapping a gene causing cerebral cavernous malformation to 7q11.2-q21. *Proceedings of the National Academy of Sciences of the United States of America* 1995; **92**: 6620–6624.

17. Holmes JF, Miller PQ, Panacek EA, et al. Epidemiology of thoracolumbar spine injury in blunt trauma. *Academic Emergency Medicine* 2001; **8**(9): 866–872.

18. Ilaslan H, Sundaram M, Unni KK, & Shives TC. Primary vertebral osteosarcoma: imaging findings. *Radiology* 2004; **230**(3): 697–702.

19. Jung HS, Lee WH, McCauley TR, Ha KY, & Choi KH. Discrimination of metastatic from acute osteoporotic compression spinal fractures with MR imaging. *Radiographics* 2003; **23**: 179–187.

20. Khosla A & Wippold FJ. CT myelography and MR imaging of extramedullary cysts of the spinal canal in adult and pediatric patients. *American Journal of Radiology* 2002; **178**: 201–207.

21. Koeller KK, Rosenblum R, & Morrison AL. Neoplasms of the spinal cord and filum terminale: radiologic-pathologic correlation. *Radiographics* 2000; **20**: 1721–1749.

22. Lacout A, Rousselin B, & Pelage J. CT and MRI of spine and sacroiliac involvement in spondyloarthropathy. *American Journal of Radiology* 2007; **191**: 1016–1023.

23. Lemole GM, Henn JS, Riina HA, et al. Spinal cord cavernous malformations. *Seminars in Cerebrovascular Diseases and Stroke* 2002; **2**(3): 227–235.

24. Liu PR, Chivers FS, Roberts CC, Schultz CJ, & Beauchamp CP. Imaging of osteoid osteoma with dynamic gadolinium-enhanced MR imaging. *Radiology* 2003; **227**(3): 691–700.

25. Llauger J, Palmer J, Amores S, Bague S, & Camins A. Primary tumors of the sacrum. *American Journal of Roentgenology* 2000; **174**: 417–424.

26. Major NM, Helms CA, & Richardson WJ. The "mini brain": plasmacytoma in a vertebral body on MR imaging. *American Journal of Radiology* 2000; **175**: 261–263.

27. Mawad ME, Rivera V, Crawford S, Ramirez A, & Breitbach W. Spinal cord ischemia after resection of thoracoabdominal aortic aneurysms: MR findings in 24 patients. *American Journal of Neuroradiology* 1990; **11** (5): 987–991.

28. Mehta RC, Marks MP, Hinks RS, Glover GH, & Enzmann DR. MR evaluation of vertebral metastases: T1-weighted, short-inversion-time inversion recovery, fast spin-echo, and inversion-recovery fast spin-echo sequences. *American Journal of Neuroradiology* 1995; **16**(2): 281–288.

29. Miyanji F, Furlan JC, Aarabi B, Arnold PM, & Fehlings MG. Acute cervical traumatic spinal cord injury: MR imaging findings correlated with neurologic outcome – prospective study with 100 consecutive patients. *Radiology* 2007; **243**(3): 820–827.

30. Modic MT, Steinberg PM, Ross JS, et al. Degenerative disk disease: assessment of changes in vertebral body marrow with MR imaging. *Radiology* 1988; **166**: 193–199.

31. Murphey MD, Andrews CL, Flemming DJ, Temple HT, Smith WS, et al. Primary tumors of the spine: radiologic-pathologic correlation. *Radiographics* 1996; **16**: 1131–1158.

32. Murphey MD, Smith WS, Al-Assir I, & Shekitka KM. MR imaging of giant cell tumor of bone: signal intensity characteristics with radiologic-pathologic correlation. *Radiology* 1995; **197**(P): 195.

33. Nabors MW, Piat TG, Byrd EB, et al. Updated assessment and current classification of spinal meningeal cysts. *Journal of Neurosurgery* 1988; **68**(3): 366–377.

34. Nathan, H. Osteophytes of the vertebral column: an anatomical study of their development according to age, race, and sex with consideration as to their etiology and significance; *Journal of Bone and Joint Surgery* 1962; **44**: 243–268.

35. Nievelstein RA, Valk J, Smit ME, & Vermeij-Keers C. MR of the caudal regression syndrome: embryologic implications. *American Journal of Neuroradiology* 1994; **15**: 1021–1029.

36. Papac RJ. Bone marrow metastases: a review. *Cancer* 1994; **74**(9): 2403–2413.

37. Plank C, Koller A, Mueller-Mang C, Bammer R, & Thurnher MM. Diffusion-weighted MR imaging (DWI) in the evaluation of epidural spinal lesions. *Neuroradiology* 2007; **49**(12): 977–985.

38. Rahme R & Moussa R. The Modic vertebral endplate and marrow changes: pathologic significance and relation to low back pain and segmental instability of the lumbar spine. *American Journal of Neuroradiology* 2008; **29**: 838–842.

39. Rodallec MH, Marteau V, Gerber S, Desmottes L, & Zins M. Craniocervical arterial dissection: spectrum of imaging findings and differential diagnosis. *Radiographics* 2008; **28**: 1711–1728.

40. Rossi A, Cama A, Piatelli G, et al. Spinal dysraphism: MR imaging rationale. *Journal of Neuroradiology* 2004; **31**: 3–24.

41. Sethi MK, Schonfeld AJ, Bono CM, & Harris MB. The evolution of thoracolumbar injury classification systems. *Spine* 2009; **9**: 780–788.

42. Sioutos PJ, Arbit E, Meshulam CF, & Galicich JH. Spinal metastases from solid tumors. Analysis of factors affecting survival. *Cancer* 1995; **76**(8): 1453–1459.

43. Smith SE, Murphey MD, Motamedi K, et al. From the archives of the AFIP: radiologic spectrum of Paget disease of bone and its complications with pathologic correlation. *Radiographics* 2002; **22**: 1191–1216.

44. Spetzler RF, Detwiler PW, Riina HA, et al. Modified classification of spinal cord vascular lesions. *Journal of Neurosurgery* 2002; **96**(2 suppl): 145–156.

45. Stull MA, Kransdorf MJ, & Devaney KO. From the archives of the AFIP: Langerhans cell histiocytosis of bone. *Radiographics* 1992; **12**: 801–823.

46. Vaccaro AR, Hulbert RJ, Patel AA, et al. The subaxial cervical spine injury classification system: a novel approach to recognize the importance of morphology, neurology, and integrity of the disco-ligamentous complex. *Spine* 2007; **32**(21): 2365–2374.

47. Wang PY, Shen WC, & Jan JS. MR imaging in radiation myelopathy. *American Journal of Neuroradiology* 1992; **13**(4): 1049–1055.

48. Wittenberg A. The rugger jersey spine sign. *Radiology* 2004; **230**: 491–492.

49. Wyndaele M & Wyndaele JJ. Incidence, prevalence and epidemiology of spinal cord injury: what learns a worldwide literature survey? *Spinal Cord* 2006; **44**: 508–523.

50. Yamauchi H. Epidemiological and pathological study of ossification of the posterior longitudinal ligament of the cervical spine. Investigation Committee 1977 report on the ossification of the spinal ligaments of the Japanese Ministry of Public Health and Welfare. 1978; pp 21–25.

51. Yuh WT, Marsh EE, Wang AK, et al. MR imaging of spinal cord and vertebral body infarction. *American Journal of Neuroradiology* 1992; **13**(1): 145–154.

Appendix: Dictation templates

Brain

Normal CT head without intravenous contrast
CT head without intravenous contrast

Clinical indication: [. . .]

Technique: This examination was performed in the axial plane utilizing the multidetector/helical technique from base to vertex without the administration of intravenous contrast. Images were reviewed at bone, soft tissue, subdural, and stroke windows.

Prior examination: [. . .]

Findings

Examination through the posterior fossa demonstrates the fourth ventricle to be midline in position. There is no evidence of focal brainstem, cerebellar, or cerebellopontine angle abnormality.

Supratentorially the third and lateral ventricles are normal in size and position. No shift. No hydrocephalus. Normal gray matter–white matter differentiation. No evidence of acute hyperdense intracranial hemorrhage or other acute focal intracranial pathology. No evidence of intracranial mass or localized areas of positive mass effect on this unenhanced examination. No extracerebral fluid collections. Basal cisterns are open.

Bone windows are unremarkable. The paranasal sinuses as visualized are clear. Mastoid air cells and tympanic cavities are well aerated. Visualized portions of the orbits are unremarkable. The scalp and surrounding soft tissues are unremarkable.

Impression
Normal CT head without contrast.

Normal CT head without and with intravenous contrast
CT head without and with intravenous contrast

Clinical indication: [. . .]

Technique: This examination was performed in the axial plane utilizing multidetector/helical technique from base to vertex without and with the intravenous administration of contrast. Images were reviewed at bone, soft tissue, subdural, and stroke windows.

Prior examination: [. . .]

Contrast utilized: [. . .]

Findings

Examination through the posterior fossa demonstrates the fourth ventricle to be midline in position. No evidence of focal brainstem, cerebellar, or cerebellopontine angle abnormality.

Supratentorially the third and lateral ventricles are normal in size and position. No shift. No hydrocephalus. Normal gray matter–white matter differentiation. No evidence of acute hyperdense intracranial hemorrhage or other acute focal intracranial pathology. No focal areas of pathologic contrast enhancement. No evidence of intracranial mass or localized areas of positive mass effect. No extracerebral fluid collections. Basal cisterns are open.

Bone windows are unremarkable. The paranasal sinuses as visualized are clear. Mastoid air cells and tympanic cavities are well aerated. Visualized portions of the orbits are unremarkable. The scalp and surrounding soft tissues are unremarkable.

Impression
Normal CT head without and with contrast.

CT head without intravenous contrast in the elderly
CT head without intravenous contrast

Clinical indication: [. . .]

Technique: This examination was performed in the axial plane utilizing multidetector/helical technique from base to vertex without the administration of intravenous contrast. Images were reviewed at bone, soft tissue, subdural, and stroke windows.

Prior examination: [. . .]

Findings
[Mild, moderate, severe] cortical involutional changes (atrophy) and proportionate ventricular enlargement are seen.

Examination through the posterior fossa demonstrates the fourth ventricle to be midline in position. No evidence of focal brainstem, cerebellar, or cerebellopontine angle abnormality. Elongation and tortuosity of the vertebrobasilar system are seen.

Supratentorially the third and lateral ventricles are normal in position. No shift.

[Mild, moderate, severe] patchy, nonspecific areas of hypodensity are seen within the white matter of both cerebral hemispheres which, given the patient's age, likely represent areas of microvascular ischemic change, although the appearance is non-specific. Old lacunar infarcts are seen in the lentiform nuclei bilaterally and in the right frontal and left parietal corona radiata. An area of macrocystic and microcystic encephalomalacia is seen in the cortical and subcortical white matter in the left occipital lobe consistent with an area of old infarction.

No acute hyperdense intracranial hemorrhage or shift. No localized areas of positive mass effect. Widening of the subarachnoid spaces is seen diffusely, consistent with the cortical involutional (atrophic) changes. No subdural or epidural fluid collection is seen.

Basal ganglia and intracranial vascular calcifications are seen.

Bone windows demonstrate numerous normal appearing intradiploic vascular channels. No focal lytic or blastic changes. Paranasal sinuses are clear. Mastoid air cells and tympanic cavities are well aerated. Focal soft tissue densities in the external auditory canals are seen bilaterally, likely representing cerumen.

Visualized portions of the orbits are unremarkable. The scalp and surrounding soft tissues are unremarkable.

Impression
1. [Mild, moderate, severe] cortical involutional (atrophic) changes and proportionate ventricular enlargement for the patient's age.
2. Probable [mild, moderate, severe] microvascular ischemic changes and areas of old infarction, as noted previously.
3. No acute hyperdense intracranial hemorrhage or other acute focal intracranial pathology and no midline shift.

Please see previous comments above for details.

Normal MRI brain without and with intravenous contrast
MRI brain without and with contrast

Clinical indication: [. . .]

Technique: This examination was performed in the sagittal, axial, and coronal planes utilizing multiple pulse sequences that produce images with T1 and variable T2 weighting. Diffusion weighted images were obtained. Post-gadolinium T1 weighted images were obtained.

Prior examination: [. . .]

Contrast utilized: [. . .]

Findings
No areas of diffusion restriction.

Examination through the posterior fossa demonstrates the fourth ventricle to be midline in position. No evidence of focal brainstem, cerebellar, or cerebellopontine angle abnormality. The internal auditory canals are grossly symmetric. Grossly symmetric signal intensity is seen arising from the membranous labyrinth regions. There is normal absence of signal from the mastoid regions.

Supratentorially the third and lateral ventricles are normal in size and position. No shift. No hydrocephalus.

There is normal gray matter–white matter differentiation. No focal regions of parenchymal signal abnormality. No focal areas of pathologic contrast enhancement. No evidence of intracranial mass or areas of localized positive mass effect. No extracerebral fluid collections. Flow void is identified within the main proximal intracranial arterial vascular pedicles.

The pituitary gland and craniovertebral junction are within normal limits.

The visualized paranasal sinuses are clear. Visualized portions of the orbits are unremarkable. The scalp and surrounding soft tissues are unremarkable.

Impression

1. Normal MRI brain without and with contrast.
2. No significant interval change since the previous examination.

Please see previous comments above for details.

MRI brain without intravenous contrast in the elderly
MRI brain without contrast

Clinical indication: [. . .]

Technique: This examination was performed in the sagittal, axial, and coronal planes utilizing multiple pulse sequences that produce images with T1 and variable T2 weighting. Diffusion weighted images were obtained.

Prior examination: [. . .]

Findings
No areas of diffusion restriction.

[Mild, moderate, severe] generalized cortical involutional changes (atrophy) and proportionate ventricular enlargement are seen for age.

Examination through the posterior fossa demonstrates the fourth ventricle to be midline in position. No evidence of focal brainstem, cerebellar, or cerebellopontine angle abnormality. The internal auditory canals are grossly symmetric. Grossly symmetric signal intensity is seen arising from the membranous labyrinth regions. There is normal absence of signal from the mastoid regions.

Supratentorially the third and lateral ventricles are normal in position. No shift. [Mild, moderate, severe] multifocal, patchy, and confluent areas of abnormal increased T2 signal are seen within the white matter of both cerebral hemispheres. Given the patient's age, these likely represent areas of microvascular ischemic changes, but the appearance is nonspecific. Old lacunar infarcts are seen scattered within the basal ganglia/internal capsule and thalamic regions bilaterally.

No localized areas of positive mass effect. No extracerebral fluid collections. Attention to the arterial vascular flow voids demonstrates elongation, tortuosity, and ectasia of the intracranial arterial vasculature.

The pituitary gland and craniovertebral junction are within normal limits. Visualized portions of the orbits are unremarkable. The scalp and surrounding soft tissues are unremarkable.

Impression

1. [Mild, moderate, severe] generalized cortical involutional changes (atrophy) and proportionate ventricular enlargement for age.
2. Probable [mild, moderate, severe] microvascular ischemic changes with multiple, old lacunar infarcts, as noted.
3. No evidence of acute infarction on diffusion weighted images.

Please see previous comments above for details.

Normal MRI brain/internal auditory canals
MRI brain/internal auditory canals

Clinical indication: [. . .]

Prior examination: [. . .]

Technique: This examination was performed in the sagittal, axial, and coronal planes utilizing multiple pulse sequences that produce images with T1 and variable T2 weighting. Diffusion weighted images were obtained. High resolution thin section imaging through the internal auditory canals was obtained prior to and after the intravenous administration of gadolinium. Post-gadolinium T1 weighted images through the entire brain were obtained.

Contrast utilized: [. . .]

Findings

No areas of diffusion restriction.

Examination through the posterior fossa demonstrates the fourth ventricle to be midline in position. No evidence of focal brainstem, cerebellar, or cerebellopontine angle abnormality. The internal auditory canals appear symmetrically normal. There is a normal appearance to the seventh and eighth cranial nerve complexes bilaterally. No evidence of a vestibular schwannoma or other intracanalicular or cerebellopontine angle cistern mass. Symmetrically normal signal intensity is seen arising from the membranous labyrinth regions bilaterally. There is normal absence of signal from the mastoid regions bilaterally.

Supratentorially the third and lateral ventricles are normal in size and position. No shift. No hydrocephalus. No significant areas of parenchymal signal abnormality. Normal gray matter–white matter differentiation. No focal areas of pathologic contrast enhancement. No localized areas of positive mass effect. No extracerebral fluid collections. Flow void is identified within the major proximal intracranial arterial vascular pedicles.

The pituitary gland and craniovertebral junction are within normal limits. Visualized paranasal sinuses are clear. Visualized portions of the orbits are unremarkable. The scalp and surrounding soft tissues are unremarkable.

Impression

1. Normal MRI brain.
2. Specifically, normal MRI internal auditory canals.

Please see previous details.

Normal MRI brain/pituitary gland
MRI brain/pituitary gland

Clinical indication: [. . .]

Prior examination: [. . .]

Technique: This examination was performed in the sagittal, axial, and coronal planes utilizing multiple pulse sequences that produce images with T1 and variable T2 weighting. Diffusion weighted images were obtained. High resolution thin section T1 weighted images through the region of the sella turcica were obtained prior to and after the intravenous administration of gadolinium. Post-gadolinium T1 weighted images through the entire brain were obtained.

Contrast utilized: [. . .]

Findings

No areas of diffusion restriction.

Examination through the posterior fossa demonstrates the fourth ventricle to be midline in position. No evidence of focal brainstem, cerebellar, or cerebellopontine angle abnormality. The internal auditory canals are grossly symmetric. There is normal absence of signal from the mastoid regions bilaterally.

Supratentorially the third and lateral ventricles are normal in size and position. No shift. No hydrocephalus. No significant areas of parenchymal signal abnormality. Normal gray matter–white matter differentiation. No focal areas of pathologic contrast enhancement. No localized areas of positive mass effect. No extracerebral fluid collections. Flow void is identified within the major proximal intracranial arterial vascular pedicles.

High resolution imaging through the sella turcica demonstrates the pituitary gland to be within normal limits in size. The infindibulum is midline in position. No evidence of intrasellar, parasellar, or suprasellar abnormality. Specifically, no evidence of a pituitary micro- or macroadenoma.

The craniovertebral junction is within normal limits. Visualized paranasal sinuses are clear. Visualized portions of the orbits are unremarkable. The scalp and surrounding soft tissues are unremarkable.

Impression

1. Normal MRI brain.
2. Specifically, normal MRI pituitary gland.

Please see previous comments above for details.

Spine

CT cervical spine without contrast
[Order reason for study]

Comparison: [none]

Technique: multiple, non-contrasted axial CT images were obtained from the skull base to the cervicothoracic junction and reformatted in the sagittal and coronal planes.

Findings

[There is a normal cervical lordosis]. [There is preservation of vertebral body and disc space height]. [The craniocervical junction is normal]. [The posterior elements are normal in appearance and alignment]. [The soft tissues of the neck and lung apices are normal].

Impression

[No evidence of acute fracture or malalignment].

CT thoracic spine without contrast
[Order reason for study]

Comparison: [none]

Technique: multiple, non-contrasted axial CT images were obtained from the cervicothoracic junction to the thoracolumbar junction and reformatted in the sagittal and coronal planes.

Findings

[There is a normal thoracic kyphosis with preservation of vertebral body and disc space height]. [Alignment is maintained]. [There is no significant neuroforaminal or central canal stenosis].

[The visualized solid and hollow organs are normal in appearance].

Impression

[No evidence of acute fracture or malalignment involving the thoracic spine].

CT lumbar spine without contrast
[Order reason for study]

Comparison: [none]

Technique: multiple, non-contrasted axial CT images were obtained from the thoracolumbar junction to the sacrum and reformatted in the sagittal and coronal planes.

Findings

[There is a normal lumbar lordosis with preservation of vertebral body and disc space height]. [Alignment is maintained]. [There is no significant neuroforaminal or central canal stenosis].

[The visualized solid and hollow organs are normal in appearance].

Impression

[No evidence of acute fracture or malalignment involving the lumbar spine].

MRI cervical spine without contrast
[Order reason for study]

Comparison: [. . .]

Technique: multiplanar, multisequence MR images of the cervical spine were obtained without intravenous contrast.

Findings

[There is a normal cervical lordosis]. [The craniocervical junction is normal]. [Vertebral body and disc space height are maintained]. [Vertebral marrow and intervertebral disc space signal are normal]. [Cord signal is normal]. [The visualized posterior fossa structures are normal].

Impression

[Normal MRI cervical spine].

MRI cervical spine with and without contrast
[Order reason for study]

Comparison: [. . .]

Technique: multiplanar, multisequence MR images of the cervical spine were obtained prior to and following the uneventful intravenous administration of [. . .] mL of Multihance.

Findings

[There is a normal cervical lordosis]. [The craniocervical junction is normal]. [Vertebral body and disc space height are maintained]. [Vertebral marrow and intervertebral disc space signal are normal]. [Cord signal is normal]. [The visualized posterior fossa structures are normal]. [There is no evidence of abnormal enhancement within the cervical spine].

Impression

[Normal MRI cervical spine].

MRI thoracic spine without contrast
[Order reason for study]
Comparison: [. . .]

Technique: multiplanar, multisequence MR images of the thoracic spine were obtained without intravenous contrast.

Findings

[There is a normal thoracic kyphosis]. [Vertebral body and intervertebral disc space height are normal]. [Vertebral marrow and intervertebral disc signal are normal]. [Cord signal is normal]. [There is no evidence of significant neural foraminal stenosis or canal compromise].

Impression

[Normal MRI thoracic spine].

MRI thoracic spine with and without contrast
[Order reason for study]
Comparison: [. . .]

Technique: multiplanar, multisequence MR images of the thoracic spine were obtained prior to and following the uneventful intravenous administration of [. . .] mL of Multihance.

Findings

[There is a normal thoracic kyphosis]. [Vertebral body and intervertebral disc space height are normal]. [Vertebral marrow and intervertebral disc signal are normal]. [Cord signal is normal]. [There is no evidence of significant neural foraminal stenosis or canal compromise]. [There is no evidence of abnormal enhancement within the thoracic spine].

Impression

[Normal MRI thoracic spine].

MRI lumbar spine without contrast
[Order reason for study]
Comparison: [. . .]

Technique: multiplanar, multisequence MR images of the lumbar spine were obtained without intravenous contrast.

Findings

[There is normal lumbar lordosis]. [There is preservation of vertebral body and disc space height]. [Vertebral marrow and intervertebral disc signal are normal]. [Cord signal is normal]. [The conus medullaris is normal in signal characteristics and morphology and terminates at the [L1–2] level]. [There is no significant neural foraminal stenosis or central canal compromise throughout the lumbar spine].

Impression

[Normal MRI lumbar spine].

MRI lumbar spine with and without contrast
[Order reason for study]
Comparison: [. . .]

Technique: multiplanar, multisequence MR images of the lumbar spine were obtained prior to and following the uneventful intravenous administration of [. . .] mL of Multihance.

Findings

[There is normal lumbar lordosis]. [There is preservation of vertebral body and disc space height]. [Vertebral marrow and intervertebral disc signal are normal]. [Cord signal is normal]. [The conus medullaris is normal in signal characteristics and morphology and terminates at the [L1–2] level]. [There is no significant neural foraminal stenosis or central canal compromise throughout the lumbar spine]. [There is no evidence of abnormal enhancement within the lumbar spine].

Impression

[Normal MRI lumbar spine].

Index